Atlas of Dermatological Manifestations of Gastrointestinal Disease

George Y. Wu • Nathan Selsky • Jane M. Grant-Kels
Editors

Atlas of Dermatological Manifestations of Gastrointestinal Disease

Springer

Editors
George Y. Wu
Department of Medicine
Gastroenterology Division
University of Connecticut Health Center
Farmington, CT, USA

Nathan Selsky
Department of Medicine
University of Connecticut
West Hartford, CT, USA

Jane M. Grant-Kels
Department of Dermatology
University of Connecticut Health Center
Farmington, CT, USA

ISBN 978-1-4939-5241-0 ISBN 978-1-4614-6191-3 (eBook)
DOI 10.1007/978-1-4614-6191-3
Springer New York Heidelberg Dordrecht London

Printed on acid-free paper

Springer is part of Springer Science+Business Media (www.springer.com)

To my best friend, love of my life, and husband Barry Kels; to my children (Joanna and Luke Albright and Charlie and Lori Kels) and to my grandchildren (G. Grant Kels, Landon Kels, and Charlotte Albright) who have given my life joy; and to the memory of my parents, George and Charlotte Grant, whom I miss every day.

Jane M. Grant-Kels

This book is dedicated to the many students whose stimulating questions led to the conception of the atlas, to my friend and mentor Dr. Irwin M. Arias who has been an inspiration and an unflagging supporter through the many years of our happy association, to my parents and family for their confidence and encouragement through the years, and to Roy Lopata and his family whose generosity and kindness have made it possible for me to engage in educational projects such as this.

George Y. Wu

For my parents, my brothers, and the Beez, who was kept awake.

Nathan Selsky

Preface

The idea for the atlas arose from a need made apparent by frequent questions from students and residents. It is not uncommon for diseases to present with abnormalities in more than one organ system. Depending on which organ system is most involved, symptoms may point in a particular direction. Such conditions often present with bewildering signs and symptoms, however, that initially appear to be unrelated, but are actually manifestations of the same condition. There are perhaps few fields in which this is more true than in gastroenterology and dermatology.

The purpose was to produce an atlas that will provide a comprehensive compendium of digestive tract diseases with dermatological manifestations. The book is arranged by digestive symptoms, with sections based on the specific digestive disease etiology. Each section will contain paired subsections of text, one on gastrointestinal manifestations and the other on dermatological manifestations. Text will include clinical presentations, pathophysiology, differential diagnosis, diagnostic tests/procedures, pathology, and references.

We think this text will provide an important resource for the dermatologist, gastroenterologist, or internist struggling with what appear to be unrelated digestive and skin complaints. Hopefully, it will also stimulate investigation into the pathogenetic mechanisms that are responsible for the involvement of the two organ systems.

Farmington, CT, USA — George Y. Wu
West Hartford, CT, USA — Nathan Selsky
Farmington, CT, USA — Jane M. Grant-Kels

Acknowledgment

George Y. Wu, Nathan Selsky and Jane M. Grant-Kels would like to express their appreciation to their authors and colleagues for their contributions and for sharing their expertise.

Contents

Part II Weight Loss Malabsorption

Part III Gastrointestinal Bleeding

Contributors

Justin Finch Department of Dermatology, University of Connecticut Health Center, Farmington, CT, USA

Faripour Forouhar Department of Pathology, University of Connecticut Health Center, Farmington, CT, USA

Jane M. Grant-Kels Department of Dermatology, University of Connecticut Health Center, Farmington, CT, USA

Laura Nieves Department of Internal Medicine, University of Connecticut Health Center, Farmington, CT, USA

Marcy Qureshi Department of Internal Medicine, University of Connecticut Health Center, Farmington, CT, USA

Marti J. Rothe Department of Dermatology, University of Connecticut Health Center, Farmington, CT, USA

Nathan Selsky Department of Medicine, University of Connecticut, West Hartford, CT, USA

Omar Shahbaz Department of Internal Medicine, University of Connecticut Health Center, Farmington, CT, USA

Michael Tadros Department of Internal Medicine, University of Connecticut Health Center, Farmington, CT, USA

Jameel Uddeen Department of Internal Medicine, University of Connecticut Health Center, Farmington, CT, USA

Marie Lourdes Ynson Department of Internal Medicine, University of Connecticut Health Center, Farmington, CT, USA

Liam Zakko Yale Department of Internal Medicine, Yale New Haven Hospital, New Haven, CT, USA

Part I

Dysphagia

1 Oropharyngeal Cancer: Gastrointestinal Features

Laura Nieves

Oropharyngeal cancer comprises the malignant pathologies involving the tissues of the oropharynx. This includes the tongue, tonsils, soft palate, and walls of the pharynx. These cancers are generally divided into those that are human papillomavirus (HPV)-positive and those HPV-negative (generally related to smoking or alcohol). The gastrointestinal (GI) symptoms include [1, 2]:

- Persistent sore throat
- Unusual bleeding, swelling, pain, or numbness in mouth
- Taste abnormalities
- Dysphagia
- Odynophagia
- Otalgia
- Hoarseness

The most frequent clinical signs and findings are [1, 2]:

- Nonhealing sores or ulcers in oral cavity (pain or painless)
- Red or white lesion with an irregular, fungating growth; surface ulcerations; easy bleeding (*see* Fig. 1.1)
- Cervical lymphadenopathy
- Associated conditions:
  - Bazex's syndrome (acrokeratosis paraneoplastica), rare, erythematous to violaceous psoriasiform plaques in acral areas. Palmoplantar keratoderma, alopecia, and nail dystrophy are common. Has also been associated with other malignancies.

The pathogenesis involves the usual risk factors for upper GI malignancy [3]:

- Chronic inflammation (thought to be precipitating factor)
  - Tobacco and alcohol (major risk factors), HPV infection
- Series of somatic or epigenetic changes allow resistance to growth-inhibitory signals, autonomous proliferation, avoidance of apoptosis, unlimited replication, angiogenesis, invasion and metastasis.

The pathology shows typical features of mucosal malignancy [4]:

- Squamous cell carcinoma
  - Classic pattern: infiltration of neoplastic squamous epithelial cells into supporting connective tissue stroma, which may be chronically inflamed with abundance of plasma cells and lymphocytes.

The diagnosis is made by considering the following [2, 4, 5]:

- Initial assessment by careful examination of oral cavity
- Confirmed by biopsy
- Panendoscopy (including laryngoscopy, esophagoscopy, and possible bronchoscopy) looking for other head and neck tumors
- Magnetic resonance imaging (MRI), computed tomography (CT) scan, and positron emission tomography (PET) scan for staging

The differential diagnosis of oropharyngeal cancer should include [2, 4, 5]:

- Aphthous ulcers
- Oral candidiasis
- Lichen planus
- Pyogenic granuloma
- Kaposi's sarcoma
- Minor salivary gland tumors
- Oral leukoplakia
- Metastatic tumors

The treatment involves usual modalities for the treatment of malignancy [6]:

- Multimodal—depends on staging and location
  - Principal treatment modalities are surgery and radiation therapy (RT)
  - Post-surgical chemoradiation (platinum-based) for advanced disease
  - Radiotherapy plus cetuximab has survival benefit over RT alone
  - Cessation of risk factors (alcohol and tobacco)

L. Nieves (✉)
Department of Internal Medicine, University of Connecticut Health Center, Farmington, CT, USA
e-mail: lnieves@resident.uchc.edu

G.Y. Wu et al. (eds.), *Atlas of Dermatological Manifestations of Gastrointestinal Disease*,
DOI 10.1007/978-1-4614-6191-3_1, © Springer Science+Business Media New York 2013

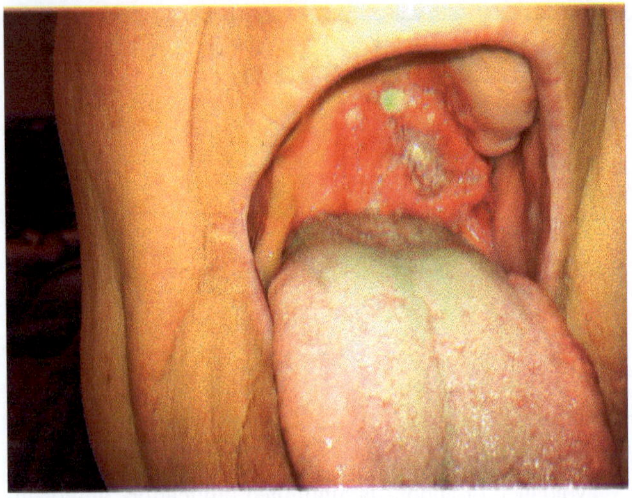

Fig. 1.1 Extensive oropharyngeal carcinoma associated with Bazex's syndrome

References

1. Moore RL, Devere TS. Epidermal manifestations of internal malignancy. Dermatol Clin. 2008;26:17–29.
2. European Society for Medical Oncology (ESMO). Squamous cell carcinoma of the head and neck: ESMO Clinical Recommendations for diagnosis, treatment and follow-up. Ann Oncol. 2007;18:ii65–6.
3. Kupferman ME, Myers JN. Molecular biology of oral cavity squamous cell carcinoma. Otolaryngol Clin N Am. 2006;39:229–34.
4. Greer R. Pathology of malignant and premalignant oral epithelial lesions. Otolaryngol Clin N Am. 2006;39:249–75.
5. Chen AY. Cancer of the oral cavity. Dis Mon. 2001;47:275–361.
6. Scottish Intercollegiate Guidelines Network (SIGN). Diagnosis and management of head and neck cancer. A national clinical guideline. Edinburgh, Scotland): Scottish Intercollegiate Guidelines Network (SIGN); 2006

Bazex's Syndrome: Dermatological Features (Acrokeratosis Paraneoplastica)

2

Liam Zakko, Justin Finch, Marti J. Rothe, and Jane M. Grant-Kels

Clinical signs and features include:

- Paraneoplastic syndrome characterized by acral psoriasiform lesions: red violaceous hyperkeratotic plaques with ill-defined borders; nail changes including subungual hyperkeratosis, onycholysis, longitudinal streaks, yellow pigmentation; hyperkeratotic plaques at pressure points (knees, elbows); and hyperkeratotic plaques on the ears, nose, and cheeks [1–3]
- Particular findings include violet discoloration and bulbous enlargement of the distal phalanges; lesions only on the helix of the ear (not entire ear like psoriasis) [1]
- Three clinical stages: (1) poorly circumscribed skin lesions on the helices of the ears, nose, cheeks, fingers, toes, and nails associated with asymptomatic carcinomas most commonly of the upper aerodigestive tract (see Fig. 2.1b); (2) lesions which spread to the palms and soles with a locally symptomatic malignancy (see Fig. 2.1a); (3) With an untreated malignancy, erythema and scale spread to the knees, elbows, and trunk [3]
- Hyperpigmentation is the main cutaneous feature in patients with type IV to VI skin [4]
- Most common associated neoplasm is squamous cell carcinoma of the upper aerodigestive tract or tumors with cervical/mediastinal lymph node spread [2]
- Other neoplasms that have caused this syndrome include: colon adenocarcinoma, small cell lung carcinoma, lung adenocarcinoma, Hodgkin's disease, T-cell lymphoma, multiple myeloma, hepatocellular carcinoma, thymoma, cutaneous squamous cell carcinoma, prostate adenocarcinoma, vulva/uterine/bladder carcinoma [1, 2]
- The cutaneous lesions precede the underlying malignancy in almost 70% of cases [3]

Pathogenesis of this disease is unclear but hypotheses include:

- An immunologic reaction with IgA, IgG, IgM, and/or C3 deposited on the basement membrane zone, perhaps related to a squamous cell carcinoma antigen
- Secreted from the underlying neoplasm [1]

Histopathological features include:

- Hyperkeratosis with foci of parakeratosis, acanthosis, isolated necrosis of keratinocytes, and a superficial perivascular lymphohistiocytic dermal inflammatory infiltrate (see Fig. 2.2) [1]

The diagnosis is made using a combination of:

- Based on high clinical suspicion as cutaneous manifestations often precede the neoplasm; the goal is to identify the causative cancer [1]
- Work-up based on a detailed clinical history and physical examination—with specific emphasis on lymph node exam [1]
- Next obtain an ear, nose, and throat examination, chest radiograph, complete blood count, erythrocyte sedimentation rate, basic chemistries, tumor markers, and a guaiac stool test [1]
- If patient is guaiac test positive and has anemia then obtain a colonoscopy [1]
- If patient is guaiac test negative and has a negative colonoscopy obtain an esophagogastroduodenoscopy [1]
- If all examinations are negative, obtain a computed tomography scan of patient's chest/abdomen/pelvis [1]

L. Zakko (✉)
Yale Department of Internal Medicine, Yale New Haven Hospital, 20 York Street, New Haven, CT 06510, USA
e-mail: liam.zakko@yale.edu

J. Finch • M.J. Rothe • J.M. Grant-Kels
Department of Dermatology, University of Connecticut Health Center, 21 South Road, Farmington, CT 06030, USA
e-mail: finch@uchc.edu; rothe@uchc.edu; grant@uchc.edu

G.Y. Wu et al. (eds.), *Atlas of Dermatological Manifestations of Gastrointestinal Disease*, DOI 10.1007/978-1-4614-6191-3_2, © Springer Science+Business Media New York 2013

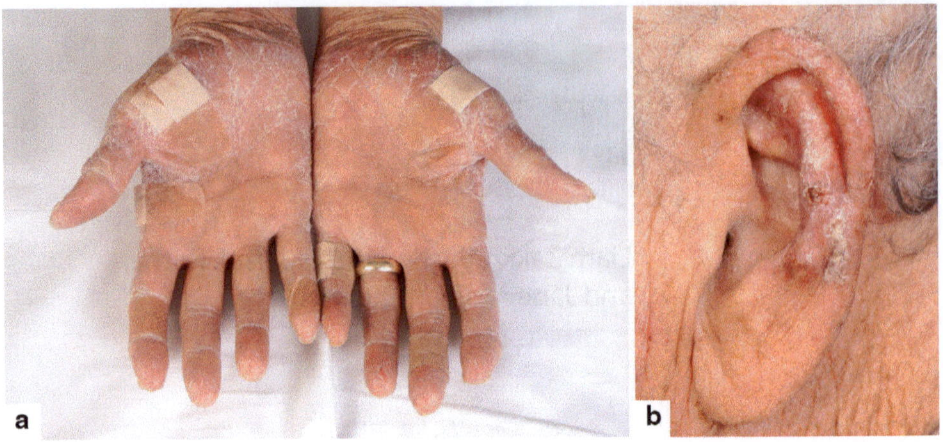

Fig. 2.1 Acrokeratosis paraneoplastica. Scaly, psoriasiform plaques involving the hands (**a**) and ears (**b**) (Image courtesy of Howard Pride, MD)

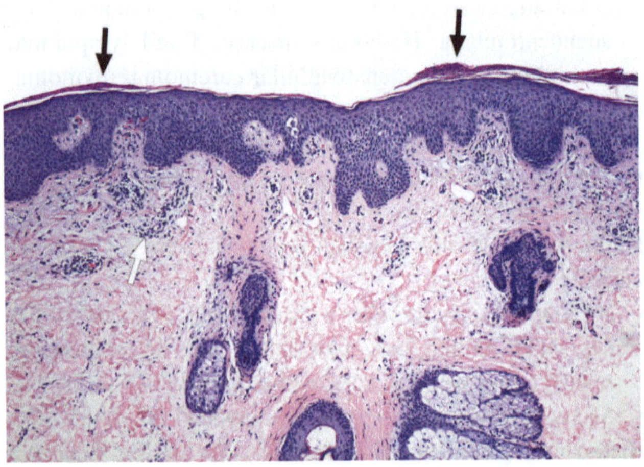

Fig. 2.2 Acrokeratosis paraneoplastica. A photomicrograph showing psoriasiform hyperplasia, confluent parakeratosis, and a superficial perivascular infiltrate of predominantly lymphocytes. Hematoxylin–eosin (H&E) stain

- If all examinations are negative but clinical suspicion remains high, repeat testing in 3 months [1]

The differential diagnosis should include:

- Psoriasis
- Eczematous dermatitis
- Fungal infection

Treatment options include:

- Treatment of underlying neoplasm leads to regression of cutaneous signs [1–3]
- Rarely is there remission of cutaneous features without treatment of the cancer [1]
- Recurrence of cutaneous disease indicates recurrence of cancer or development of metastases [4]

References

1. Valdivielso M, Longo I, Suarez R, et al. Acrokeratosis paraneoplastica (Bazex syndrome). J Eur Acad Dermatol Venereol. 2005; 19:340–4.
2. Sharma V, Sharma NL, Ranjan N, et al. Acrokeratosis paraneoplastic (Bazex syndrome): case report and review of literature. Dermatol Online J. 2006;12:11. http://dermatology.cdlib.org/121/case_reports/bazex/sharma.html. Accessed December 14, 2011.
3. Khachemoune A, Yalamanchili R, Rodriguez C. Bazex syndrome (paraneoplastic acrokeratosis). Cutis. 2004;74:289–92.
4. Bolognia JL, Brewer YP, Cooper DL. Bazex syndrome (acrokeratosis paraneoplastica). An analytic review. Medicine (Baltimore). 1991; 4:269–80.

3 Plummer-Vinson Syndrome: Gastrointestinal Features

Liam Zakko

Plummer-Vinson syndrome consists of the triad of dysphagia, esophagitis, and iron deficiency anemia. The disease is more common in women than in men and often occurs in the menopausal period after age 50. The gastrointestinal symptoms [1] associated with this disease are:

- Intermittent dysphagia to solids that progresses over years
- Occasionally weight loss

The classic clinical signs and findings include [1]:

- Triad of dysphagia, iron deficiency anemia, upper esophageal webs (see Fig. 3.1)
- Signs and symptoms of iron deficiency often predominate
- Esophageal webs are smooth, thin, and gray with a central lumen. Usually extend from the anterior wall laterally and are found in the proximal part of the esophagus
- More common in Caucasians
- Incidence decreases with improved nutrition
- Typically presents in women in fourth to seventh decades of life

The pathogenesis of Plummer-Vinson syndrome is unclear [1]:

- Iron deficiency is important, but it is neither necessary nor sufficient to cause the syndrome

The pathology of mucosal biopsies will show [1]:

- One or more thin horizontal membranes consisting of squamous epithelium and submucosa

The diagnosis is made by finding [1]:

- One or more esophageal webs in a patient with postcricoid dysphagia and iron deficiency anemia
- Esophageal webs can be visualized by barium swallow or upper endoscopy
- Endoscopy needs to begin under direct visualization in order not to push through and rupture the webs

The differential diagnosis of Plummer-Vinson syndrome should include [1, 2]:

- Malignant tumors
- Esophageal strictures
- Diverticula
- Motility disorders
- Scleroderma
- Gastroesophageal reflux disease
- Diabetes mellitus
- Neuromuscular disorders
- Skeletal muscle disorders

The treatment involves [1]:

- Iron replacement to treat iron deficiency
- Determination of the cause of iron deficiency

L. Zakko (✉)
Yale Department of Internal Medicine, Yale New Haven Hospital,
20 York Street, New Haven, CT 06510, USA
e-mail: liam.zakko@yale.edu

G.Y. Wu et al. (eds.), *Atlas of Dermatological Manifestations of Gastrointestinal Disease*,
DOI 10.1007/978-1-4614-6191-3_3,

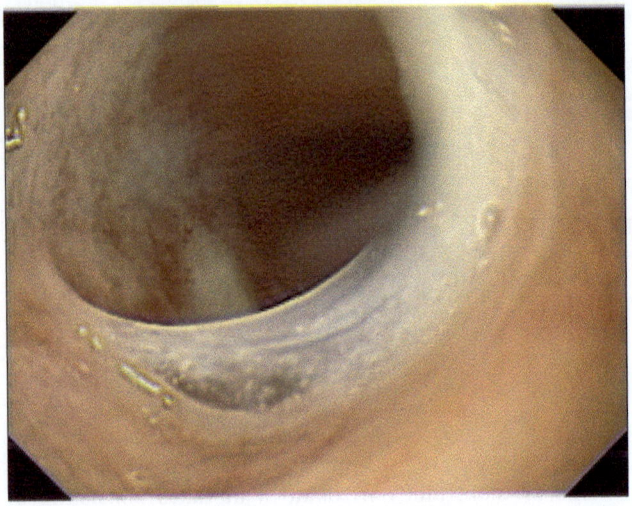

Fig. 3.1 An endoscopic view of an esophageal web in Plummer-Vinson syndrome. A thin membranous constriction is typical (Courtesy of Connecticut Gastroeatology Institute)

References

1. Novacek G. Plummer-Vinson syndrome. Orphanet J Rare Dis. 2006;1:36.
2. Baron R, Darber RPR, Hanske E, et al. Text atlas of nail disorders: techniques, investigation, and diagnosis. 3rd ed. London: Martin Dunitz/Taylor & Francis; 2003. p. 23–7. Chapter 2, section 2, Koilonychia. Available at www.rusmedserv.com/mycology/html/Atlas_of_Nail_Disorders.pdf. Accessed June 5, 2012.

Plummer-Vinson Syndrome: Dermatological Features

4

Liam Zakko, Justin Finch, Marti J. Rothe, and Jane M. Grant-Kels

Clinical signs and features include:

- Classic triad of dysphagia, iron deficiency anemia (symptoms of this often predominate), upper esophageal webs [1]
- More common in Caucasians [1]
- Incidence decreases with improved nutrition [1]
- Typically presents in women in the fourth to seventh decades of life [1]
- Skin findings related to iron deficiency; most common is koilonychia—nails that flatten and thin and then eventually form a spoon shape (see Fig. 4.1) [1]

Pathogenesis of this disease is unclear but hypotheses include:

- Plummer-Vinson Syndrome's etiology is unclear; clearly iron deficiency is important but it is neither necessary nor sufficient to cause the syndrome [1]

Histopathological features include:

- Nails with koilonychia are firmly attached to the bone by vertical dermal connective tissue bundles in the subungual area that bind directly to the boney periosteum [2]

The diagnosis is made using a combination of:

- Identify classic triad of iron deficiency (including the skin findings), dysphagia, and esophageal webs [1]

The differential diagnosis of koilonychias should include [2]:

- Physiological
- LEOPARD syndrome
- Ectodermal dystrophy
- Trichothiodystrophy
- Iron deficiency
- Acromegaly
- Hemochromatosis
- Porphyria
- Secondary to dialysis/transplant
- Thyroid disease
- Dermatic- or inflammatory-induced nail changes
- Alopecia create
- Darier's disease
- Lichen planus
- Psoriasis
- Raynaud's
- Occupational-induced nail changes
- Onychomycosis
- Syphilis
- Trauma

Treatment options include:

- Iron replacement to treat iron deficiency and determination of cause of iron deficiency [1]

References

1. Novacek G. Plummer-Vinson syndrome. Orphanet J Rare Dis. 2006;1:36.
2. Baron R, Darber RPR, Hanske E, et al. A text atlas of nail disorders: techniques, investigation, and diagnosis. 3rd ed. London: Martin Dunitz/Taylor & Francis; 2003. p. 23–7. Chapter 2, section 2, Koilonychia. Available at www.rusmedserv.com/mycology/html/Atlas_of_Nail_Disorders.pdf. Accessed June 5, 2012.

L. Zakko (✉)
Yale Department of Internal Medicine, 20 York Street,
Yale New Haven Hospital, New Haven, CT 06510, USA
e-mail: liam.zakko@yale.edu

J. Finch • M.J. Rothe • J.M. Grant-Kels
Department of Dermatology,
University of Connecticut Health Center,
21 South Road, Farmington, CT 06030, USA
e-mail: finch@uchc.edu; rothe@uchc.edu; grant@uchc.edu

G.Y. Wu et al. (eds.), *Atlas of Dermatological Manifestations of Gastrointestinal Disease*,
DOI 10.1007/978-1-4614-6191-3_4, © Springer Science+Business Media New York 2013

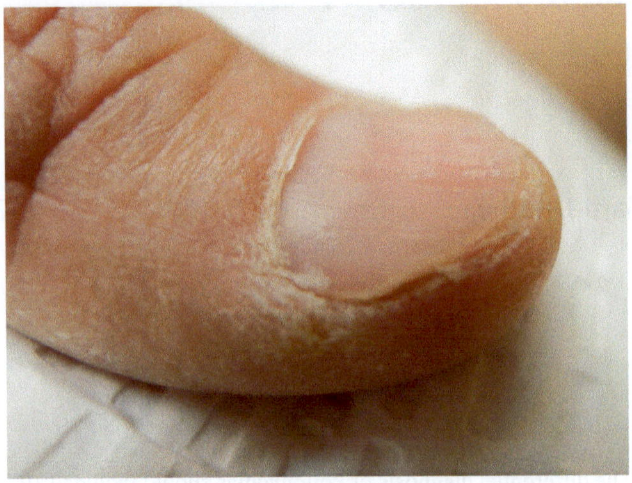

Fig. 4.1 Koilonychia

5 Esophageal Cancer: Gastrointestinal Features

Laura Nieves

Esophageal cancers comprise all the malignant lesions of the esophagus, but primarily consist of squamous cell carcinoma worldwide, and adenocarcinoma in the United States. Symptoms can vary widely depending on stage, and prognosis is largely dependent on the stage at which the tumor is detected. Late-stage lesions typically portend a poor prognosis [1].

Gastrointestinal symptoms include [1,2]:

- Dysphagia (predominant symptom) initially to solids progressing to liquids
- Anorexia, vomiting, cough, gastroesophageal reflux disease, hematemesis or hemoptysis
- Odynophagia
- Hoarseness
- Back pain if mediastinal invasion is present
- Chest pain

The clinical signs and findings include [1–3]:

- Aspiration pneumonia may occur due to stricture, partial or complete obstruction (see Fig. 5.1)
- Cervical or supraclavicular lymphadenopathy (see Fig. 5.2)
- Associated conditions
  - Achalasia
  - Celiac sprue
  - Plummer-Vinson syndrome
  - Tylosis-inherited form (Howel-Evans Syndrome): 95% of affected individuals develop esophageal squamous cell carcinoma by age 65
  - Barrett's esophagus: strongest risk factor for esophageal adenocarcinoma
  - Scleroderma
  - Zollinger-Ellison syndrome
  - Obesity

The pathogenesis is not clear, but includes [1–3]:

- Chronic inflammation (thought to be a precipitating factor)
  - Squamous cell carcinoma (SCC): toxins (alcohol, cigarettes, aflatoxin B1)
  - Adenocarcinoma (AC): acid and bile reflux
- Series of somatic or epigenetic changes allow resistance to growth-inhibitory signals, autonomous proliferation, avoidance of apoptosis, unlimited replication, angiogenesis, invasion, and metastasis

The pathology typically shows [2,3]:

- SCC and adenocarcinoma main two histologic subtypes
  - SCC predominant in proximal esophagus and midesophagus
  - Adenocarcinoma in distal esophagus and gastroesophageal junction

The differential diagnosis of esophageal cancer should include [1–3]:

- Achalasia
- Diffuse esophageal spasm
- GERD
- Scleroderma
- Leiomyoma and other benign tumors of the esophagus
- Gastric cancer

The diagnosis is made with [1–3]:

- Biphasic barium esophagography
- Upper endoscopy with biopsy to confirm diagnosis
- Chest computed tomography (CT) scan, endoscopic ultrasound, and positron emission tomography (PET) for preoperative staging.

Treatment, dependent on TNM stage, is usually multimodal and includes [4]:

- Surgical resection for early stages
- Neoadjuvant chemotherapy
- Chemoradiation superior to radiotherapy alone
- Palliative therapy: stenting, brachytherapy, and esophageal dilatation.

L. Nieves (✉)
Department of Internal Medicine, University of Connecticut Health Center, Farmington, CT, USA
e-mail: lnieves@resident.uchc.edu

G.Y. Wu et al. (eds.), *Atlas of Dermatological Manifestations of Gastrointestinal Disease*,
DOI 10.1007/978-1-4614-6191-3_5, © Springer Science+Business Media New York 2013

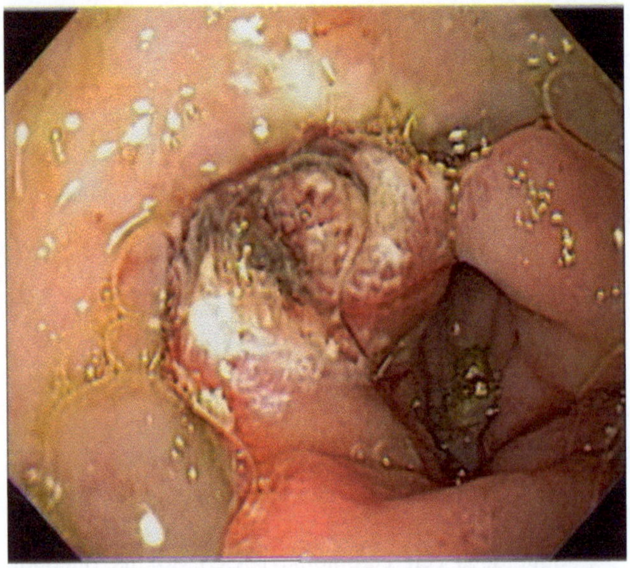

Fig. 5.1 An endoscopic view of an ulcerated circumferential esophageal malignancy, partially obstructing the esophageal lumen

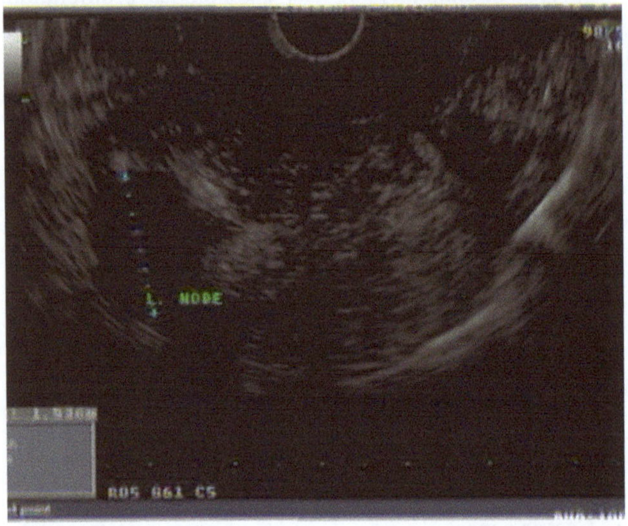

Fig. 5.2 A radial endoscopic ultrasound image of an enlarged lymph node in a patient with esophageal malignancy. The lack of an esophageal serosal surface is thought to facilitate the spread of esophageal malignancies to local lymphatics and nodes

References

1. Khushalani NI. Cancer of the esophagus and stomach. Mayo Clin Proc. 2008;83:712–22.
2. Stahl M, Oliveira J. Esophageal cancer: ESMO clinical recommendations for diagnosis, treatment and follow-up. Ann Oncol. 2009; 20:32–3.
3. Bird-Lieberman EL, Fitzgerald RC. Early diagnosis of oesophageal cancer. Br J Cancer. 2009;101:1–6.
4. Wolf MC, Stahl M, Krause BJ, et al. Curative treatment of oesophageal carcinoma: current options and future developments. Radiat Oncol. 2011;6:55.

Howel-Evans Syndrome: Dermatological Features (Familial Keratoderma with Carcinoma of the Esophagus)

6

Liam Zakko, Justin Finch, Marti J. Rothe, and Jane M. Grant-Kels

Clinical signs and features include:
- Genodermatosis associated with carcinoma of the esophagus [1, 2]
- Leukoplakia (see Fig. 6.1) [1]
- Palmoplantar keratoderma (PPK): thickening of the skin on the palms and soles with pruritus and deep, painful fissures; focal hyperkeratotic skin related to physical activity and with regression on bed rest (see Fig. 6.2) [1]
- PPK begins in the second decade [3, 4]
- Associated risk of esophageal squamous cell cancer with 90% developing by age 65 and usually earlier at age 45 [3]
- Two families in the United Kingdom and one family in the United States have been found with the condition to date [1]

Pathogenesis of this disease involves:
- Autosomal dominant with complete penetrance by teen years [1]
- Appears related to 17q25 gene with loss of heterozygosity of the tylosis with esophageal carcinoma gene—*TOC*, a tumor suppressor gene [1]

Histopathological features include:
- Prominent hyperkeratosis of the palms and soles. Underlying epidermis can be acanthotic. In addition hypertrophy of the sweat glands and their ducts have been reported [4].

The diagnosis is made using a combination of:
- Clinical with tylosis and esophageal carcinoma extensively seen on a family tree [1, 4]

The differential diagnosis should include:
- Ectodermal dysplasia
- Tylosis
- Bazex Syndrome

Treatment options include:
- Urea cream or 50% propylene glycol in water under occlusive plastic dressing for the thickened skin [1, 2]
- Systemic retinoids [2]
- Early and frequent screening for esophageal cancer [1]

References

1. Sroa N, Witman P. Howel Evans syndrome: a variant of ectodermal dysplasia. Cutis. 2010;85:183–5.
2. Genetics/genomics competency center. Genetic and rare diseases information center. Available at http://www.g-2-c-2.org/search_detail.php. Accessed 6 June 2012.
3. Merger BS, Merger D. Carcinoma of the esophagus and tylosis: a lethal genetic combination. Cancer. 1993;72:17–9.
4. Howel-Evans W, McConnell RB, Clarke CA, Sheppard PM. Carcinoma of the oesophagus with keratosis palmaris et plantaris (tylosis). Q J Med. 1958;27:413–9.

L. Zakko (✉)
Yale Department of Internal Medicine, 20 York Street, Yale New Haven Hospital, New Haven, CT 06510, USA
e-mail: liam.zakko@yale.edu

J. Finch • M.J. Rothe • J.M. Grant-Kels
Department of Dermatology, University of Connecticut Health Center, 21 South Road, Farmington, CT 06030, USA
e-mail: finch@uchc.edu; rothe@uchc.edu; grant@uchc.edu

G.Y. Wu et al. (eds.), *Atlas of Dermatological Manifestations of Gastrointestinal Disease*, DOI 10.1007/978-1-4614-6191-3_6, © Springer Science+Business Media New York 2013

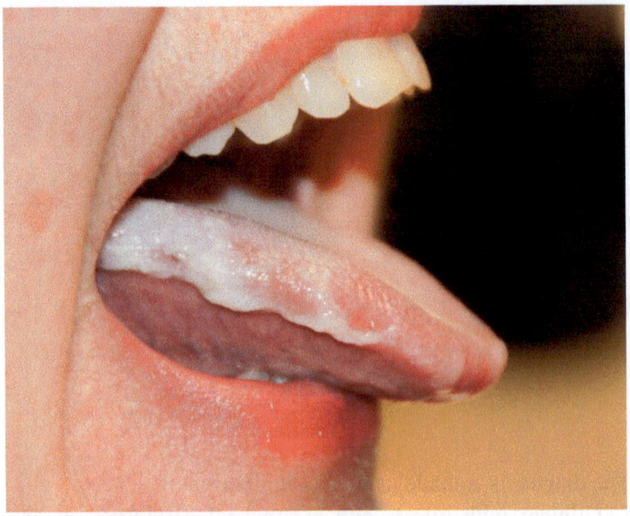

Fig. 6.1 Leukoplakia. Shaggy white plaque on the lateral tongue

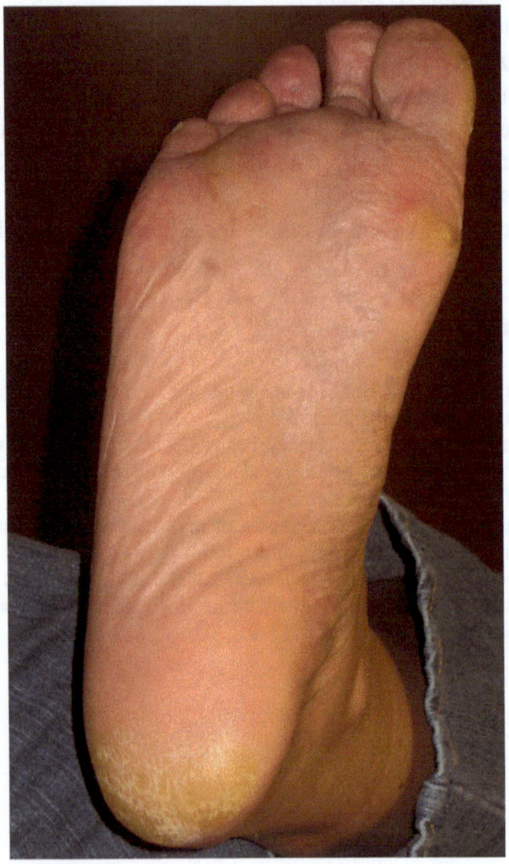

Fig. 6.2 Focal keratoderma of the plantar foot

Scleroderma: Gastrointestinal Features

7

Liam Zakko

Scleroderma is an autoimmune disease characterized by associated autoantibodies, vascular alterations, and fibrosis. The skin is most commonly affected, although any organ can be involved. Prognosis is determined by the extent of disease and involvement of the lung.

The gastrointestinal (GI) symptoms include [1, 2]:

- Pain, dysphagia, heartburn, vomiting, diarrhea, fecal incontinence, constipation, weight loss
- The GI tract is possibly the second most common site of systemic sclerosis (SSc) organ disease
- GI symptoms occur with limited cutaneous SSc (lcSSc) and diffuse cutaneous SSc (dcSSc) depending on the location and extent of skin involvement
- These symptoms severely impact prognosis and quality of life (6–12% mortality attributed to GI involvement)
- Any part of the GI tract can be affected—although esophagus is most common, it is disease at other sites that is more likely to lead to morbidity and mortality

The typical GI clinical signs and findings are [2, 3]:

- Esophagus—affected in 70–90% of patients with SSc; can present with heartburn, dysphagia, or early on can be asymptomatic; early diagnosis is essential to limit effects of the disease
  - Esophageal dysmotility, classically an aperistaltic tubular esophagus with low resting pressure of lower esophageal sphincter—may be associated with interstitial lung disease
  - Gastroesophageal reflux disease (GERD)—occurs due to a weakened lower esophageal sphincter and loss of peristaltic function—resulting in reflux and stasis of gastric contents (see Fig. 7.1), and if untreated leads to erosive esophagitis, and then frank ulceration, strictures (see Figs. 7.2 and 7.3), Barrett's esophagitis (see Fig. 7.4), fistulae, and an achalasia-like syndrome [3]
- Gastric manifestations
  - Gastroparesis—leads to solid food intolerance and worsening GERD; more common in patients with dcSSc and esophageal dysmotility
  - Gastric antral vascular ectasia (GAVE)—"watermelon stomach"—multiple, parallel longitudinal columns of red vessels (see Fig. 7.5); key cause of chronic bleeding in SSc patients
- Intestinal manifestations
  - Small intestine—hypomotility—pseudoobstruction (see Fig. 7.6) and bacterial overgrowth
  - Colonic—early constipation; later, diarrhea (from bacterial overgrowth and reduced rectal compliance), colonic telangiectasia, pseudodiverticulum, and rectal prolapsed
  - Fecal incontinence: effects 38% of SSc patients

The pathogenesis is based on autoimmune damage to vasculature resulting in increased connective tissue and scarring, and autonomic nervous system dysfunction [2, 3]:

- Abnormal deposition of type I and III collagen in the extracellular matrix (ECM) likely due to abnormal cytokine and growth factors
- Dysmotility due to collagen disruption which first disrupts enteric neuronal pathways and then disrupts enteric smooth muscle—the order is based on studies showing first dysmotility is due to inappropriate contraction pattern (neuron failure) with normal contraction strength (smooth muscles active), and then due to a contraction (smooth muscle) failure
- Etiology of GAVE is unknown

The pathology generally shows [2, 3]:

- Increased collagen deposition
- In esophagus, most commonly see signs of esophagitis; may see Barrett's esophagus; columnar intestinal epithelium in the esophagus

The diagnosis is based on a combination of findings [2, 3]:

- Initially based on skin findings and antibody testing

L. Zakko (✉)
Yale Department of Internal Medicine, Yale New Haven Hospital, New Haven, CT, USA

Yale Primary Care Clinic, 789 Howard Avenue, New Haven, CT 06519-1304, USA
e-mail: zakko@yale.edu

G.Y. Wu et al. (eds.), *Atlas of Dermatological Manifestations of Gastrointestinal Disease*, DOI 10.1007/978-1-4614-6191-3_7, © Springer Science+Business Media New York 2013

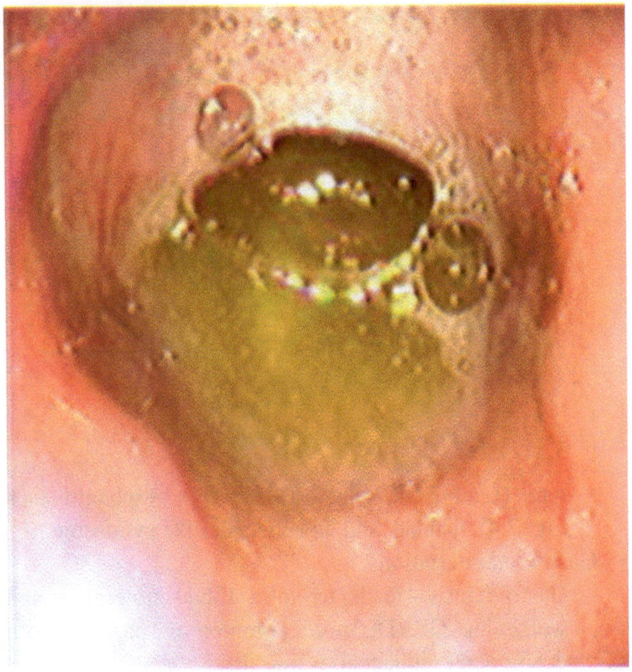

Fig. 7.1 An endoscopic view of the esophagus showing stasis of bile-stained gastric refluxate due to weakening of the lower esophageal sphincter and loss of esophageal peristalsis (Image courtesy of the CT GI Institute)

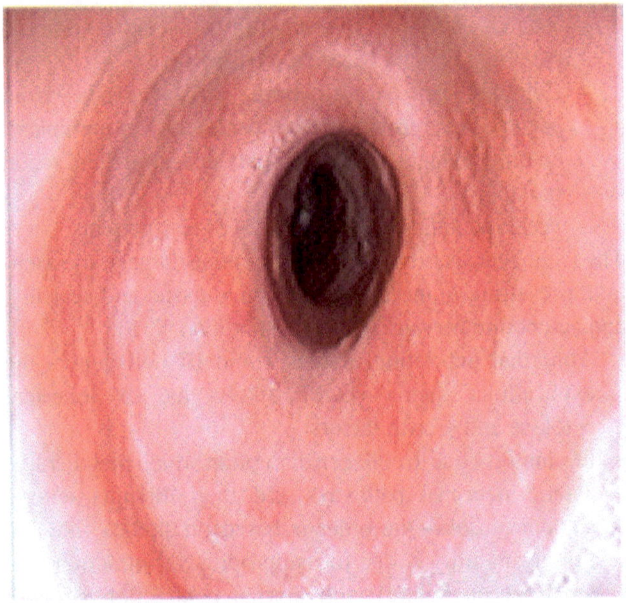

Fig. 7.2 An endoscopic view of a gradually tapered stricture of the mid-esophagus in SSc (Image courtesy of the CT GI Institute)

- Esophagus: combination of upper GI endoscopy, ambulatory pH monitoring, and esophageal manometry
- Delayed gastric emptying: gastric emptying study
- GAVE: upper endoscopy
- Small intestine hypomotility: can consider manometry
- Fecal incontinence—endosonography; detects loss of internal anal sphincter

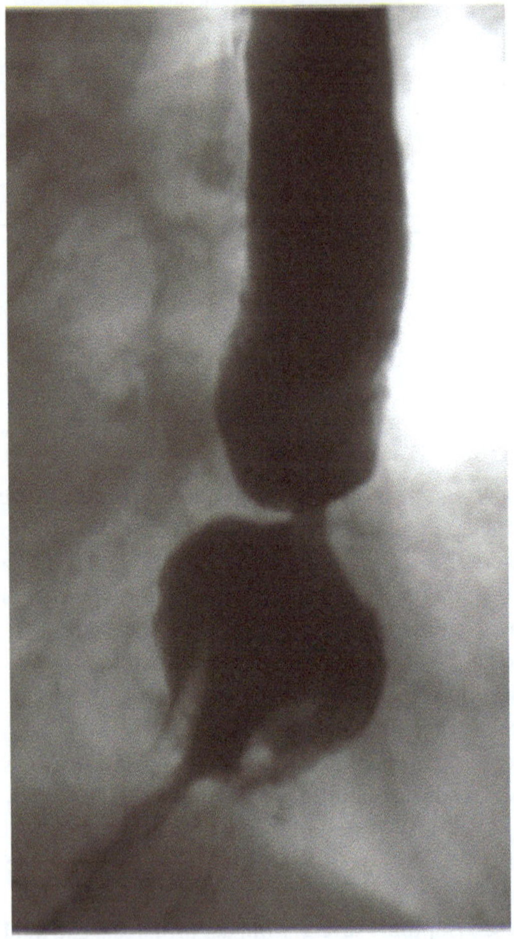

Fig. 7.3 A barium swallow showing a short stricture of the distal esophagus in a patient with SSc (Reprinted from Domsic et al. [2]; with permission)

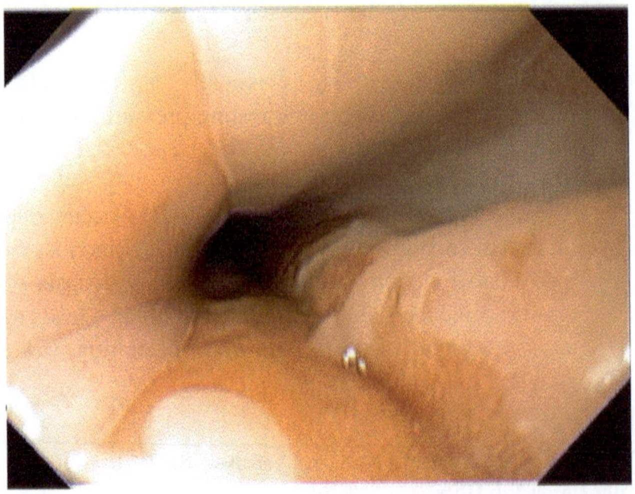

Fig. 7.4 An endoscopic view of tongues and islands of inflammation in the midesophagus consistent with the presence of Barrett's epithelium in a patient with SSc.(Image courtesy of the CT GI Institute)

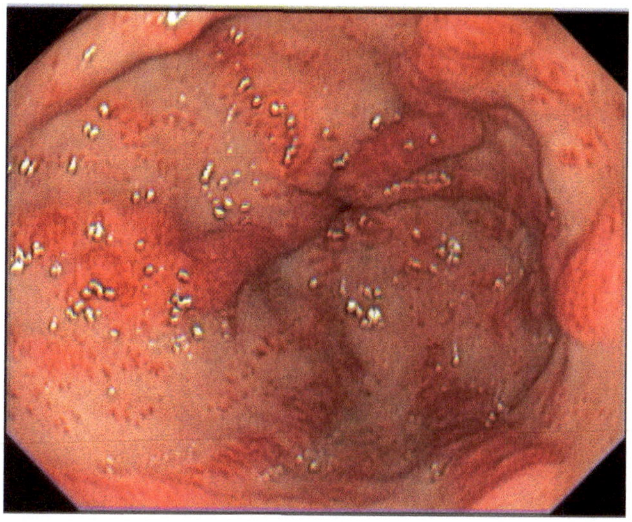

Fig. 7.5 An endoscopic view of vascular ectasias in parallel columns in the gastric antrum, often called "watermelon" stomach because of the pattern (Image courtesy of the CT GI Institute)

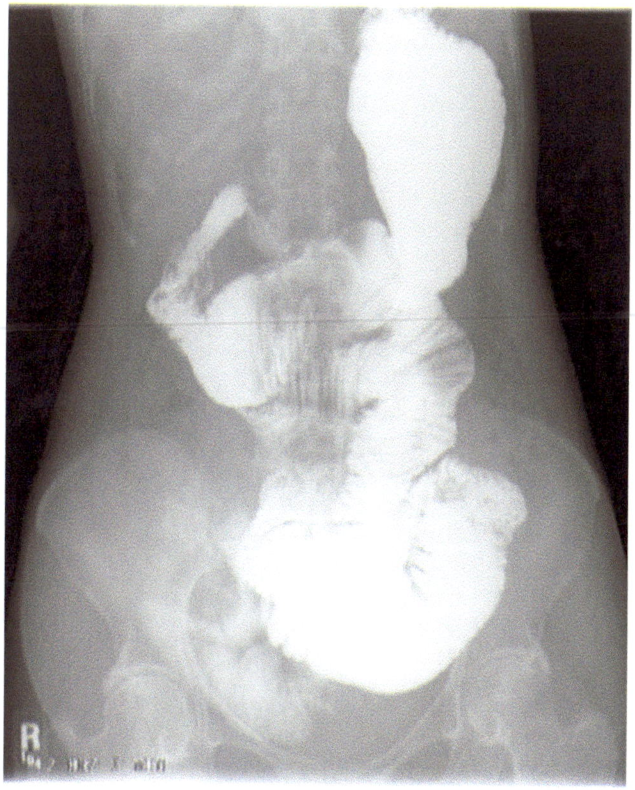

Fig. 7.6 An upper GI series showing distended small bowel loops (Reprinted from Domsic et al. [2]; with permission)

- Carcinoid syndrome
- Insulin-dependent diabetes
- Infiltrating carcinomas
- Mixed connective tissue disease
- Amyloidosis
- Eosinophilic esophagitis

There is no cure for this disease but symptomatic treatment involves [2, 3]:

- Esophageal disease: GERD—behavioral changes (elevate head of bed, avoid eating before sleep, smoking cessation) and long-term proton pump inhibitor therapy
- Delayed gastric emptying—dietary modifications—small meals, low fat; promotility agents—erythromycin, reglan, domperidone; gastric pacemaker; percutaneous jejunal tube placement for feedings
- GAVE—blood transfusion, iron supplementation, argon plasma coagulation
- Intestinal dysmotility/pseudoobstruction—octreotide; nightly tube feedings; severe disease total parenteral nutrition
- Fecal incontinence —sphincter muscle training; sacral nerve stimulation

References

1. Black CM. Scleroderma—clinical aspects. J Intern Med. 1993; 234: 115–8.
2. Domsic R, Fasanella K, Bielefeldt K. Gastrointestinal manifestations of systemic sclerosis. Dig Dis Sci. 2008;53:1163–74.
3. Forbes A, Marie I. Gastrointestinal complications: the most frequent internal complications of systemic sclerosis. Rheumatol. 2008; 48: 36–9.

Scleroderma: Systemic Sclerosis

8

Liam Zakko, Justin Finch, Marti J. Rothe, and Jane M. Grant-Kels

Clinical signs and features include:

- Ranges from localized cutaneous scleroderma (morphea) to systemic disease [1]
- Usually begins from 25 to 60 years of age with female:male ratio 4:1 [1]
- Heterogeneity in clinical presentation and course [2]
- Cutaneous involvement is almost universal [2], but also can have pulmonary, cardiac, renal, and gastrointestinal (especially esophageal) organ involvement [1]
- Often preceded by Raynaud's phenomenon [2]
- Skin disease is characterized by loss of cutaneous elasticity followed by thickening/hardening of the skin; three phases of skin disease: (1) skin edema and itching with hyper- or hypopigmentation; (2) fibrotic phase; (3) atrophic phase [1]
- Limited cutaneous scleroderma (LcSSc) (CREST syndrome): primarily vascular disease characterized by Raynaud's phenomenon for years; skin involvement limited to the hands, face, feet, and forearms (often notice puckering/wrinkling in the face first); late onset of pulmonary hypertension (with or without interstitial lung disease [ILD]), trigeminal neuralgia, skin calcification, and telangiectasia; dilated nailfold capillaries without drop out [1]
- LcSSc: early stage (first 10 years)—mild skin involvement with nonpitting edema of the fingers leading to sclerosis (sclerodactyly), Raynaud's, digital ulcers from local ischemia, GERD; late stage (after 10 years)—increased vascular disease with telangiectasia and digital tip ulcers, wide spread calcinosis, pulmonary hypertension, and esophageal disease with strictures [1]
- Diffuse cutaneous scleroderma (DcSSc): characterized by onset of Raynaud's within 1 year of skin changes; truncal and acral skin involvement; early onset ILD, oliguric renal failure, diffuse gastrointestinal disease, and myocardial involvement; nailfold capillary dilation and destruction [1]
- DcSSC: early stage (first 5 years)—fatigue, decreased weight, rapidly progressive skin disease, increased risk of renal failure, early onset ILD, arthritis/myositis/tendonitis; late stage (after 5 years)—constitutional symptoms resolve, stable skin symptoms, no new organ involvement, progression of disease in those organs with involvement, no active musculoskeletal involvement but deformities from previous involvement [1] (see Fig. 8.1)

Pathogenesis of this autoimmune disease involves:

- Abnormal deposition of type I and III collagen in the extracellular matrix (ECM) [2]
- Cytokines and growth factors play an important role particularly transforming growth factor beta (TGF-β) that increases fibroblast activity and connective tissue growth factor (CTGF), which sustains fibroblast activity [2]
- ET-1 also plays a role in vasoconstriction and ECM remodeling by activating the cell adhesion molecules and moderating the inflammatory response, which activates myofibroblasts that make sclerodermal changes [2]

L. Zakko (✉)
Yale Department of Internal Medicine, 20 York Street, Yale New Haven Hospital, New Haven, CT 06510, USA
e-mail: liam.zakko@yale.edu

J. Finch • M.J. Rothe • J.M. Grant-Kels
Department of Dermatology, University of Connecticut Health Center, 21 South Road, Farmington, CT 06030, USA
e-mail: finch@uchc.edu; rothe@uchc.edu; grant@uchc.edu

G.Y. Wu et al. (eds.), *Atlas of Dermatological Manifestations of Gastrointestinal Disease*, DOI 10.1007/978-1-4614-6191-3_8, © Springer Science+Business Media New York 2013

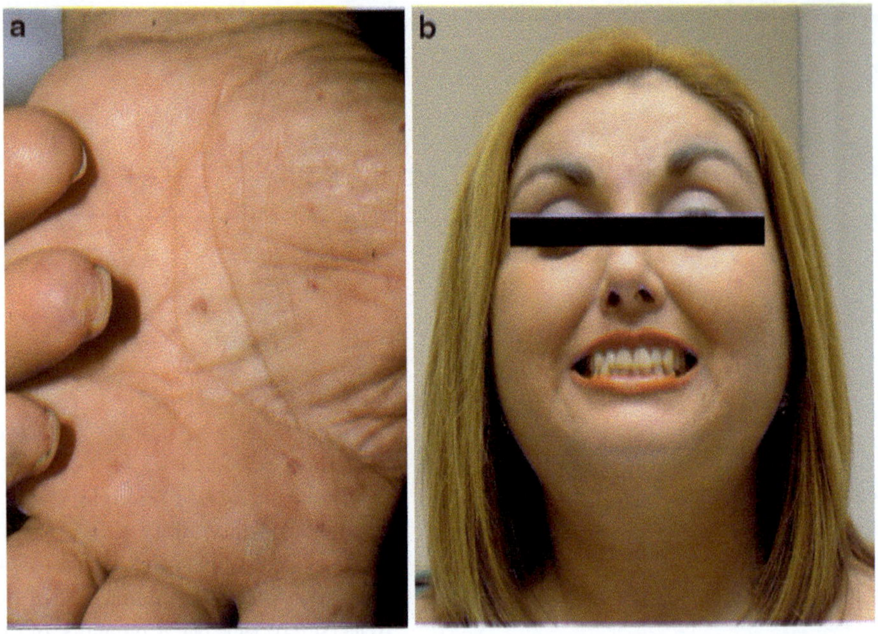

Fig. 8.1 Scleroderma. (**a**) Mat telangiectasias and pitting of the digital pulp. (**b**) Mask-like, expressionless facies of scleroderma, with pinched appearance of the nose

Histopathological features include:

- Early: cellular stage—thickened collagen bundles within the reticular dermis that run parallel to the skin surface and predominantly lymphocytic (occasionally with eosinophils) inflammatory cell infiltrate between the collagen bundles and around blood vessels. Thickened collagen bundles often replace the subcutaneous fat and trap eccrine glands [2]
- Late: avascular stage—after 12–18 months little inflammation or inflammatory cells. Evidence of sclerosis with collagen replacing fat and no remaining adnexal structures [2] (*see* Fig. 8.2)

The diagnosis is made using a combination of:

- Clinical based on above findings [1, 2]
- Role for antibody testing: anticentromere antibody—LcSSc (60% sensitivity; 100% specificity); anti-topoisomerase I—DcSSc (38% sensitivity; 100% specificity) [1]

The differential diagnosis should include:

- Scleromyxedema
- Carcinoid syndrome
- Insulin-dependent diabetic cheiroarthropathy
- Lichen sclerosis et atrophicus
- Infiltrating carcinomas
- Mixed connective tissue disease
- Morphea
- Nephrogenic fibrosing dermopathy
- Amyloidosis

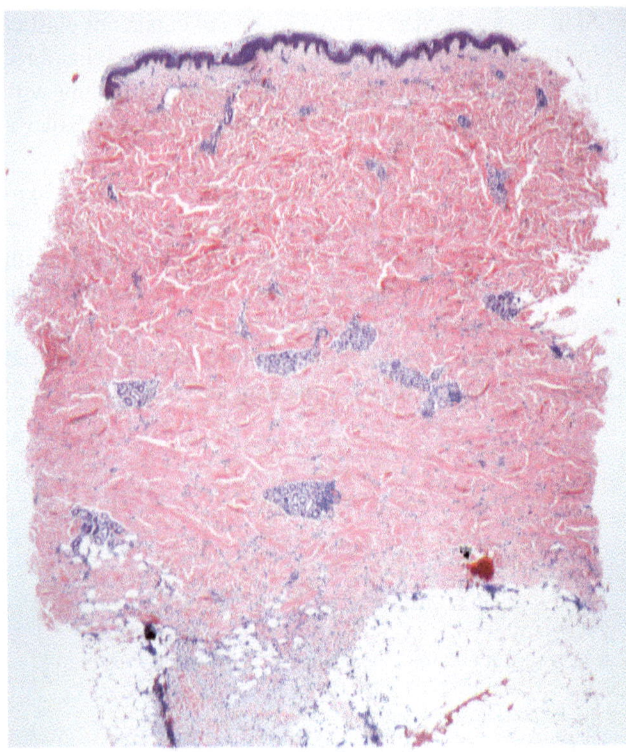

Fig. 8.2 Scleroderma. Squared biopsy shape due to the thickened collagen. Normal epidermis with hyalinized dermis. Adnexal structures are sparse and appear bound-down by the surrounding collagen (20×)

- Eosinophilic fasciitis
- Scleredema

Treatment options include:

- Physical therapy to maintain strength and flexibility [2]
- Limit exposure to cold [2]
- Drug therapies: topical steroids, topical calcineurin inhibitors, systemic steroids, pulsed IV steroids with mycophenolate mofetil, cyclosporine, methotrexate, cyclophosphamide, D-penicillamine [2]
- Therapy for digital ulcers: intravenous iloprost, bosentan and losartan, dressings [2]
- Therapy for calcinosis cutis: bisphosphonates, rituximab, diltiazem, minocycline, warfarin, IVIg, intralesional steroids, laser, surgical excision, lithotripsy [3]
- Laser for telangiectasias [2]
- PUVA, UVA1 to decrease skin hardening [2]

References

1. Black CM. Scleroderma: clinical aspects. J Intern Med. 1993;234:115–8.
2. Krieg T, Takehara K. Skin disease: a cardinal feature of systemic sclerosis. Rheumatology. 2009;48:14–8.
3. Daoussis D, Antonopoulos I, Liossis SN, et al. Treatment of systemic sclerosis-associated calcinosis: a case report of rituximab-induced regression of CREST-related calcinosis and review of the literature. Semin Arthritis Rheum. 2012;41:822–9.

Epidermolysis Bullosa Acquisita: Gastrointestinal Features

9

Liam Zakko

Epidermolysis bullosa acquisita is an inherited connective tissue disease that causes blistering of the skin and mucous membranes. The incidence is estimated at 1/50,000, with severity ranging from mild to debilitating. Acquisita occurs in 0.2–0.5/million persons/year, with increased incidence in persons of sub-Saharan African descent. Mean age of onset is 50.

The gastrointestinal (GI) symptoms associated with this disease include [1, 2]:

- Dysphagia, chronic constipation, fecal impaction

Gastrointestinal clinical signs and findings include [1–4]:

- Mucosal involvement in 20% of cases: mostly oral but also laryngeal and conjunctival
- Esophagus can have blisters, erosions, scars, webs, ulcers, and strictures (see Fig. 9.1), which can lead to esophageal shortening and narrowing particularly in the dystrophic form (these symptoms are thought to be more prevalent in the dystrophic form because it presents earlier in life with a more narrow esophagus than acquisita) (see Fig. 9.2)
- Also may have pyloric stenosis and malabsorption from GI epithelial disruption in the dystrophic form

Pathogenesis is thought to be due to [5]:

- In the acquisita form, the deposition of autoantibodies against collagen type VII, a major component of the anchoring fibrils, in the basement membrane zone (BMZ) of stratified squamous epithelium; specifically, antibodies react with NC1 zone of collagen type VII, which interacts with extracellular matrix components to stabilize the BMZ; antibodies reduce the number of anchoring fibrils and, thus, the strength of the epithelial-lamina propria links leading to cleavage between the two layers
- In the dystrophic form, mutations in the *COL7A1* gene lead to changes in the amount or structure of collagen type VII

Typical pathologic features include [5]:

- Acquisita
  - Light microscopy-subepidermal blisters with intact epidermis and dermal inflammatory infiltrate
  - Direct immunofluorescence: IgG lines deposit only on BMZ
  - Indirect IgG: antibodies recognizing BMZ, although often negative with low titers
- Dystrophica
  - Collagen type VII usually strongly reduced or absent
  - Blister formation below the lamina propria

Diagnosis involves [3–5]:

- Routine tests (standard pathology/direct immunofluorescence) allow the diagnosis of autoimmune subepidermal blistering disease, but do not specify epidermolysis bullosa
- Immunoblotting/enzyme-linked immunosorbent assay (ELISA) can confirm antibodies against type VII collagen for acquisita type
- Gold standard for aquisita: direct immunoelectron microscopy—confirm immunodeposits against anchoring fibrils under lamina densa; dystrophica: immunofluorescence mapping for location of blister and number of collage type VII molecules, blood testing for *COL7A1* mutations

The differential diagnosis of epidermolysis bullosa should include [3–5]:

- Porphyria cutanea tarda
- Bullous amyloidosis
- Bullous pemphigoid
- Cicatricial pemphigoid

Treatment for this disease includes [6, 7]:

- Acquisita treatment is based on disease severity. Mild: steroids and colchicine, dapsone; moderate: steroids and colchicine, dapsone; severe: steroids (consider intravenous) and colchicine, dapsone/cyclosporine/mycophenolate, consider rituximab, plasmapheresis, and intravenous immunoglobulin

L. Zakko (✉)
Yale Department of Internal Medicine, 20 York Street, Yale New Haven Hospital, New Haven, CT 06510, USA
e-mail: Liam.zakko@yale.edu

G.Y. Wu et al. (eds.), *Atlas of Dermatological Manifestations of Gastrointestinal Disease*, DOI 10.1007/978-1-4614-6191-3_9,

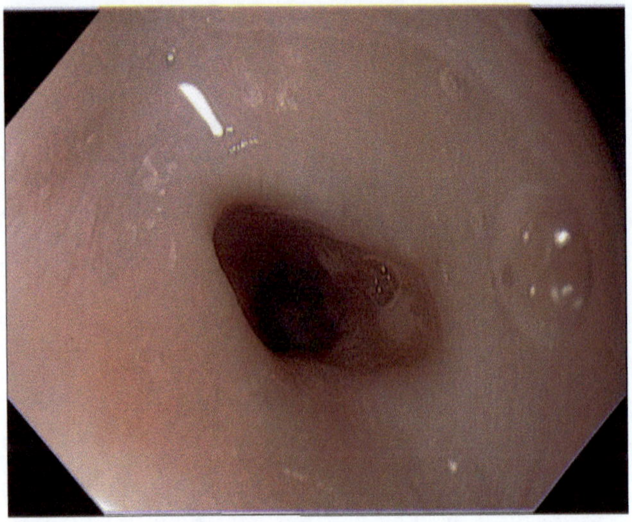

Fig. 9.1 An endoscopic view of an esophageal stricture with distal esophagitis and a shallow ulcer as can be seen in epidermolysis bullosa

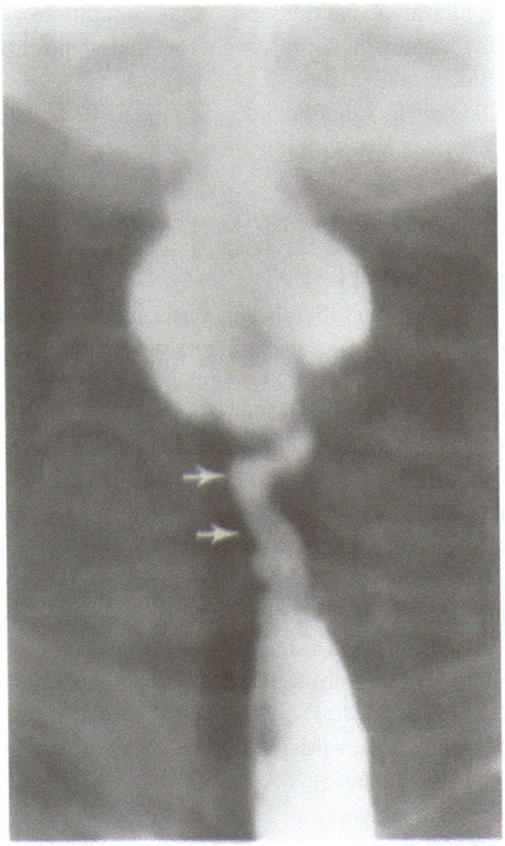

Fig. 9.2 Epidermolysis bullosa dystrophica. A spot film from a barium swallow demonstrates a luminal narrowing in the cervical esophagus (*arrows*), which was pliable but aperistaltic (Reprinted from Jones et al. [8]; with permission)

- Dystrophica treatment includes symptomatic treatment for esophageal lesions

References

1. Bruckner-Tuderman L. Dystrophic epidermolysis bullosa. Dermatol Clin. 2010;28:107–14.
2. Bübl R, Schön B. Dysphagia in dermatologic disease. Dysphagia. 1993;8:85–90.
3. Caux F. Diagnosis and clinical features of epidermolysis bullosa acquisita. Dermatol Clin. 2011;29:485–91.
4. Das BB, Sahoo S. Dystrophic epidermolysis bullosa. J Perinatol. 2004;24:41–7.
5. Gammon WR. Epidermoylsis bullosa acquisita: a disease of autoimmunity to type VII collagen. J Autoimmun. 1991;4:59–71.
6. Intong LRF, Murrel DF. Management of epidermolysis bullosa acquisita. Dermatol Clin. 2011;29:643–7.
7. Trattner A, David M, Sandbank M. Esophageal manifestations in autoimmune bullous diseases. Int J Dermatol. 1992;31:687–91.
8. Jones B, Ravich WJ, Donner MW. Dysphagia in systemic disease. Dysphagia. 1993;8:368–83.

Epidermolysis Bullosa Acquisita: Dermatological Features

10

Liam Zakko, Justin Finch, Marti J. Rothe, and Jane M. Grant-Kels

Clinical signs and features include [1, 2]:

- Incidence: 0.2–0.5/million persons/year [1]; increased in persons of sub-Saharan African descent (African Americans) [1]; mean onset is age 50
- Classic: skin fragility, tense blisters on trauma prone extensor surfaces, noninflamed skin with milia cysts and atrophic scars when healed, scarring alopecia, nail dystrophy, rare oral mucosal involvement (see Figs. 10.1 and 10.2)
- Inflammatory: widespread tense blisters surrounded by urticarial plaques associated with pruritus
- Cicatricial pemphigoid like form: mucosal involvement with lesions in the mouth, conjunctiva, nose, larynx, genitalia, anus, and esophagus (strictures in proximal third leading to dysphagia)
- Brunsting/Perry pemphigoid-like form: vesicles and blisters only on the head, neck, and upper aspect of the trunk, with no mucosal involvement
- IgA disease: severe pruritus; varied skin findings including urticarial plaques, vesicles, bullae, erythema multiforme-like rash, erosions; oral mucosal disease in 30% of patients; atrophic scars and milia are rare
- Multiple disease associations have been reported; systemic lupus erythematosus and Crohn's disease are the most well-substantiated disease associations

L. Zakko (✉)
Yale Department of Internal Medicine, 20 York Street, Yale New Haven Hospital, New Haven, CT 06510, USA
e-mail: liam.zakko@yale.edu

J. Finch • M.J. Rothe • J.M. Grant-Kels
Department of Dermatology, University of Connecticut Health Center, 21 South Road, Farmington, CT 06030, USA
e-mail: finch@uchc.edu; rothe@uchc.edu; grant@uchc.edu

Pathogenesis of this autoimmune disease involves [1, 3]:

- Deposition of autoantibodies against type VII collagen, a major component of the anchoring fibrils, in the basement membrane zone (BMZ) of stratified squamous epithelium
- Specifically antibodies react with NC1 zone of collagen VII, which interacts with extracellular matrix components to stabilize the BMZ to the dermis
- Antibodies reduce the number of anchoring fibrils and thus reduce the strength of the dermal–epidermal link leading to cleavage between the two layers

Histopathological features include:

- Light microscopy: subepidermal blister with intact epidermis and a variable dermal inflammatory infiltrate; spectrum includes noninflammatory lesions with little or no inflammation to inflammatory lesions with neutrophils, eosinophils, or lymphocytes (see Fig. 10.3)
- Direct immunofluorescence: most commonly IgG with complement as a linear deposition at the BMZ
- Indirect IgG: antibodies recognizing BMZ though often negative with low titers

The diagnosis is made using a combination of [4]:

- Routine tests (standard pathology/direct immunofluorescence) that allow the diagnosis of autoimmune subepidermal blistering disease but do not specify epidermolysis bullosa acquisita
- Specific tests including localizing autoantibodies to dermal side of salt-skin split specimen
- Immunoblotting/enzyme-linked immunosorbent assay (ELISA) that can confirm antibodies against type VII collagen
- Gold standard: direct immunoelectron microscopy that confirms immune deposits against anchoring fibrils under lamina densa

The differential diagnosis should include:

- Dystrophic bullous epidermolysis
- Porphyria cutanea tarda

G.Y. Wu et al. (eds.), *Atlas of Dermatological Manifestations of Gastrointestinal Disease*,
DOI 10.1007/978-1-4614-6191-3_10, © Springer Science+Business Media New York 2013

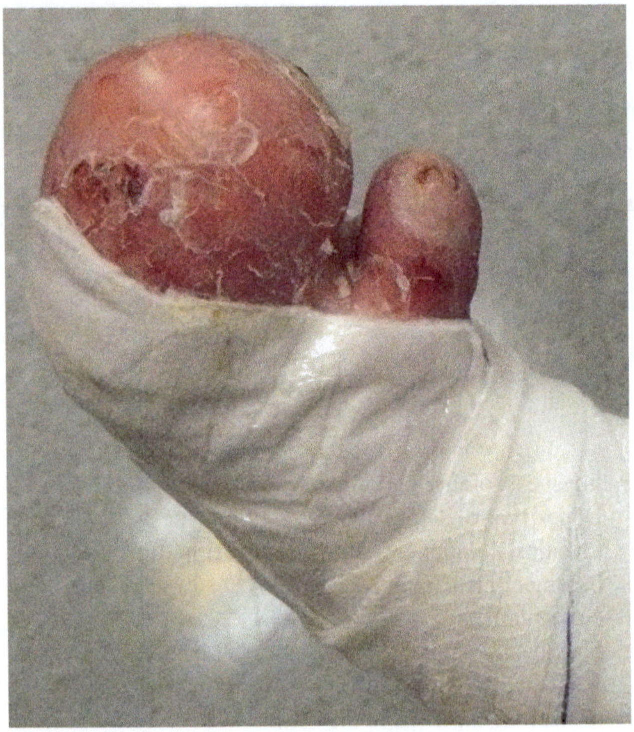

Fig. 10.1 Recessive dystrophic epidermolysis bullosa. Mitten deformity caused by repetitive severe scarring and resultant syndactyly

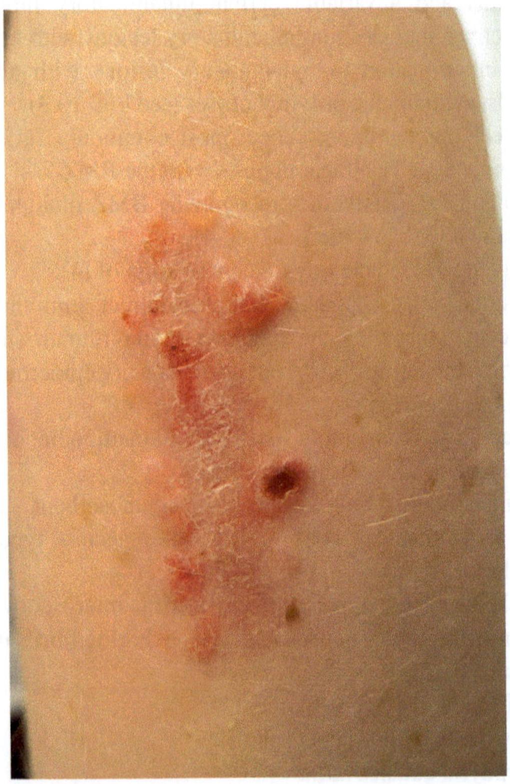

Fig. 10.2 Epidermolysis bullosa acquisita. Pauci-inflammatory subepidermal blister

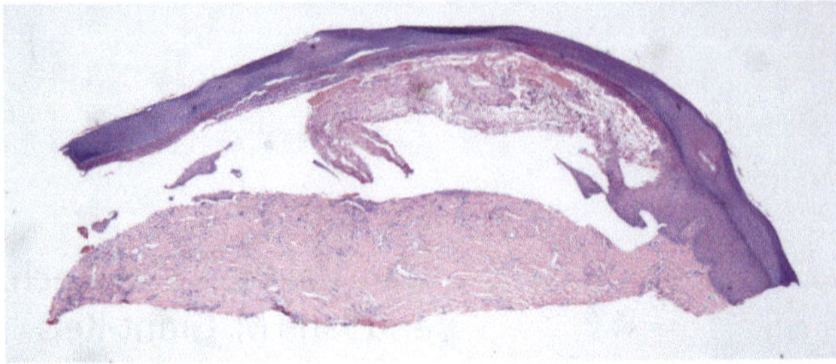

Fig. 10.3 EB Aquisita. Pauci-inflammatory subepidermal blister

- Bullous amyloidosis
- Bullous pemphigoid
- Cicatricial pemphigoid
- Bullous lupus erythematosus

Treatment options include:

- Local wound care, trauma avoidance, protective padding for extensor surfaces
- Based on disease features: colchicine can be effective for both classical mechanobullous epidermolysis bullosa acquisita (EBA) and inflammatory EBA; systemic corticosteroids can be effective for inflammatory EBA but not for mechanobullous EBA [2]
- Based on disease severity, mild: oral steroids and colchicine ± dapsone; moderate: oral steroids and colchicine ± dapsone; severe: steroids (consider intravenous) and colchicine ± dapsone/cyclosporine/mycophenolate with consideration for rituximab, plasmapheresis, and intravenous immunoglobin [4]
- Recommended dosages of oral steroids and colchicine are higher for more severe disease than for more mild disease

References

1. Caux F. Diagnosis and clinical features of epidermolysis bullosa acquisita. Dermatol Clin. 2011;29:485–91.
2. Gupta R, Woodley DT, Chen M. Epidermolysis bullosa acquisita. Clin Dermatol. 2012;30:60–9.
3. Gammon WR. Epidermolysis bullosa acquisita: a disease of autoimmunity to type VII collagen. J Autoimmun. 1991;4:59–71.
4. Intong LRA, Murrel DF. Management of epidermolysis bullosa acquisita. Dermatol Clin. 2011;29:643–7.

Pemphigus Vulgaris: Gastrointestinal Features

11

Liam Zakko

Pemphigus vulgaris is a chronic autoimmune disease due to antibodies against proteins involved in cell-to-cell binding within the epidermis. There is an equal gender distribution with the disease often manifesting itself in the fifth or sixth decade. Incidence has been estimated at 0.1/100,000 persons, but it is more common in the Middle East and Asia. Mucous membranes are usually affected before any cutaneous lesions manifest [1].

- The most common gastrointestinal symptoms include [1, 2]: Odynophagia, dysphagia, emesis, hematemesis
- Oral ulcers, then cutaneous manifestations
- May involve: oropharynx, skin, esophagus, conjunctiva, nasal mucosa, larynx, urethra, vulva, cervix
- Esophageal involvement is often asymptomatic but may present with esophagitis (see Fig. 11.1)
- Rarely can cause dissection and exfoliation of the esophageal mucosa in all layers leading to esophageal dissecans superficialis—a condition in which the patient vomits a mucosal cast of the esophagus
- Stomach and duodenal involvement, although may also be secondary to steroid treatment
- Rare reports of colonic involvement

Pathogenesis is not entirely clear, but appears to involve altered immunity [3]:

- Antibody to desmoglein 3 (DSG3), a glycoprotein cadherin responsible for cell-to-cell adhesion, leads to damage to intracellular adhesion structures leading to loss of cell-to-cell attachment
- Triggers appear to be medications, pesticides, malignancy, ultraviolet radiation, stress, and foods with allium, phenol, or urushiol groups
- More likely to occur in persons with HLA-DR4 or HLA-DR6

Pathology studies of mucosal biopsies can show [2, 3]:

- Acantholysis in visible lesions
- Direct immunofluorescence will show antibody deposition of IgG and C3 throughout the intercellular spaces of the esophageal epithelium even if there is no visual evidence of disease

Diagnosis is made by considering [1–3]:

- Clinical symptoms with histological findings as listed above
- Detection of tissue and circulating autoantibodies, DSG3 and desmoglein 1 (DSG1) antibody in some patients with skin involvement
- Acute disease: anti-DSG3—IgG4, IgA, IgE; chronic disease: anti-DGS3: IgG1 and IgG4
- Enzyme-linked immunosorbent assay (ELISA) to monitor disease activity and response to treatment, although ELISA can be positive without any blistering condition
- Upper endoscopy to diagnose esophageal disease

The differential diagnosis of pemphigus vulgaris should include [1–3]:

- Bullous pemphigoid
- Herpes gestationis
- Mucous membrane pemphigoid
- Linear IgA dermatosis
- Epidermolysis bullosa acquisita
- Bullous lupus
- Dermatitis herpetiformis
- Pemphigus foliaceus
- Aphthous ulcers
- Lichen planus
- Systemic lupus erythematosus

Although not curative, treatment should involve [4]:

- Corticosteroids have a central role: with prednisolone should see a response in 1 week to 1 month
- Role of other systemic immunomodulating agents (azathioprine, cyclophosphamide, cyclosporine, dapsone,

L. Zakko (✉)
Yale Department of Internal Medicine, Yale New Haven Hospital, 20 York Street New Haven, CT 06510, USA
e-mail: liam.zakko@yale.edu

G.Y. Wu et al. (eds.), *Atlas of Dermatological Manifestations of Gastrointestinal Disease*,
DOI 10.1007/978-1-4614-6191-3_11, © Springer Science+Business Media New York 2013

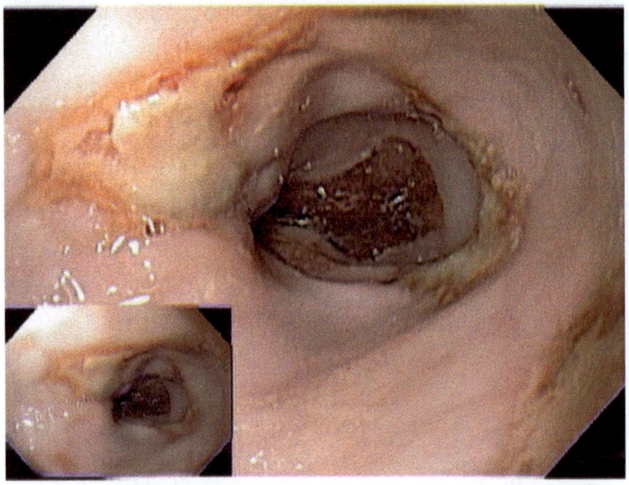

Fig. 11.1 An endoscopic view of ulceration and early exfoliation of portions of the esophageal mucosa in a patient with pemphigus. *Inset* shows more esophageal involvement by positioning the endoscope more proximally (Image courtesy of the Connecticut Gastrointestinal Institute)

mycophenolate) is unclear; if no complete response, azathioprine is often used as second line with corticosteroids

References

1. Fukuchi H, Otake S, Naitoh H, et al. A case of exfoliative esophagitis with pemphigus vulgaris. Dis Esophagus. 2011;24:23–5.
2. Narashima RP, Samarth A, Aurangabadkar SJ, et al. TSS: study of upper gastrointestinal tract involvement in pemphigus by esophago-gastro-duodenoscopy. Indian J Dermatol Venereol Leprol. 2006;72:421–4.
3. Trattner A, Lurie R, Leiser A, et al. Esophageal involvement in pemphigus vulgaris: a clinical, histologic and immunopathologic study. J Am Acad Dermatol. 1991;24:233–6.
4. Martin LK, Werth VP, Villaneuva EV, Murrel DF. A systemic review of randomized control trials for pemphigus vulgaris and pemphigus foliaceus. J Am Acad Dermatol. 2011;64:903–8.

12 Pemphigus Vulgaris: Dermatological Features

Liam Zakko, Justin Finch, Marti J. Rothe, and Jane M. Grant-Kels

Clinical signs and features include [1]:

- Intraepithelial blister formation secondary to acantholysis (loss of cell to cell adhesion of keratinocytes)
- Incidence 0.1–0.5/100,000 persons: more common in patients of Jewish descent and most common autoimmune bullous disease in Middle East and Asia
- Presents as oral ulcers then cutaneous manifestations
- May involve: oropharynx, esophagus, conjunctiva, nasal mucosa, larynx, urethra, vulva, cervix
- Skin lesions have a predilection for the trunk, gingiva, axillae, scalp, face, and pressure points
- Flaccid, nonscarring, fragile vesicles, and bullae develop and rupture, causing painful erosions (see Fig. 12.1)
- Characterized by Nikolsky's sign: direct—press on blister extends blister to adjacent skin; indirect—rub clinically normal skin and get shearing

Pathogenesis of this disease involves [1]:

- Initially, when involvement is limited to the oral mucosa, antibody to desmoglein 3 (DSG3), a glycoprotein cadherin responsible for cell to cell adhesion, leads to damage to intracellular adhesion structures leading to loss of cell to cell attachment
- Later, antibodies against desmoglein 1 (DSG1) develop when skin becomes involved
- Triggers appear to be medications, pesticides, malignancy, ultraviolet radiation, stress, and foods with allium, phenol, thiol, or urushiol groups
- After trigger, more likely to occur in persons with HLA-DR4 or HLA-DR6

Histopathological features include:

- Light microscopy: suprabasilar loss of adhesion of keratinocytes with acantholytic or rounded-up keratinocytes identified in the blister cavity. The basal keratinocytes remain attached to the basement membrane due to the lack of involvement of hemidesmosomes. However, the basal cells lose attachment to adjacent (overlying and lateral) keratinocytes and therefore have been described as appearing as a "row of tombstones." Often there is an inflammatory infiltrate-containing eosinophils and/or neutrophils in addition to lymphocytes (see Fig. 12.2)
- Direct Immunofluorescence: IgG/C3 binding to intercellular areas in predominantly the mid-lower epidermis
- Indirect immunofluorescence: serum autoantibodies against desmosomal antigens

The diagnosis is made using a combination of:

- Clinical symptoms with histological findings as listed above
- Tzanck preparation reveals acantholytic keratinocytes
- Detection of tissue and circulating autoantibodies: DSG3 and DGS1 antibodies in some patients with skin involvement
- Can use enzyme-linked immunosorbent assay (ELISA) stains to monitor disease activity and response to treatment, though ELISA can be positive without any blistering condition
- Immunoblot analysis shows in acute disease: anti-DSG3—IgG4, IgA, IgE, and in chronic disease shows anti-DSG3—IgG1 and IgG4 [1]

The differential diagnosis should include:

- Bullous pemphigoid
- Herpes gestationis

L. Zakko (✉)
Yale Department of Internal Medicine, Yale New Haven Hospital, 20 York Street New Haven, CT 06510, USA
e-mail: liam.zakko@yale.edu

J. Finch • M.J. Rothe • J.M. Grant-Kels
Department of Dermatology, University of Connecticut Health Center, 21 South Road, Farmington, CT 06030, USA
e-mail: finch@uchc.edu; rothe@uchc.edu; grant@uchc.edu

G.Y. Wu et al. (eds.), *Atlas of Dermatological Manifestations of Gastrointestinal Disease*,
DOI 10.1007/978-1-4614-6191-3_12, © Springer Science+Business Media New York 2013

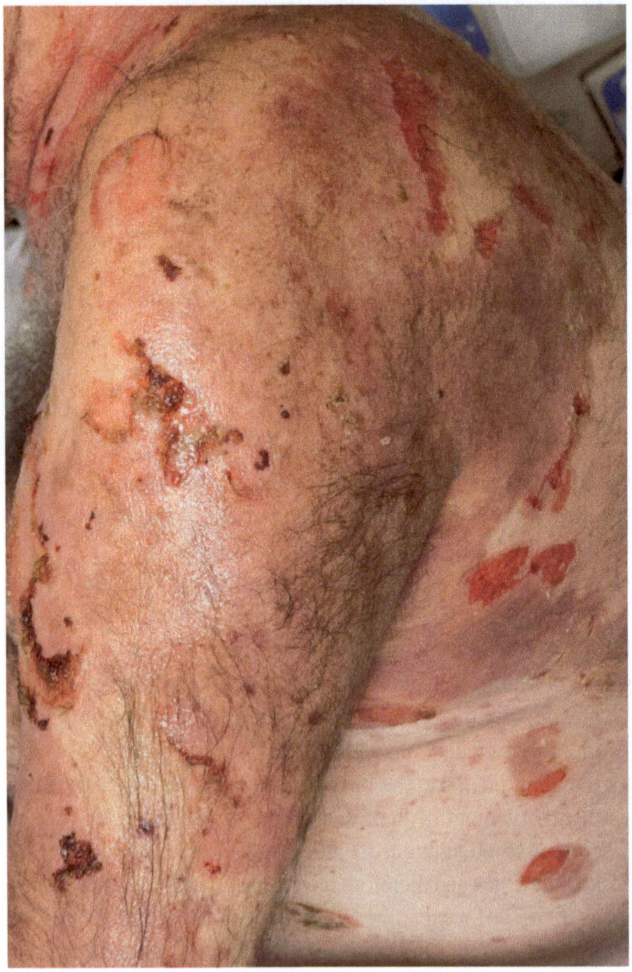

Fig. 12.1 Pemphigus vulgaris. Flaccid bullae and large plaques of denuded skin

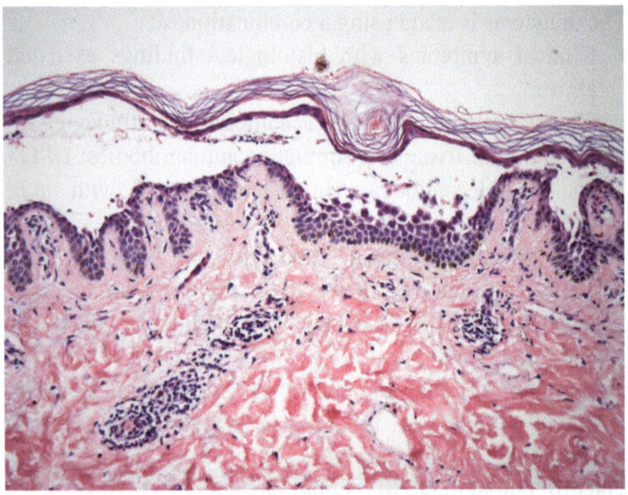

Fig. 12.2 Pemphigus vulgaris. Histology demonstrates a suprabasilar split in the epidermis, with acantholysis ("tombstoning") of the basal keratinocytes (100×)

- Mucous membrane pemphigoid
- Linear IgA dermatosis
- Epidermolysis bullosa acquisita
- Bullous systemic lupus erythematosus
- Dermatitis herpetiformis
- Pemphigus foliaceus
- Paraneoplastic pemphigus
- Aphthous ulcers
- Lichen planus (bullous type, oral lichen planus)

Treatment options include [2]:

- Systemic corticosteroids have a central role
- Standard of care is to prescribe a steroid sparing agent (azathioprine, cyclophosphamide, cyclosporine, dapsone, mycophenolate) in conjunction with systemic corticosteroid taper, but the best therapeutic protocol remains unclear
- Rituximab alone or with intravenous immunoglobin for refractory cases

References

1. Venugopal SS, Murrell DF. Diagnosis and clinical features of pemphigus vulgaris. Dermatol Clin. 2011;29:373–80.
2. Martin LK, Werth VP, Villaneuva EV, Murrel DF. A systematic review of randomized control trials for pemphigus vulgaris and pemphigus foliaceus. J Am Acad Dermatol. 2011;64:903–8.

13 Dermatomyositis: Gastrointestinal Features

Laura Nieves

Dermatomyositis is a connective tissue disease associated with inflammation of the muscles and skin. The exact cause remains unknown. There is evidence that the disease is autoimmune in origin but may also have components of viral infection and can be drug-induced, as well. Although the presentation is mainly with skin rash and proximal muscle weakness, the disease can affect multiple organs [1].

Gastrointestinal (GI) symptoms of dermatomyositis include [1, 2]:

- Dysphagia, dysmotility, megaesophagus (see Fig. 13.1) [3]
- Nasal regurgitation and nasal speech
- Aspiration
- Malabsorption
- Ulceration, perforation, or hemorrhage anywhere along GI tract (rare)
- Pancreatitis, cholestasis, and hepatomegaly have been reported in juvenile diabetes mellitus

Clinical signs and findings include [1, 2]:

- Paraneoplastic syndrome associated with colon cancer, and non-Hodgkin's lymphoma, ovarian cancer, breast cancer, and melanoma

The pathogenesis likely involves autoimmune mechanisms [2, 4]:

- Antibodies to specific autoantigens
- Hypoxia hypothesis: microvessel involvement and loss leading to tissue hypoxia and fatigue

The pathology will show [1, 2, 4]:

- Perifascicular atrophy, muscle infarcts (necrosis), and capillary necrosis with membrane attack, complex deposition on vessel walls
- Reduced capillary density
- Degenerating/regenerating fibers, fiber size variation, and mononuclear inflammatory infiltrate

The diagnosis is made by considering the following [1, 2, 4]:

- Laboratory: creatine kinase (CK), lactate dehydrogenase (LDH), aldolase, aspartate
- Aminotransferase (AST), alanine aminotransferase (ALT), antinuclear antibodies (ANA), anti-signal recognition particle (SRP), anti-Jo-1
- Anti-Mi-2 antibodies
- Electromyography
- Skin biopsy
- Muscle biopsy
- Magnetic resonance imaging

The differential diagnosis of dermatomyositis should include [1, 2, 4]:

- Polymyositis
- Inclusion body myositis
- Drug-induced myopathy
- Polymyalgia rheumatica
- Hypothyroidism
- Neuromuscular disorders (myasthenia gravis, Eaton-Lambert syndrome)

Although not curative, the treatment involves [1, 2, 5]:

- First-line: high-dose corticosteroids (up to 90% response)
- Second-line: immunomodulators (azathioprine, methotrexate, cyclosporine A), intravenous immunoglobulin, alkylating agents (cyclophosphamide, chlorambucil), mycophenolate mofetil, and biologics (rituximab, etanercept, infliximab).

References

1. Khan S, Christopher-Stine L. Polymyositis, dermatomyositis, and autoimmune necrotizing myopathy: clinical features. Rheum Dis Clin North Am. 2011;37:143–58.
2. Ramanan AV, Feldman BM. Clinical features and outcomes of juvenile dermatomyositis and other childhood onset myositis syndromes. Rheum Dis Clin North Am. 2002;28:833–57.

L. Nieves (✉)
Department of Internal Medicine, University of Connecticut Health Center, Farmington, CT, USA
e-mail: lnieves@resident.uchc.edu

G.Y. Wu et al. (eds.), *Atlas of Dermatological Manifestations of Gastrointestinal Disease*,
DOI 10.1007/978-1-4614-6191-3_13, © Springer Science+Business Media New York 2013

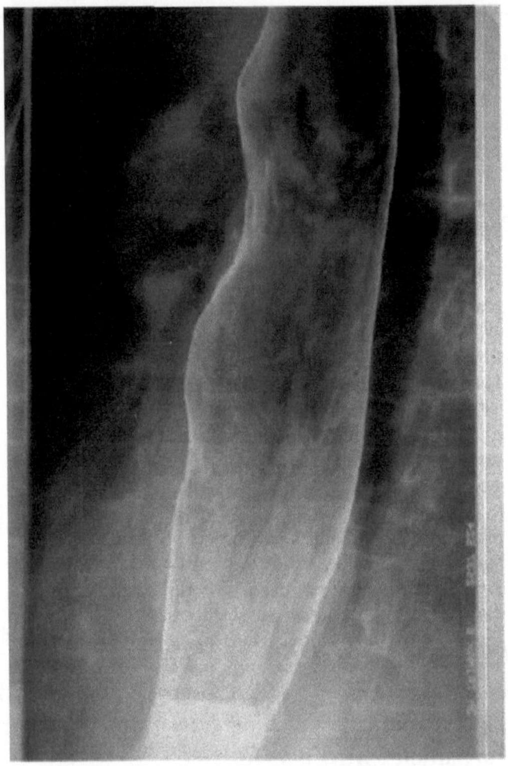

Fig. 13.1 A radiograph showing a markedly dilated (megaesophagus) in a patient with dermatomyositis (Reprinted from Caramaschi et al. [3]; with permission)

3. Caramaschi E, Biasi D, Carletto A, et al. Megaoesophagus in a patient affected by dermatomyositis. Clin Rheumatol. 1997;16:106–7.
4. Nagaraju K, Lundberg IE. Polymyositis and dermatomyositis: pathophysiology. Rheum Dis Clin North Am. 2011;37:159–71.
5. Iorizzo LJ, Jorizzo JL. The treatment and prognosis of dermatomyositis: an updated review. J Am Acad Dermatol. 2008;59:99–112.

Dermatomyositis: Dermatological Features

14

Liam Zakko, Justin Finch, Marti J. Rothe, and Jane M. Grant-Kels

Clinical signs and features include:

- Bimodal incidence pattern—childhood and then age 50–70s; four to ten new cases per million; more common in women [1]
- Associated with internal malignancy in about 25 % [2] of cases, especially adenocarcinoma of ovary, lung, and gastrointestinal tract in Western countries and nasopharyngeal carcinomas in South East Asia, Southern China, and North Africa [3]; the diagnosis of dermatomyositis may be made prior to, concurrently, or after the diagnosis of malignancy; age-appropriate malignancy surveillance is recommended
- Muscle symptoms: symmetric proximal muscle and truncal weakness that develops relatively slowly over the course of weeks to months, occasionally associated with myalgias and muscle tenderness early in the disease course. It is atypical for muscle disease to precede skin manifestations.
- Also can have joint, gastrointestinal tract, pulmonary (interstitial lung disease), and cardiac involvement: the latter two are associated with a worse prognosis [1]
- Types of dermatomyositis: adult, juvenile, associated with malignancy, dermatomyositis overlap syndrome, amyopathic dermatomyositis (dermatologic disease without muscle findings)
- Cutaneous symptoms: precede myositis by up to 2 years; can be most active part of condition and not respond to treatment that improves muscle symptoms; often photosensitive [1]
  - Gottron papules: pathognomonic—violaceous, flat-topped papules and plaques located over dorsal aspect of interphalangeal or metacarpophalangeal joints that over time may develop atrophic, depressed, white centers with prominent telangiectasias
  - Heliotrope sign: highly characteristic—periorbital violaceous erythema with or without associated edema of the eyelids and periorbital tissue; rash can become more confluent and involve the entire face (see Fig. 14.1a)
  - Gottron sign: characteristic—violaceous erythema with or without edema overlying the dorsal aspect of the interphalangeal or metacarpophalangeal joints, olecranon processes, patella, and medial malleoli (see Fig. 14.1b)
  - Macular violaceous erythema: shawl sign (nape of shoulders, upper back); V sign (V of neck and upper chest), linear extensor erythema
  - Mechanic's hands: hyperkeratosis, scaling, horizontal fissuring of the palms and fingers bilaterally
  - Also see nail fold telangiectasia, periungual erythema, cuticular hypertrophy, pruritus, calcinosis cutis, non-scarring alopecia, poikiloderma, Raynaud's; rare findings include erythroderma, livedo reticularis, flagellate erythema, cutaneous vasculitis
  - Wong type of dermatomyositis is a rare variant showing hyperkeratotic, follicular, erythematous papules that occur in a linear distribution over the dorsal aspect of the hands and feet over bony prominences, resembling pityriasis rubra pilaris; can evolve into full blown dermatomyositis; may be more common in Asian patients.

L. Zakko (✉)
Yale Department of Internal Medicine, Yale New Haven Hospital, 20 York Street New Haven, CT 60510, USA
e-mail: liam.zakko@yale.edu

J. Finch • M.J. Rothe • J.M. Grant-Kels
Department of Dermatology, University of Connecticut Health Center, 21 South Road, Farmington, CT 06030, USA
e-mail: finch@uchc.edu; rothe@uchc.edu; grant@uchc.edu

G.Y. Wu et al. (eds.), *Atlas of Dermatological Manifestations of Gastrointestinal Disease*, DOI 10.1007/978-1-4614-6191-3_14, © Springer Science+Business Media New York 2013

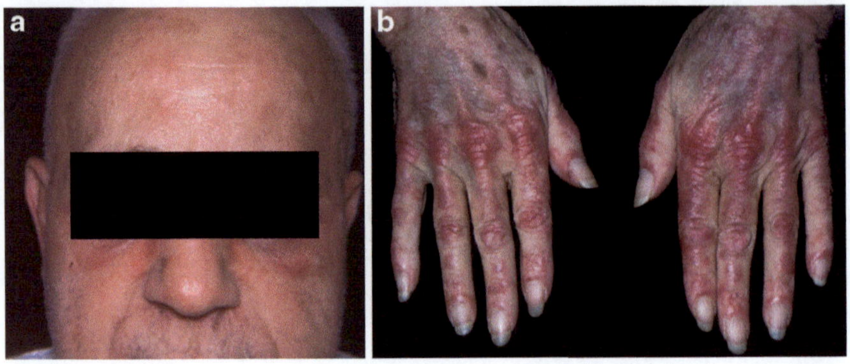

Fig. 14.1 Dermatomyositis. Gottron's papules (**a**); Heliotrope sign (**b**) (Image courtesy of Yale Residency Collection)

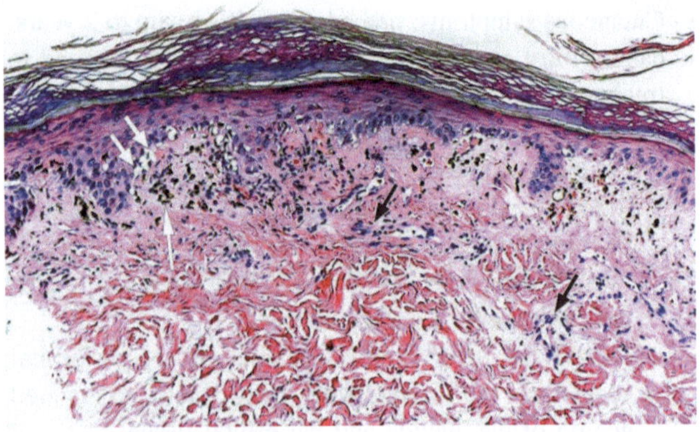

Fig. 14.2 Dermatomyositis. Liquefaction degeneration, with vacuolization of the basal layer (*short white arrows*). Melanin incontinence (*long white arrow*). Sparse perivascular lymphocytes (*black arrows*) (40×)

Pathogenesis of this autoimmune disease involves:

- Likely autoimmune as associated with specific autoantibodies and presence of B-cells and plasma cells in the muscle tissue inflammatory infiltrates [4]
- Hypothesis that etiology is an immune response to cancer with crossover to muscle antigens [3]

Histopathological features include:

- Cell poor, vacuolar interface dermatitis with a sparse infiltrate of lymphocytic inflammatory cells (see Fig. 14.2)
- Dermal, perivascular infiltrate with T-cells with interstitial mucin
- Epidermis may be atrophic or acanthotic (as in Gottron's papules)
- Muscle biopsy usually demonstrates muscle fiber atrophy in association with evidences of regeneration, necrosis, and hypertrophy with lymphocytic perivascular and perifascicular inflammation.

The diagnosis is made using a combination of:

- Bohan and Peter Classification Criteria: symmetrical proximal muscle weakness; increase of serum skeletal muscle enzyme levels including CK and aldolase
- Electromyography: polyphasic, short, small motor unit potentials; fibrillation; positive sharp waves; increased insertional irritability; and repetitive high-frequency discharges
- Muscle biopsy with findings of degeneration and regeneration, necrosis, and interstitial mononuclear infiltrate
- Magnetic resonance imaging, ultrasound, computed tomography may be utilized to assess myositis
- Cutaneous manifestations: heliotrope rash or Gottron sign

The differential diagnosis should include:

- Contact dermatitis
- Psoriasis
- Systemic lupus erythematosus
- Polymyalgia rheumatic
- Metabolic myopathy
- Polyarteritis
- Drug-induced myositis
- Myasthenia gravis
- Lambert-Eaton syndrome

Treatment options include:

- First-line treatment: high-dose oral prednisone with slow taper and consider intravenous immunoglobin (IVIG) with severe systemic complications [5]
- If first-line fails, then methotrexate, azathioprine, or IVIG if cytotoxic agents contraindicated [5]
- Third line: combined methotrexate and azathioprine, mycophenolate mofetil (but three patients in a series of ten treated with mycophenolate had serious opportunistic infections leading to one death [6]), rituximab, cyclosporine, cyclophosphamide, tacrolimus [5]

- Treatment specifically for the skin manifestations include sun protection, topical steroids, antimalarials, low-dose weekly methotrexate [7], and topical calcineurin inhibitors [8]

References

1. Khan S, Christopher-Stine L. Polymyositis, dermatomyositis, and autoimmune necrotizing myopathy: clinical features. Rheum Dis Clin North Am. 2011;37:143–58.
2. Ramos-E-Silva M, Carvalho JC, Carneiro SC. Cutaneous paraneoplasia. Clin Dermatol. 2011;29:541–7.
3. Zahr ZA, Baer AN. Malignancy in myositis. Curr Rheumatol Rep. 2011;13:208–15.
4. Nagaraju K, Lundberg IE. Polymyositis and dermatomyositis: pathophysiology. Rheum Dis Clin North Am. 2011;37:159–71.
5. Marie I, Mouthon L. Therapy of polymyositis and dermatomyositis. Autoimmun Rev. 2011;11:6–13.
6. Rowin J, Amato AA, Deisher N, et al. Mycophenolate mofetil in dermatomyositis: is it safe? Neurology. 2006;66:1245–7.
7. Dawkins MA, Jorizzo JL, Walker FO, et al. Dermatomyositis. A dermatology-based case series. J Am Acad Dermatol. 1998;38:397–404.
8. Kim JE, Jeong MG, Lee HE, et al. Successful treatment of cutaneous lesions of dermatomyositis with topical pimecrolimus. Ann Dermatol. 2011;23:348–51.

Part II

Weight Loss Malabsorption

Pernicious Anemia: Gastrointestinal Features

15

Michael Tadros

Pernicious anemia is one of the many megaloblastic anemias. It is due to a deficiency of vitamin B_{12}, which is itself due loss of gastric parietal cells capable of secreting intrinsic factor. Although often applied to any type of vitamin B_{12}—related anemia, the *pernicious anemia* specifically refers to the disease associated with atrophic gastritis, parietal cell loss, and lack of intrinsic factor. Because of the location of the disease, there are multiple gastrointestinal (GI) symptoms including [1, 2]:

- Burning and soreness on anterior portion of the tongue
- Change in bowel habits
- Anorexia and weight loss
- Nonspecific GI symptoms: nausea, vomiting, pyrosis, and a sense of distention
- Abdominal pain can occur rarely due to spinal cord damage

Clinical signs and findings include [1, 2]:

- Painful beefy red tongue with loss of papillae
- Signs and symptoms of megaloblastic anemia from vitamin B_{12} deficiency and indirect hyperbilirubinemia from ineffective erythropoiesis
- There is increased risk of gastric polyps and cancer
- Neurologic manifestations from axonal demyelination and degeneration of peripheral nerves and dorsal and lateral columns, resulting in paresthesias, weakness, ataxia, and sphincter dysfunction
- Higher association with other autoimmune disorders as diabetes type 1, vitiligo, thyroid dysfunction, and polyglandular autoimmune deficiency syndrome

The pathogenesis appears to involve an autoimmune process [3, 4]:

- Autoimmune disorder characterized by antibodies to parietal cell antigens, most notably the proton pump (H^+,K^+-ATPase) and to intrinsic factor leading to:
  - B_{12} malabsorption
  - Achlorhydria or hypochlorhydria, and hypergastrinemia
- T-cells plays a major role in the autoimmune destruction of the gastric mucosa; Th17 cells are associated with the most destructive disease
- There is some evidence for the role of *Helicobacter pylori* in this disease

The pathology typically shows [1, 2]:

- Histological: autoimmune destruction and inflammation of body and fundus of the stomach with loss of the partial and chief cells
- Gross: flatting of the gastric folds and thinning of the gastric mucosa with prominent vasculature (*see* Fig. 15.1).

The diagnosis is made on the basis of a combination of tests [1, 2]:

- Antiparietal and intrinsic factor antibodies
- Complete blood count (CBC) will show anemia and/or pancytopenia, with oval macrocytes and hypersegmented granulocytes on peripheral smear.
- Elevated indirect bilirubin and lactate dehydrogenase (LDH)
- Decreased gastric secretions leading to achlorhydria and hypergastrinemia
- Low levels of vitamin B_{12} and elevated methylmalonic acid and homocysteine
- Schilling test
- Upper endoscopy with multiple gastric biopsies

The differential diagnosis of pernicious anemia should include [1, 2]:

- Helicobacter pylori gastritis
- Gastric cancer
- Hypergastrinemia (Zollinger–Ellison disorder, and chronic protein pump inhibitor use)
- Other causes of vitamin B_{12} deficiency (malabsorption syndromes)
- Other causes of anemia (myeloproliferative disorders)

The treatment consists of vitamin replacement [1, 2]:

- Parenteral vitamin B_{12} replacement with monitoring of adequate response
- Rarely blood transfusion is needed

M. Tadros (✉)
Department of Internal Medicine, University of Connecticut Health Center, Farmington, CT, USA

560 Hudson Street, Apt 750, Hartford, CT 06106, USA
e-mail: MTadros@resident.uchc.edu

G.Y. Wu et al. (eds.), *Atlas of Dermatological Manifestations of Gastrointestinal Disease*, DOI 10.1007/978-1-4614-6191-3_15, © Springer Science+Business Media New York 2013

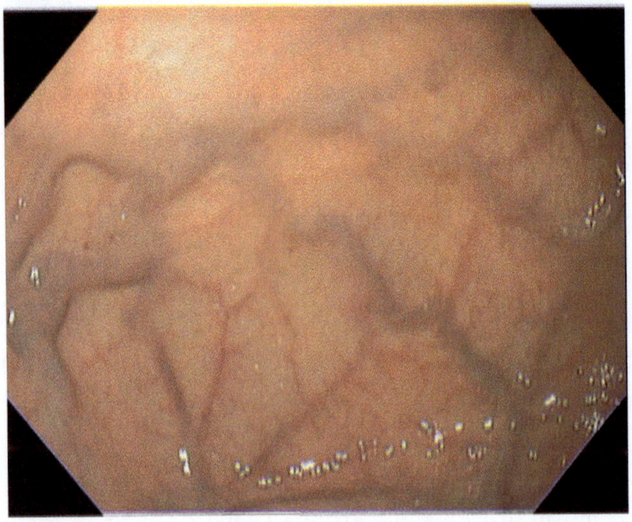

Fig. 15.1 An endoscopic view of atrophic gastritis seen in pernicious anemia. Rugae are flattened and the gastric mucosa is thin, allowing vessels to be easily visualized through the mucosa

- Endoscopic surveillance for gastric cancer (although no clear guidelines)

References

1. Feldman M, Friedman LS, Brandt LJ. Sleisenger and Fordtran's gastrointestinal and liver disease. 9th ed. Philadelphia: Saunders; 2010.
2. El-Zimaity H. Gastritis and gastric atrophy. Curr Opin Gastroenterol. 2008;24:682–6.
3. Huter EN, Stummvoll GH, DiPaolo RJ, et al. Pre-differentiated Th1 and Th17 effector T cells in autoimmune gastritis: Ag-specific regulatory T cells are more potent suppressors than polyclonal regulatory T cells. Int Immunopharmacol. 2009;9:540–5.
4. Lahner E, Annibale B. Pernicious anemia: new insights from a gastroenterological point of view. World J Gastroenterol. 2009;15:5121–8.

Vitiligo

16

Liam Zakko, Justin Finch, Marti J. Rothe, and Jane M. Grant-Kels

Clinical signs and features include:

- Well-circumscribed depigmented macules and patches, which often increase with time
- Often occurs at typically hyperpigmented sites (face, dorsal surface of the hands, nipples, axillae, umbilicus, sacrum, inguinal, anogenital regions) [1]
- Lesions occasionally may itch, all have a propensity for sunburn, may exhibit Koebner phenomenon developing in areas of friction (elbows, knees, digits, flexor wrists) [1]
- Localized—focal, segmental (dermatomal) or mucosal—often in trigeminal dermatome (see Fig. 16.1) [1]
- Generalized: acrofacial, vulgaris, mixed [1]
- Universal: >80% of the body [1]
- Ponctué: rare, discrete, confetti macules [1]
- Trichrome: tan zone of varying width between normal and depigmented skin [1]
- Quadrichrome: additional marginal or perifollicular hyperpigmentation [1]
- Blue vitiligo: blue-gray hue [1]
- Inflammatory: erythema at border of depigmented macules [1]
- Presents as early as 6 weeks old, 50% present by age 20, earlier in women than men; affects 0.5–1% of the population (although some areas have increased prevalence, e.g, India) [1]
- 15% to 20% of patients have one or more affected first-degree relative [1]
- Link with other autoimmune diseases: Addison's disease, thyroid disease, diabetes mellitus, 20% with hearing loss, pernicious anemia—1.9% of persons with vitiligo (13-fold increase over the general population) [1]

Vitiligo probably represents a heterogeneous group of disorders with multifactorial pathogenesis, including:

- Loss of functioning epidermal and sometimes hair follicle melanocytes [1]
- Current hypothesis is that vitiligo is a group of heterogeneous pathophysiologic disorders with a similar phenotype; although systemic autoimmune processes may underlie generalized vitiligo, more localized processes (dysregulation of the nerve system or cytotoxic stress) may underlie focal segmental or focal vitiligo [1]

Histopathological features include:

- Few or no melanocytes within the lesion; melanocytes on the edge of the lesion are large, with long dendritic processes filled with melanin (see Fig. 16.2) [1]
- Perivascular inflammatory infiltrate is occasionally seen with focal areas of adjacent vacuolar alteration of the dermal epidermal junction [1]
- Pan melanoma cocktail (HMB45 + tyrosinase + MART) can maximize yield of detecting active and/or inactive melanocytes [1]
- Trichome variant: increased melanocytes in tan area
- Blue vitiligo: an absence of epidermal melanocytes with an increased number of melanophages [1]

L. Zakko (✉)
Yale Department of Internal Medicine, Yale New Haven Hospital, 20 York Street New Haven, CT 06510, USA
e-mail: liam.zakko@yale.edu

J. Finch • M.J. Rothe • J.M. Grant-Kels
Department of Dermatology, University of Connecticut Health Center, 21 South Road, Farmington, CT 06030, USA
e-mail: finch@uchc.edu; rothe@uchc.edu; grant@uchc.edu

G.Y. Wu et al. (eds.), *Atlas of Dermatological Manifestations of Gastrointestinal Disease*, DOI 10.1007/978-1-4614-6191-3_16,

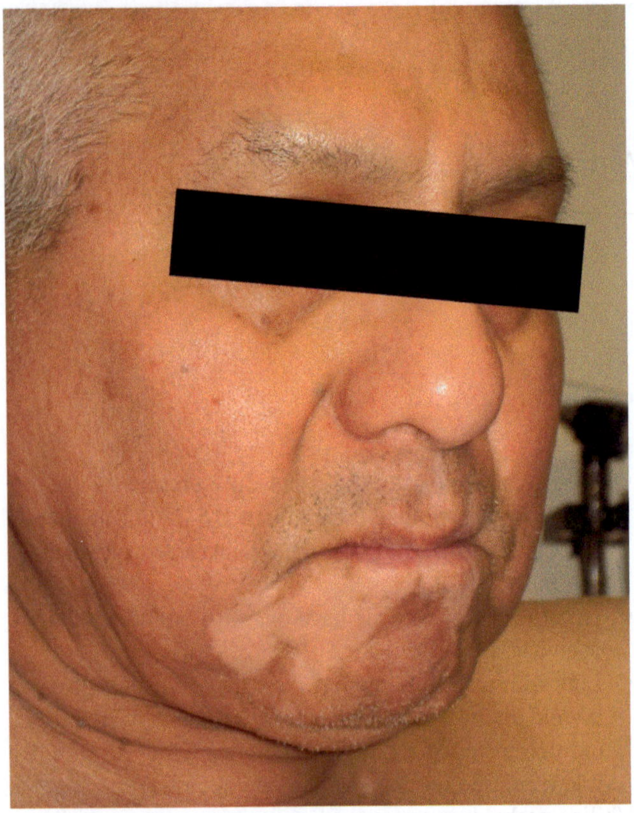

Fig. 16.1 Vitiligo. Depigmented patches in the perioral region

Vitiligo is generally a clinical diagnosis aided by:

- Wood's lamp may aid in finding extent of activity of disease and monitoring symptoms of response to treatment [1]
- Histology is useful if disease is clinically not obviously vitiligo [1]
- May check for other autoimmune diseases depending on other clinical symptoms [1]

The differential diagnosis should include:

- Chemical-induced leukoderma
- Infections with hypopigmentation (Leishmaniasis, tinea versicolor, treponematoses, leprosy)
- Genetic syndromes with hypopigmentation (tuberous sclerosis, Waardenburg syndrome, hypomelanosis of Ito, Vogt-Koyanagi-Harada syndrome)
- Post-inflammatory syndrome including pityriasis alba
- Neoplastic (amelanotic melanoma, halo nevus, hypopigmented mycosis fungoides)
- Idiopathic guttate hypomelanosis
- Lichen sclerosus et atrophicus
- Lichen striatus-like leukoderma
- Nevus anemicus, nevus depigmentosus

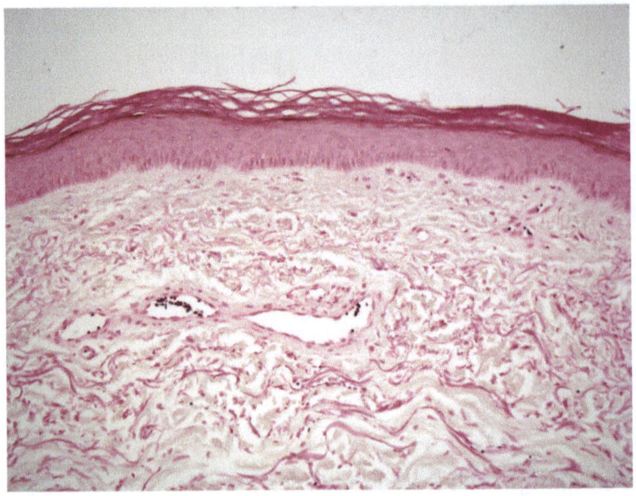

Fig. 16.2 A photomicrograph of a skin biopsy from a patient with vitiligo demonstrating an absence of melanocytes (Fontana-Masson stain, 100×)

Treatment of vitiligo is notoriously difficult. Treatment options include:

- Camouflage agents and if necessary psychotherapy; no curative therapy [1, 3]
- Sunscreen
- Initially consider topical steroids, topical calcineurin inhibitors, topical L-phenylalanine, topical antioxidants, sunlight [2]
- Second-line: ultraviolet B (UVB), narrowband UVB, or PUVA (psoralen [P] and long-wave ultraviolet radiation [UVA]) phototherapy with topical steroids; if rapidly progressive consider oral steroids [2]
- Third-line: laser treatment with steroids [2]
- Fourth-line: surgical grafts or melanocyte transplant [2]
- Depigmentation for patients who fail to repigment with therapy or have extensive disease (e.g., monobenzone) [2]

References

1. Alikhan A, Felsten LM, Daly M, Petronic-Rosic V. Vitiligo: a comprehensive overview: part I. Introduction, epidemiology, quality of life, diagnosis, differential diagnosis, associations, histopathology, etiology, and workup. J Am Acad Dermatol. 2011;65:473–91.
2. Alkhateeb A, Fain PR, Thody A, Bennett DC, Spritz RA. Epidemiology of vitiligo and associated autoimmune diseases in Caucasian probands and their families. Pigment Cell Res. 2003;16:208–14.
3. Felsten LM, Alikhan A, Petronic-Rosic V. Vitiligo: a comprehensive overview. Part II: treatment options and approach to treatment. J Am Acad Dermatol. 2011;65:493–514.

Celiac Disease: Gastrointestinal Features

17

Liam Zakko

Celiac disease, also called gluten-sensitive enteropathy, is estimated to affect up to 1% of the U.S. population. However, it is thought that only 10–15% of those with disease have been diagnosed. The diagnosis is often made by the fifth decade [1].

The most common gastrointestinal (GI) symptoms of celiac disease are [1]:

- Diarrhea (50%)
- Lactose intolerance
- Bloating
- Abdominal distension
- Weight loss
- Steatorrhea
- Dyspepsia
- Heartburn

The clinical signs and findings in celiac disease are often nonspecific [1, 2]:

- Abnormalities in motility of GI tract, gastroesophageal reflux disease (GERD)—like symptoms
- Rarely may see axonal neuropathy and cerebellar ataxia
- Osteoporosis, iron/folate deficiency, and short stature due to malabsorption
- T-cell lymphoma due to chronic inflammation
- Untreated, celiac disease increases mortality four to fivefold over general population
- Refractory celiac disease: unresponsive to 6–12 months of gluten-free diet (continued malabsorption symptoms and/or villous atrophy); increased risk of ulcerative jejunitis and T-cell lymphoma (the latter particularly with type II)
- Associated with type I diabetes, autoimmune thyroiditis, hepatobiliary disorders (primary biliary cirrhosis [PBC], autoimmune hepatitis), inflammatory bowel disease (IBD), Down's syndrome, Turner's syndrome, connective tissue autoimmune disease (Sjogren's, rheumatoid arthritis, systemic lupus erythematous), dermatitis herpetiformis, immunoglobin A (IgA) deficiency, IgA neuropathy

The pathogenesis is thought to be related to host immunological abnormalities [1, 3]:

- Inappropriate T-cell–mediated immune response to ingested gluten that causes inflammatory injury to small intestine in genetically predisposed persons resulting in malabsorption
- Increased in persons who eat gluten in first 3 months of life
- Inherited HLA-DQ2 and HLA-DQ8 are necessary but not sufficient for disease; occurs in 5–10% of children with affected parents and 10–20% of children with affected siblings
- Motility changes and other GI tract symptoms are thought to be due to decreased nutrient absorption, GI hormonal disorders due to absorption changes, and inflammation with inflammatory fragments being released into the GI lumen

The diagnosis can be difficult to make and may require evidence from several different tests [1, 3]:

- Endoscopic appearance—scalloping or notching of the mucosal folds is characteristic of the disease (see Fig. 17.1)
- Screen persons with an affected first-degree relative
- Consider HLA-DQ2/DQ8 testing in individuals with close relatives that have the disease (can avoid repeated antibody testing), patients already on a gluten-free diet without disease confirmation who may want a gluten challenge to confirm the disease, and those with histologic/serologic findings that are equivocal; this test is useful as a negative test eliminates the disease (only used to rule out disease)
- The disease is defined as villus atrophy with crypt hyperplasia and intraepithelial lymphocytosis while on a gluten-containing diet that normalizes on a gluten-free diet; endoscopic biopsy is used to confirm the disease (see Figs. 17.2 and 17.3)
- Serologic tests (serum IgA antibody to tissue transglutaminase and to transglutaminase 2), and antiendomysial antibody can be used to determine those who need a biopsy; consider anti-deamidated gliadin peptide anti-

L. Zakko (✉)
Yale Department of Internal Medicine, Yale New Haven Hospital, 20 York Street New Haven, CT 06510, USA
e-mail: Liam.zakko@yale.edu

G.Y. Wu et al. (eds.), *Atlas of Dermatological Manifestations of Gastrointestinal Disease*, DOI 10.1007/978-1-4614-6191-3_17, © Springer Science+Business Media New York 2013

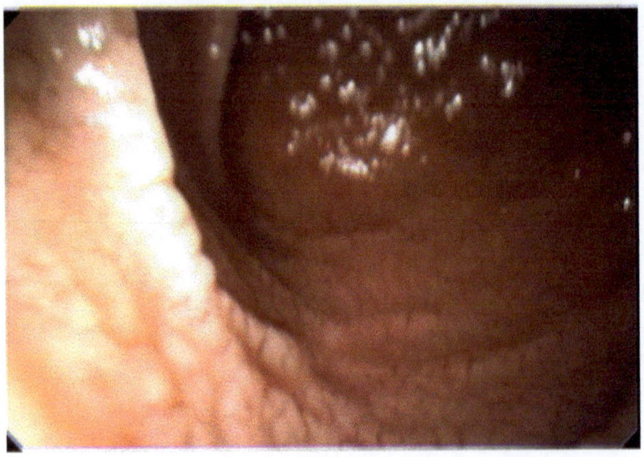

Fig. 17.1 An endoscopic view of the duodenum showing typical "scalloping" of the mucosa in celiac disease

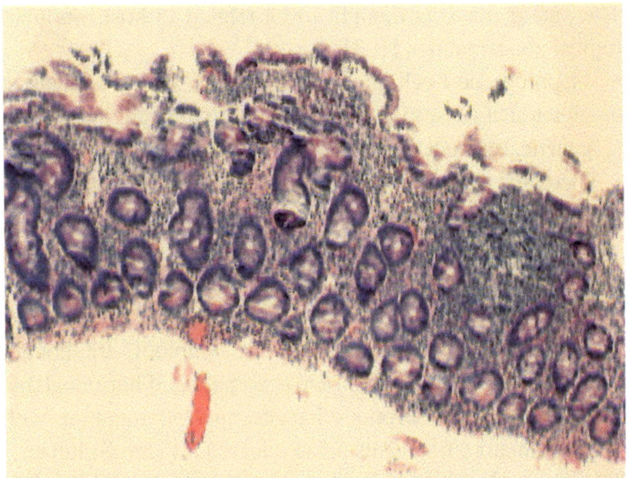

Fig. 17.2 A low-power photomicrograph of a duodenal biopsy showing submucosal inflammation. Hematoxylin and eosin (H and E)

body test although this is perhaps less sensitive and is more expensive; if patient has an IgA deficit, IgG antibodies must be checked

- Also check for vitamin deficiencies, anemia, iron deficiency, electrolyte imbalances, coagulopathies, and liver aminotransferase elevations
- In refractory celiac disease, T-cell immunohistochemistry and genetic staining for gene rearrangement must be checked; type I disease, no gene rearrangement, CD3 and CD8 positive; type II disease has gene rearrangement, only CD3 positive

Because of the protean nature of the presentation of celiac disease, the differential diagnosis is broad [1, 3]:

- Irritable bowel syndrome
- Inflammatory bowel disease
- Microscopic colitis
- Lactose intolerance

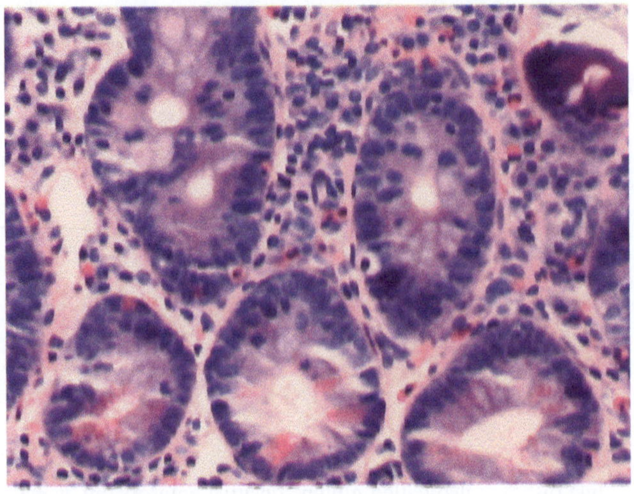

Fig. 17.3 A photomicrograph of a duodenal biopsy showing details of the intraepithelial inflammation characterized by a primarily mononuclear infiltration with eosinophils. H and E, high power

- Other carbohydrate intolerances
- Eosinophilic esophagitis [4], gastroenteritis
- Food protein-induced enteropathies
- Small intestinal bacterial overgrowth
- Giardia infection
- Intestinal lymphoma
- IgA deficiency
- Common variable immunodeficiency
- Autoimmune enteropathy
- Zollinger-Ellison syndrome

The fundamental basis of treatment is to remove the offending antigens [1, 3]:

- Important to treat early to reduce complications from disease
- Gluten-free diet: needs to be lifelong (can have continued asymptomatic inflammation even with minimal gluten intake); a nutrition consult can be very helpful
- Vitamin replacement (particularly fat soluble vitamins) as needed
- Failure of diet: first confirm adherence to diet and ensure no unknown gluten ingestion; in truly refractory celiac disease, steroids, azathioprine, 6-mercaptopurine, cyclosporine, and other immunosuppressants may be useful

References

1. Crowe SE. In the clinic: celiac disease. Ann Intern Med. 2011;154:ITC5-1–ITC5-15.
2. Green PHR, Cellier C. Celiac disease. N Engl J Med. 2007;157:1731–43.
3. Evans KE, Sanders DS. What is the use of biopsy and antibodies in coeliac disease diagnosis? J Intern Med. 2011;269:572–81.
4. Lucendo AJ. Esophageal manifestations of celiac disease. Dis Esophagus. 2010;24:470–5.

Dermatitis Herpetiformis

18

Liam Zakko, Justin Finch, Marti J. Rothe, and Jane M. Grant-Kels

There is a strong relationship between celiac disease and dermatitis herpetiformis. It affects mostly young people, 20–40 years of age, of Northern European descent with a male predominance. One third of patients with dermatitis herpetiformis have symptoms of malabsorption, and more than 90% have evidence of gluten-sensitive enteropathy on endoscopic biopsy.

Clinical signs and features include:

- Primary lesions are round erythematous papules with overlying vesicles (papulovesicles)
- Skin lesions often so pruritic that primary lesions are absent and replaced with excoriations and erosions
- Lesions are clustered (herpetiform) but not caused by a herpes virus
- Classic distribution is symmetrical and bilaterally on extensor surfaces (elbows, knees), scalp, buttocks, and nuchal area (see Fig. 18.1); rarely on face and groin
- Rarely palmoplantar purpura that affects children more commonly than adults [1]
- Patients with dermatitis herpetiformis have an increased risk of hypothyroidism, type I diabetes mellitus, vitiligo, Addison's disease, lupus, and non-Hodgkin's lymphoma (MALT lymphoma)

L. Zakko (✉)
Yale Department of Internal Medicine, Yale New Haven Hospital, 20 York Street, New Haven, CT 06510, USA
e-mail: liam.zakko@yale.edu

J. Finch • M.J. Rothe • J.M. Grant-Kels
Department of Dermatology, University of Connecticut Health Center, 21 South Road, Farmington, CT 06030, USA
e-mail: finch@uchc.edu; rothe@uchc.edu; grant@uchc.edu

There is substantial evidence that dermatitis herpetiformis is an autoimmune disease [1, 2]:

- Mediated by IgA deposition in the tips of the dermal papillae
- Linked with epidermal transglutaminase (eTG, transglutaminase 3)
- Evidence of a genetic component with family clustering and an association with HLA DQ2 and DQ8
- Associated with a gluten sensitive enteropathy in over 90% of patients

Histopathological features can be very helpful and include:

- Neutrophils and neutrophilic abscesses at the tips of dermal papillae with vesiculation at the dermal–epidermal interface (see Fig. 18.2).
- Immunomapping shows subdermal cleft within lamina lucida
- Direct immunofluorescence: 85% demonstrate granular deposition of IgA at the tips of dermal papillae along the dermal epidermal interface; 5–10% demonstrate linear IgA deposition along the basement membrane zone, which are pathognomonic. Biopsy for direct immunofluorescence should be taken from normal skin adjacent to a lesion.

The diagnosis is made using a combination of [3]:

- Physical examination findings, history of celiac disease (although often dermatitis herpetiformis is a presenting symptom of celiac disease)
- Histopathology: biopsy should be of perilesional skin for direct immunofluorescence and of lesional skin for routine histology
- Serum total IgA (can be deficient in celiac disease), IgA/IgG anti-eTG, IgA/IgG anti-tTG, IgA/IgG antiendomysial Ab
- Check thyroid function, blood glucose, and other autoimmune serologies

The differential diagnosis should include:

- Linear IgA bullous dermatosis
- Bullous pemphigoid
- Bullous lupus erythematosus
- Scabies and other arthropod bite reactions

G.Y. Wu et al. (eds.), *Atlas of Dermatological Manifestations of Gastrointestinal Disease*, DOI 10.1007/978-1-4614-6191-3_18, © Springer Science+Business Media New York 2013

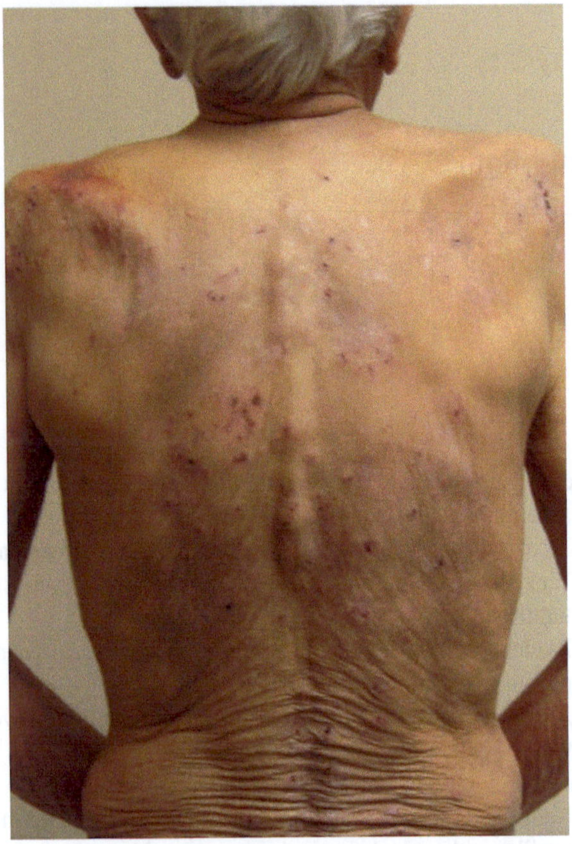

Fig. 18.1 Dermatitis herpetiformis. Minute excoriations and hemorrhagic crusts distributed on extensor surfaces

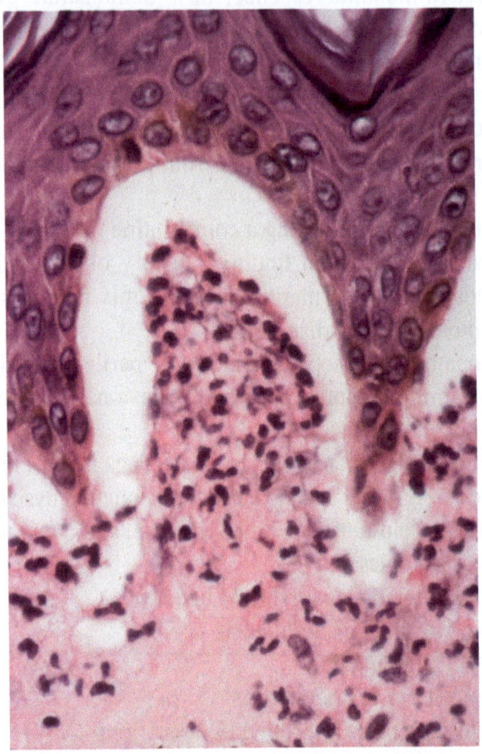

Fig. 18.2 Dermatitis herpetiformis. A photomicrograph of a skin biopsy demonstrating clusters of neutrophils in the dermal papillae. H and E (400×)

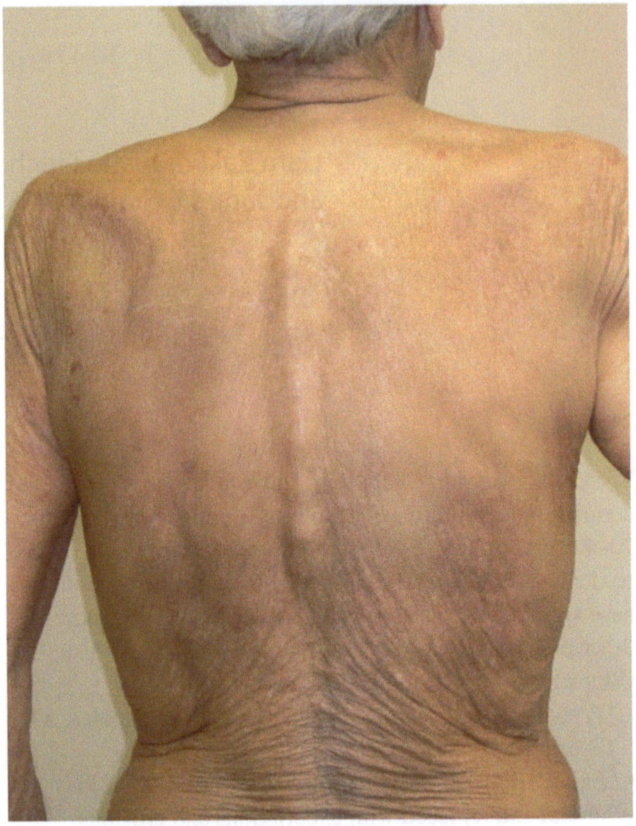

Fig. 18.3 Dramatic response after 4 weeks of oral dapsone

- Herpes simplex virus
- Urticaria
- Folliculitis
- Erythema multiforme
- Atopic/nummular/contact dermatitis

Treatment options include management of celiac disease and skin medications [3]:

- Acutely dapsone will dramatically reduce lesions and symptoms (see Fig. 18.3)
- Chronically, gluten-free diet that will decrease IgA eTG in serum and IgA in skin. By reducing this inflammation, the risk of lymphoma may also be reduced

References

1. Bolotin D, Petronic-Rosic V. Dermatitis herpetiformis. Part I. Epidemiology, pathogenesis, and clinical presentation. J Am Acad Dermatol. 2011;64:1017–24.
2. Reunala T. Dermatitis herpetiformis: coeliac disease of the skin. Ann Med. 1998;30:416–8.
3. Bolotin D, Petronic-Rosic V. Dermatitis herpetiformis. Part II. Diagnosis, management, and prognosis. J Am Acad Dermatol. 2011;64:1027–33.

Crohn's Disease: Gastrointestinal Features

19

Liam Zakko

Crohn's disease has been estimated to affect two per 1,000 individuals in the United States. It presents primarily in young adults, but can occur in the elderly. The gastrointestinal symptoms are often nonspecific, but may be debilitating [1, 2]:

- Crampy abdominal pain, commonly periumbilical
- Fatigue
- Fever
- Diarrhea that often fluctuates; chronic
- Peri-anal discomfort, drainage (33%)
- Unintentional weight loss

Clinical signs and findings include [1, 2]:

- Thirty percent small bowel involvement only (usually terminal ileum), 30% colon only, and 30% both.
- Diarrhea, malabsorption
- Microscopic intestinal tract bleeding
- Colitis, possible inflammatory and/or fibrotic strictures
- Enterocutaneous, enteroenteric fistula, and phlegmon/abscos
- Aphthous ulcers/mouth gum disease, esophagitis, gastroduodenal disease

The pathogenesis is not entirely clear, but there are several hypotheses:

- Hygiene hypothesis: decrease in gut flora diversity
- Genetic factors
  - Defects in gut epithelial barrier
  - Exaggerated immune response to normal gut flora

The pathology may show typical features:

- Gross: skip lesions, ulcers (see Figs. 19.1 and 19.2) fissures leading to fistulas (see Figs. 19.3 and 19.4), polypoid mucosal changes (cobblestone), fibrosing strictures
- Histological: focal ulcerations, transmural inflammation, noncaseating granulomas, crypt abscesses (see Fig. 19.5).

The diagnosis is made using a combination of [1, 2]:

- Laboratory: complete blood count, C-reactive protein (CRP), erythrocyte sedimentation rate (ESR), electrolytes, liver enzymes, Fe saturation, ferritin, vitamin B_{12}, anti-neutrophil cytoplasmic antibody (pANCA), anti-*Saccharomyces cerevisiae* antibody (ASCA), carotene
- Colonoscopy with examination/biopsy of the terminal ileum
- Capsule endoscopy of the small bowel
- CT with contrast; CT enterography

The differential diagnosis of Crohn's disease should include [1, 2]:

- Ulcerative colitis
- Infectious colitis (*Yersinia, Cryptosporidium, Histoplasma, Mycobacterium*)
- Ischemic colitis
- Diverticular disease
- Behçet's syndrome
- Irritable bowel syndrome

There is no cure for this disease, but several treatments have been shown to suppress symptoms and improve the quality of life [3, 4]:

- Glucocorticoids (prednisolone, prednisone, budesonide)
- Immunomodulators (azathioprine, 6-mercaptopurine, methotrexate)
- Biologics (rituximab, adalimumab, etanercept, certolizumab)
- Antibiotics (fluoroquinolone, metronidazole)

There is a strong association between Crohn's disease and erythema nodosum.

L. Zakko (✉)
Yale Department of Internal Medicine, Yale New Haven Hospital, 20 York Street New Haven, CT 06510, USA
e-mail: Liam.zakko@yale.edu

G.Y. Wu et al. (eds.), *Atlas of Dermatological Manifestations of Gastrointestinal Disease*, DOI 10.1007/978-1-4614-6191-3_19, © Springer Science+Business Media New York 2013

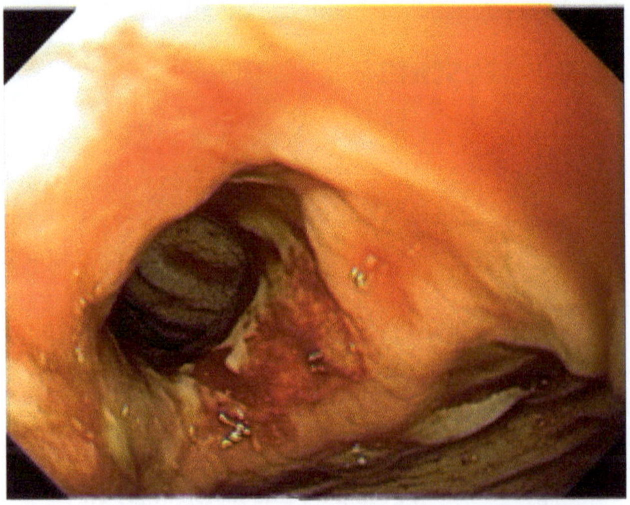

Fig. 19.1 A colonoscopic view of an ulcer in the ileocecal valve typical of Crohn's disease

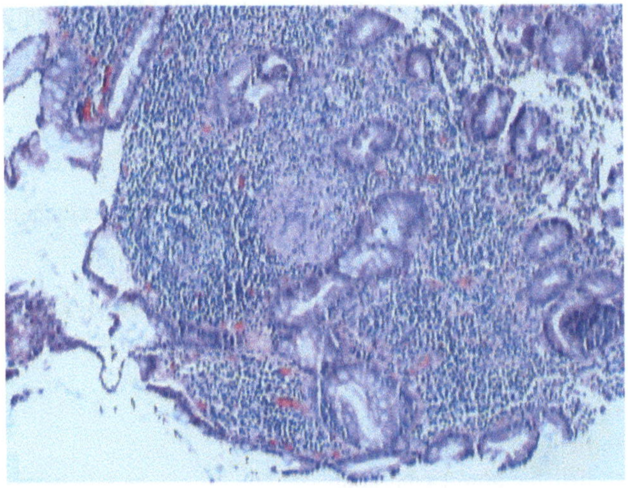

Fig. 19.2 A colonoscopic view of ulcers in the terminal ileum

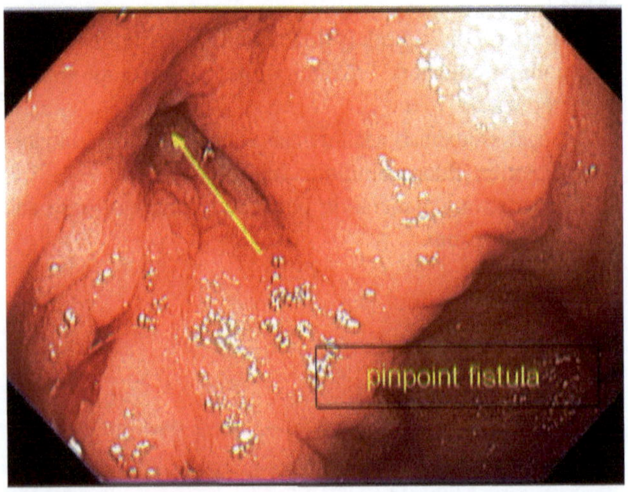

Fig. 19.3 A colonoscopic view of a fistula in the colon. *Arrow* indicates the pinpoint orifice

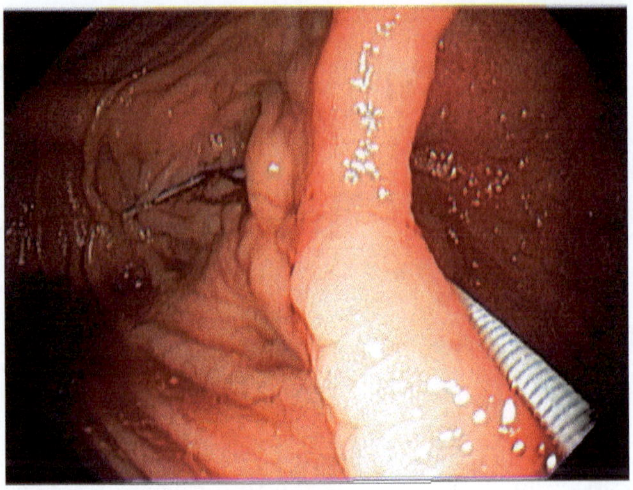

Fig. 19.4 A wire probe demonstrates the path of the enteroenteric fistula within the bowel wall

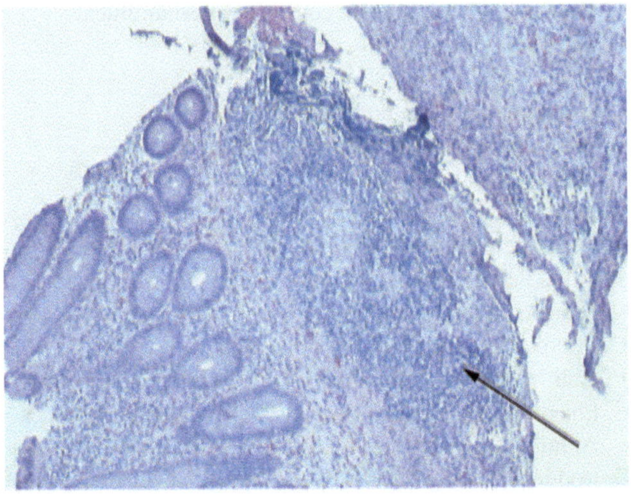

Fig. 19.5 A colonic biopsy specimen showing inflammation involving an ulcer, and a granuloma (*arrow*). Hematoxylin and eosin (H and E) staining, 100×

References

1. Abraham C, Cho JH. Inflammatory bowel disease. N Eng J Med. 2009;361:2066–78.
2. Mekhijian HS, Switz DM, Meinyk CS, et al. Clinical features and natural history of Crohn's disease. Gastroenterology. 1979;77:898–906.
3. Talley NJ, Abreu MT, Achkar JP, et al. An evidence based systematic review on medical therapies for inflammatory bowel disease. Am J Gastroenterol. 2011;106:S2–S25.
4. Vatn MH. Natural history and complications of IBD. Curr Gastroenterol Rep. 2009;11:481–7.

Cutaneous Crohn's Disease

20

Liam Zakko, Justin Finch, Marti J. Rothe, and Jane M. Grant-Kels

Clinical

- Also named acute metastatic Crohn's disease
- Noncontiguous with the intestine. This is referred to as "metastatic" Crohn's.
- Nongenital disease presents as ulcerations, nodules, plaques, papules, pustules, and abscesses on the lower extremities/plantar surface (38%); thorax (24%); upper extremities/palms (15%); face and lips (11%) (see Fig. 20.1a); flexural areas (8%); and as a generalized skin disease (4%) [1]
- Genital and nongenital lesions; 67% of pediatric and 33% of adult cases are genital
- Genital disease most often presents with erythema, edema, and ulcerations of the vulva, bilateral, or unilateral labia, clitoris, scrotum, penis, or perineum (see Fig. 20.1b). Less common are plaques, warty papules, or a pedunculated labial mass
- In adults, disease usually comes during a Crohn's exacerbation
- In children, disease can precede Crohn's colitis/ileitis by months to years [2]

Pathogenesis

- Related to intestinal Crohn's disease (pathogenesis unclear). However, it does appear to be active in some persons when their intestinal disease is controlled

Pathology

- Histology classically demonstrates sarcoidal or tuberculoid non-caseating granulomas with lymphocytes, histiocytes and occasional multinucleated histiocytes perivascularly [3] (see Fig. 20.2)
- Distinguish from sarcoid by overlying ulcerated epidermis and a denser lymphocytic infiltrate [1]

Diagnosis

- Tissue cultures, chest radiograph, purified protein derivative (PPD)
- Biopsy is characteristic; special stains (periodic acid Schiff [PAS] and acid fast bacilli [AFB]) and polarizing microscopy rule out other causes [2]
- If no intestinal symptoms at time of diagnosis, prompt gastrointestinal (GI) referral to search for subclinical Crohn's disease and treatment is beneficial [2]

Differential Diagnosis

- Cutaneous sarcoidosis
- Mycobacterial infection

L. Zakko (✉)
Yale Department of Internal Medicine, Yale New Haven Hospital, New Haven, CT, USA

Yale Primary Care Clinic, 789 Howard Avenue, New Haven, CT 06519-1304, USA
e-mail: liam.zakko@yale.edu

J. Finch • M.J. Rothe • J.M. Grant-Kels
Department of Dermatology, University of Connecticut Health Center, 21 South Road, Farmington, CT 06030, USA
e-mail: finch@uchc.edu; rothe@uchc.edu; grant@uchc.edu

G.Y. Wu et al. (eds.), *Atlas of Dermatological Manifestations of Gastrointestinal Disease*, DOI 10.1007/978-1-4614-6191-3_20, © Springer Science+Business Media New York 2013

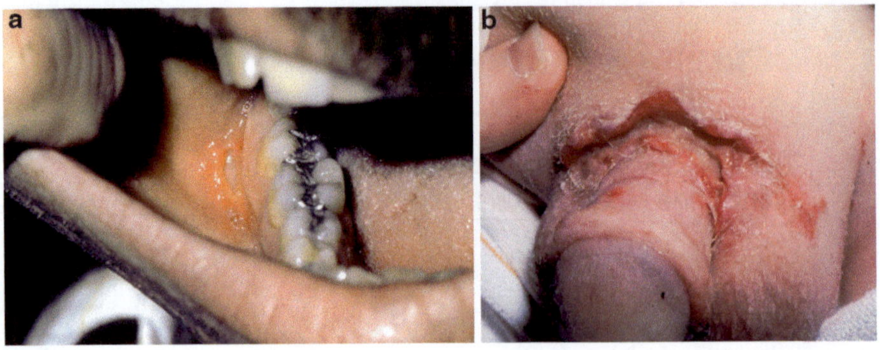

Fig. 20.1 Cutaneous Crohn's disease. (**a**) Linear fissures at the buccal-gingival margin. (**b**) Ulcers and fissures on the genitalia is a more common presentation in children

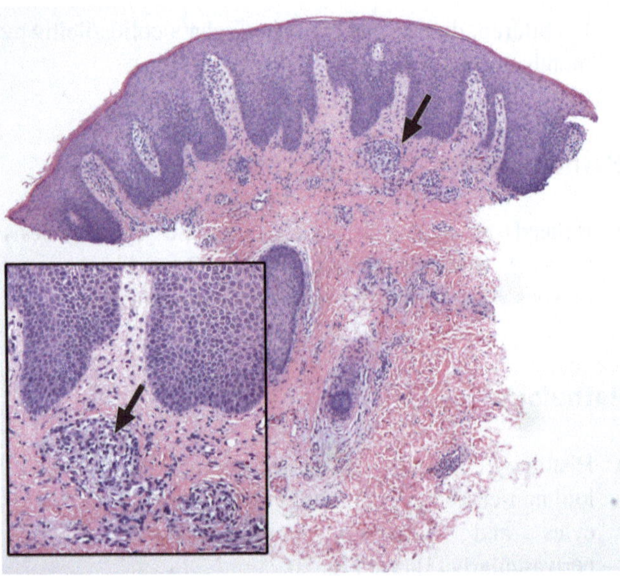

Fig. 20.2 Cutaneous Crohn's disease. A photomicrograph of a skin biopsy showing noncaseating granulomas (*black arrows*) in the superficial dermis (40×, *inset* 200×)

- Fungal infection
- Sexually transmitted diseases
- Foreign body reaction
- Lymphangioma circumscriptum
- Angioedema
- Pyoderma gangrenosum
- Hidradenitis suppurativa

Treatment

- Oral metronidazole reportedly most effective [1]
- Also try topical, intralesional, and/or oral steroids, dapsone, thalidomide, minocycline, sulfasalazine, 6-mercaptopurine, azathioprine, anti–tumor necrosis factor (TNF) alpha antibodies [2]
- Refractory disease: consider surgical debridement [2]

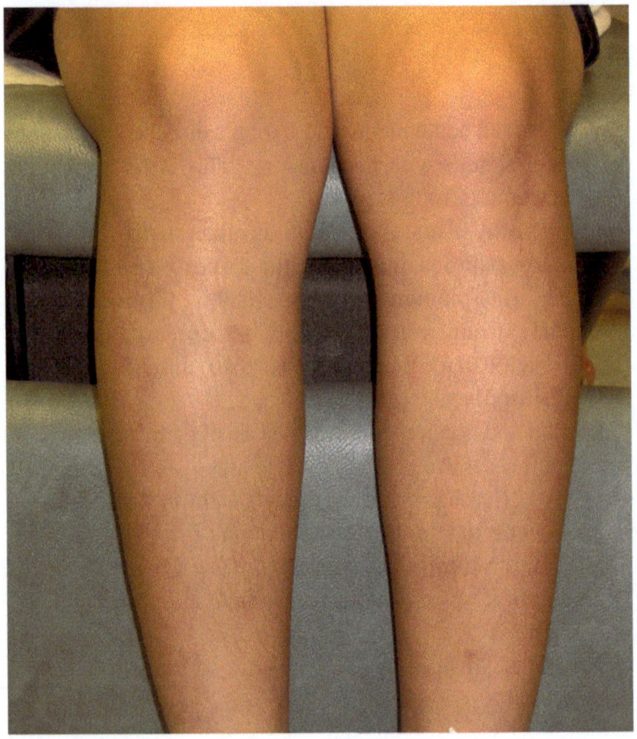

Fig. 20.3 Erythema nodosum. Tender erythematous nodules over the shins

Erythema Nodosum

Clinical

- Red, round, warm, subcutaneous, tender nodules distributed primarily over lower extremities, especially on the shins (occasionally occur elsewhere) [4, 5] (see Fig. 20.3)
- Later in course change color to bruise-like yellow [4]
- Heal spontaneously within 6 weeks [5]
- Occasionally associated with fever, arthralgias, and malaise [5]
- Often associated with an exacerbation of IBD [4]

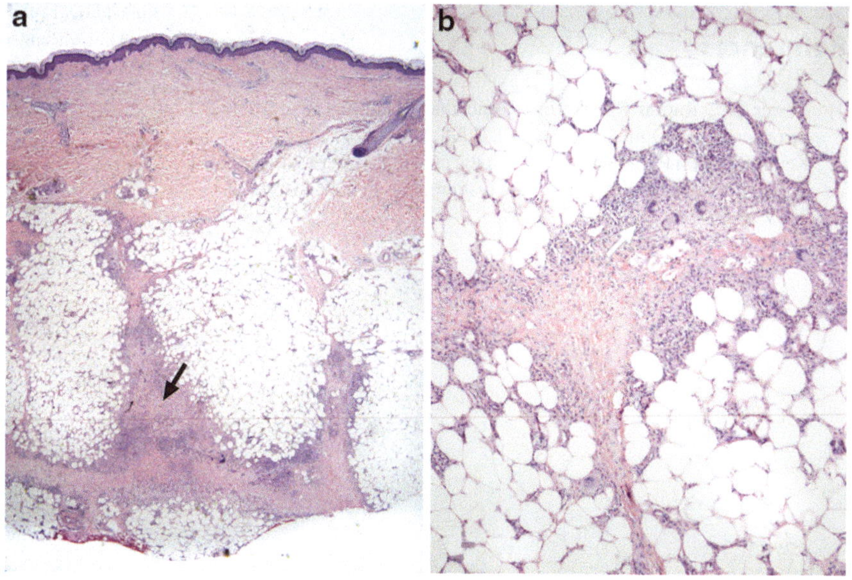

Fig. 20.4 Erythema nodosum. (**a**) A photomicrograph of a skin biopsy showing septal panniculitis with widening of septae (*black arrow*) (20×). (**b**) Mixed inflammatory infiltrate involving neutrophils, histiocytes, lymphocytes, and multinucleated giant cells. Hematoxylin and eosin (H and E) staining (200×)

- Most common dermatological manifestation of IBD; present in 2–20% of IBD patients [4, 5]
- More common in women than men [4, 5]

Pathogenesis

- Delayed hypersensitivity reaction—antigen is identified in 40% of cases [5]
- The list of reported associations is extensive and most commonly includes: IBD, Streptococcal infections, *Yersinia* enterocolitis, *Mycoplasma* pneumonia, leprosy, *Salmonella*, TB, coccidiomycosis, histoplasmosis, blastomycosis, lymphoma, leukemia, pregnancy, sarcoidosis, and medications (especially sulfonamides, OCPs, penicillin, halogens) [5]
- About half of the cases are idiopathic [4]

Pathology

- Characteristic lesions: predominantly septal panniculitis with infiltration of subcutaneous septae by neutrophils and lymphocytes without associated vasculitis. In the overlying dermis there is usually a superficial and deep perivascularly predominantly lymphohistiocytic infiltrate [5] (see Fig. 20.4).
- Early lesions show septal thickening with edema and many neutrophils.
- Later lesions show septal thickening with fibrosis and granulation tissue containing many lymphocytes, histiocytes and multinucleated histiocytes. Nodular aggregates of histiocytes radially arranged around a cleft can be identified and are known as *Miescher's radial granulomas* [5].

Diagnosis is primarily clinical. If there is any doubt, supporting tests include:

- Skin biopsy: preferably deep wedge biopsy to adequately sample subcutaneous fat
- Once the diagnosis has been established, rule-out associated inciting factors via:
  - History to rule out drugs, infection, pregnancy
  - Throat culture/anti-streptolysin antibody/erythrocyte sedimentation rate/blood culture/stool culture/chest radiograph/purified protein derivative
  - Colonoscopy if symptoms of inflammatory bowel disease
- Biopsy [5]

Differential Diagnosis

- Other panniculitis
- Subcutaneous lymphoma
- Cutaneous infection

Treatment

- Usually self-limited illness: average time to remission is 5–6 weeks [4, 5]
- Discontinue possible culprit medications; treat underlying infection
- Supportive treatment with compression stockings, leg elevation, rest [4, 5]
- In severe cases treatment with nonsteroidal anti-inflammatory drugs, prednisone, saturated solution of potassium iodide (SSKI), colchicine hydroxychloroquine [4, 5]
- In refractory cases consider infliximab, mycophenolate mofetil, cyclosporine [4, 5]

References

1. Lester LU, Rapini RP. Dermatologic manifestations of colonic disorders. Curr Opin Gastroenterol. 2008;25:66–73.
2. Keiler S, Tyson P, Tamburro J. Metastatic cutaneous Crohn's disease in children: case report and review of literature. Pediatr Dermatol. 2009;26:604–9.
3. Guest GD, Fink RLW. Metastatic Crohn's disease: case report of an unusual variant and review of the literature. Dis Colon Rectum. 2000;43:1764–6.
4. Larsen S, Bendtzen K, Nielsen OH. Extraintestinal manifestations of inflammatory bowel disease: epidemiology, diagnosis, and management. Ann Med. 2010;42:97–114.
5. Timani S, Mutasim DF. Skin manifestations of inflammatory bowel disease. Clin Dermatol. 2008;26:265–73.

21 Bowel Bypass Syndrome: Gastrointestinal Features

Michael Tadros

Bowel bypass syndrome is seen in those with chronic diarrhea and malabsorption following a bypass procedure, biliary diversion, or other gastrointestinal (GI) disorders.

GI symptoms include [1]:

- Abdominal pain
- Dyspepsia
- Rectal bleeding
- Stool incontinence

Clinical signs and findings can include [1, 2]:

- Occurrence within weeks and up to 6 years after bowel bypass surgery
- Usually acute and can be recurrent
- Fever and chills may precede its onset
- Malabsorption and fat-soluble vitamin deficiency, especially zinc deficiency
- Endoscopy can reveal the area of gastrojejunal anastomosis from previous bypass surgery (see Fig. 21.1); this also can be confirmed by a barium study of the upper GI tract (see Fig. 21.2); inspection of the colon by colonoscopy may reveal evidence of colitis.

Pathogenesis is poorly understood but some hypotheses include [1–3]:

- Possible role of bacterial overgrowth in a blind loop of the intestine where the bacterial peptidoglycans generate an immune complex reaction creating a hypersensitivity reaction
- Some surgeries can create a blind loop syndrome with subsequent bacterial overgrowth resulting in diarrhea, flatulence, and malabsorption
  - Ileojejunal bypass surgery
  - Gastric bypass surgeries (even after laparoscopic surgeries)
  - Pancreatobiliary diversion
- Inflammatory states
  - Inflammatory bowel disease (Crohn's and ulcerative colitis)
  - Appendicitis
  - Diverticulitis
  - Peptic ulcer disease

Typical pathological features include [1, 3]:

- Neutrophilic infiltrates mostly in the perivascular and interstitial areas
- Lymphocytes and histiocytes are often seen
- Leukocytoclasis and pustular vasculitis may be present

The diagnosis is made by considering the following [1, 3]:

- Historical, endoscopic, or radiologic evidence of bowel bypass surgery
- Laboratory investigation can show evidence of anemia, malabsorption, fat-soluble vitamin deficiency, and electrolyte abnormalities
- Biopsy and histopathologic examination showing neutrophilic infiltrates mostly in the perivascular and interstitial areas
- Rule out bacterial overgrowth (hydrogen breath test, serum vitamin B_{12}, and folate levels)

The differential diagnosis of bowel bypass syndrome should include [1, 3]:

- Other causes of neutrophilic dermatosis (Sweet's syndrome, pyoderma gangrenosum, neutrophilic eccrine hidradenitis, Behçet's disease)
- Serum sickness
- Gastroenteritis
- Henoch-Schönlein purpura

The treatment should include [1, 3]:

- Antibiotic therapy (metronidazole, erythromycin, tetracycline, trimethoprim-sulfamethoxazole, amoxicillin-clavulanic acid)
- Combination therapy with nonsteroidal anti-inflammatory drugs, colchicine, dapsone, and oral steroids
- Topical steroids
- Refractory cases may require surgical revision of blind loops

M. Tadros (✉)
Department of Internal Medicine, University of Connecticut Health Center, Farmington, CT, USA

560 Hudson Street, Apt 750, Hartford, CT 06106, USA
e-mail: MTadros@resident.uchc.edu

G.Y. Wu et al. (eds.), *Atlas of Dermatological Manifestations of Gastrointestinal Disease*,
DOI 10.1007/978-1-4614-6191-3_21, © Springer Science+Business Media New York 2013

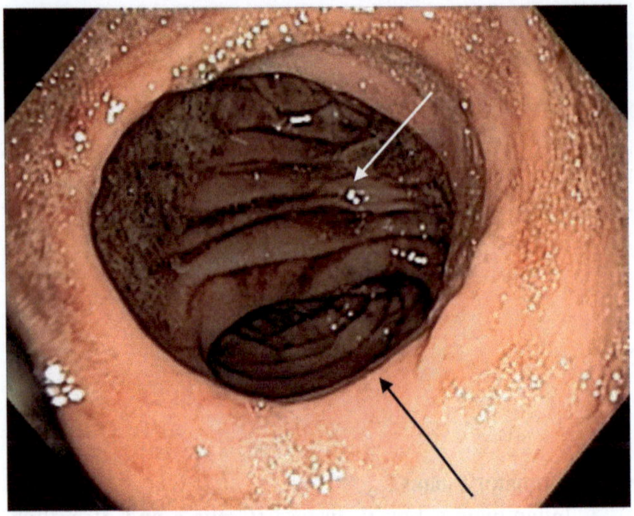

Fig. 21.1 Endoscopic view of a gastrojejunal anastomosis. *Black arrow* indicates the gastric margin of the anastomosis. *White arrow* points to the jejunal folds

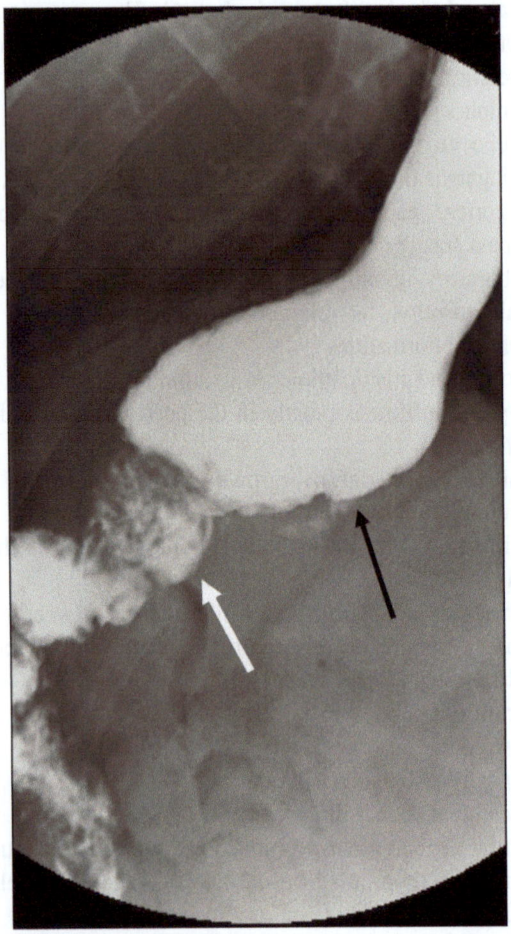

Fig. 21.2 A barium study demonstrating the anastomosis between a resected stomach and the jejunum after gastric bypass surgery. *Black arrow* indicates the gastric remnant and *white arrow* shows the jejunum

References

1. Saavedra AP, Kovacs SC, Moschella SL. Neutrophilic dermatoses. Clin Dermatol. 2006;24:470–81.
2. Tu J, Chan JJ, Yu LL. Bowel bypass syndrome/bowel-associated dermatosis arthritis syndrome post laparoscopic gastric bypass surgery. Australas J Dermatol. 2011;52:e5–7.
3. Slater GH, Kerlin P, Georghiou PR, Fielding GA. Bowel-associated dermatosis-arthritis syndrome after biliopancreatic diversion. Obes Surg. 2004;14:133–5.

Bowel-Associated Dermatosis–Arthritis Syndrome

22

Liam Zakko, Justin Finch, Marti J. Rothe, and Jane M. Grant-Kels

Clinical signs and features include:

- Seen in up to 20% of patients with jejunal-ileal bypass 3 months to 5 years following surgery; also associated with biliopancreatic diversion, Billroth II gastrectomy, occasionally inflammatory bowel disease (IBD), and rarely after laparoscopic gastric bypass surgery [1-3]
- Presents with flu-like symptoms of fevers, myalgia, and tenosynovitis with symmetrical small joint polyarthritis without deformities [1]
- Painful skin rash develops 12–36 h after flu-like symptoms with crops of small erythematous purpuric macules often on the upper trunk and extremities that progress to indurated, urticarial purpuric papules and then vesiculopustular lesions over the next 24–48 h (see Fig. 22.1). The lesions heal without scarring over the next 2 weeks [1].
- Symptoms tend to recur every 4–6 weeks [1]
- Erythema nodosum-like nodules may be present on the legs [1]

L. Zakko (✉)
Yale Department of Internal Medicine, 20 York Street, Yale New Haven Hospital, New Haven, CT 06510, USA
e-mail: liam.zakko@yale.edu

J. Finch • M.J. Rothe • J.M. Grant-Kels
Department of Dermatology, University of Connecticut Health Center, 21 South Road, Farmington, CT 06030, USA
e-mail: finch@uchc.edu; rothe@uchc.edu; grant@uchc.edu

The differential diagnosis should include other neutrophil mediated skin disorders, such as:

- Pyoderma gangrenosum
- Sweet's syndrome
- Pustular vasculitis of the hands
- Leukocytoclastic vasculitis
- Septic vasculitis
- Behçet's syndrome
- Rheumatoid neutrophilic dermatosis
- Acute generalized exanthematous pustulosis
- Erythema nodosum
- Henoch-Schönlein purpura

Pathogenesis of this disease involves:

- Bacterial overgrowth in blind loops of bowel leads to immune complexes containing peptidoglycans that circulate in the bloodstream and deposit in the skin and joints leading to the joint and skin pathology [3]

Histopathological features include:

- Neutrophilic dermatosis similar to Sweet's syndrome with leukocytoclasis and perivascular inflammation, usually without vasculitis or vessel wall destruction (see Fig. 22.2)
- Early: perivascular lymphocytic infiltrate with neutrophils, leukocytoclasis, extravasated red blood cells without fibrin depositions
- Mature: papillary dermal edema results in subepidermal blister, papillary and reticular dermal edema, and nodular neutrophilic infiltrate with nuclear dust that may include some lymphocytes and histiocytes

The diagnosis is made using a combination of:

- Clinical symptoms in a patient with appropriate clinical history
- Biopsy can help distinguish from other skin processes associated with gut pathology
- No radiographic joint changes with negative rheumatoid factor, antinuclear antibodies (ANA), immunoglobulins, uric acid

G.Y. Wu et al. (eds.), *Atlas of Dermatological Manifestations of Gastrointestinal Disease*, DOI 10.1007/978-1-4614-6191-3_22, © Springer Science+Business Media New York 2013

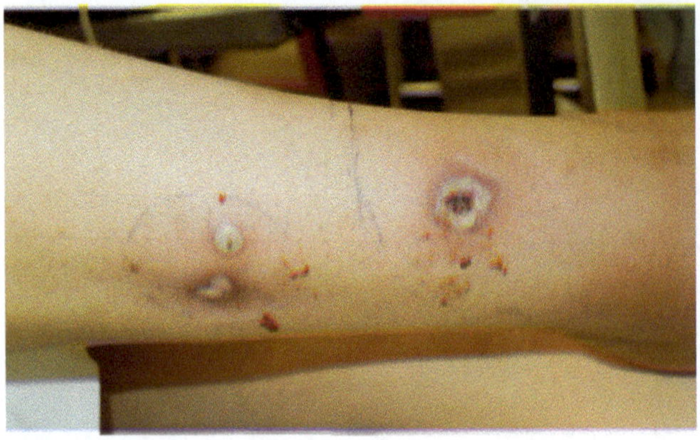

Fig. 22.1 Bowel-associated dermatosis–arthritis syndrome. Purulent nodules and ulcers

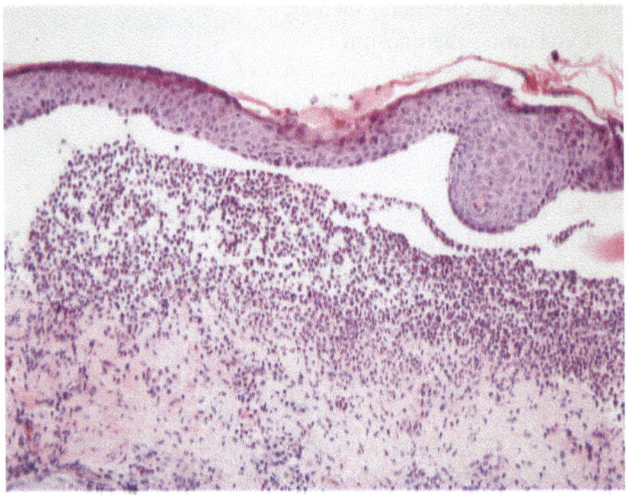

Fig. 22.2 Bowel-associated dermatosis–arthritis syndrome. Dense neutrophilic infiltrate in the superficial and mid-dermis (40×)

Treatment options include [1]:

- Systemic corticosteroids antibiotics such as tetracycline, minocycline, sulfapyridine, erythromycin, metronidazole, rifaximin although response is inconsistent
- Colchicine
- In refractory cases may need to remove blind loops surgically

Acrodermatitis Enteropathica

Clinical signs and features include:

- Acrodermatitis enteropathica can be genetic or acquired [4, 5] Zinc (Zn) deficiency
- Acrodermatitis enteropathica [4, 5]
  - Classic clinical triad of diarrhea, alopecia, and a periorificial, acral cutaneous eruption (see Fig. 22.3)
  - Genetic disease presents soon after weaning off the breast (breast milk has its own zinc binding factor) or between fourth and tenth week in formula-fed infants
  - Begins as symmetric, eczematous plaques that evolve into vesiculobullous, pustular, desquamative, and erosive plaques
  - Often periorificial with classic sparing of the upper lip: "horseshoe-shaped" or "U-shaped" configuration
  - Risk of superinfection with *Staphylococcus aureus* and *Candida albicans*
  - Alopecia with brittle and dry hair
  - Other signs: hypopigmentation, impaired wound healing, stomatitis, angular cheilitis, paronychia, photophobia, conjunctivitis, and irritability
  - Infants can be listless and apathetic; can be fatal in infants
  - Mild deficiency can lead to growth retardation in children, hypogonadism in men, dysgeusia, abnormal dark adaptation, and psoriasiform dermatitis of the hands, feet, and occasionally knees

The differential diagnosis should include:

- Other forms of deficiency dermatitis due to deficiency in amino acids (*e.g.*, Hartnup disease), fatty acids, biotin (multiple carboxylase deficiency), niacin (pellagra) [6]
- Necrolytic migratory erythema
- Necrolytic acral erythema: zinc deficiency and/or improvement of rash with zinc supplementation is observed in patients with hepatitis C and necrolytic acral erythema [7]

Pathogenesis of this disease involves:

- Genetic: autosomal recessive due to mutations SLC39A4 intestinal zinc transporter on chromosome 8q24.3 that encodes ZIP4-transporter on chromosome 8q24.3 that encodes ZIP4-transporter on enterocytes with resultant impaired zinc absorption [5]
- Acquired: decreased dietary intake; alcoholics; vegetarians and vegans; anorexia nervosa; total parenteral nutrition; diets high in cereal grain and low in animal protein; increased usage and decreased stores in premature infants; decreased absorption secondary to cystic fibrosis, gastric bypass, IBD, celiac disease, short bowel syndrome, chronic diarrhea, premature gut epithelium; increased elimination related to alcoholism, burns, malignancy, infections, pregnancy, renal disease (nephrotic syndrome), and stress; medications: penicillamine, diuretics, antimetabolites, valproate [4]

Histopathological features include:

- Psoriasiform epidermal hyperplasia with prominent confluent parakeratosis occasionally with neutrophils, pallor of keratinocytes due to intracellular edema in the superficial epidermis, leading to intraepidermal blisters, hypergranulosis, occasional acantholysis, focal dyskeratosis, edema of papillary dermis, and dilated tortuous capillaries (see Fig. 22.4)

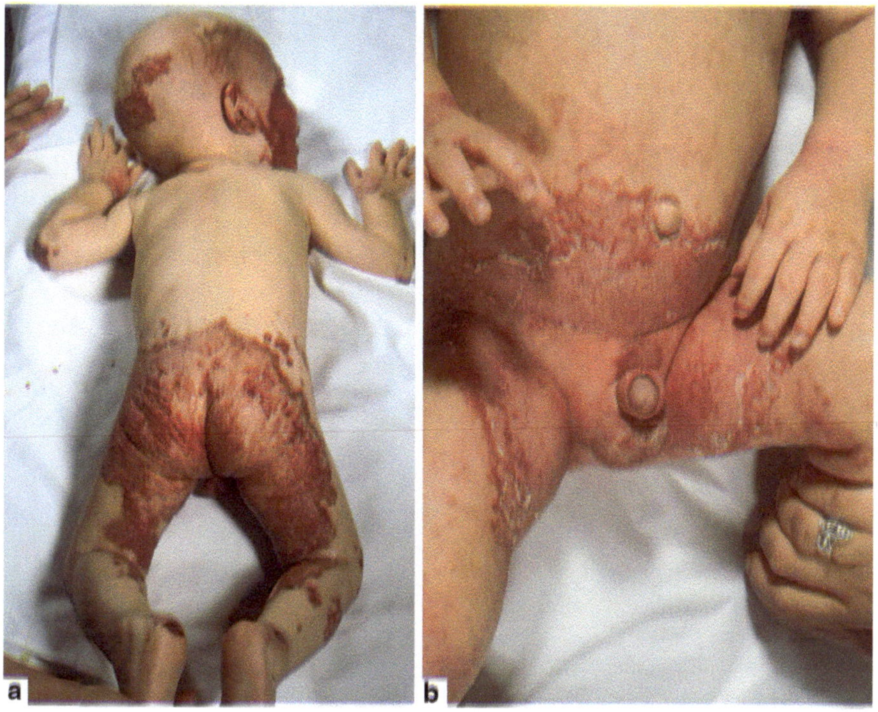

Fig. 22.3 Acrodermatitis enteropathica. Alopecia and confluent erythematous, scaly, eroded plaques involving the periorificial and diaper regions (Image courtesy of Howard Pride, MD)

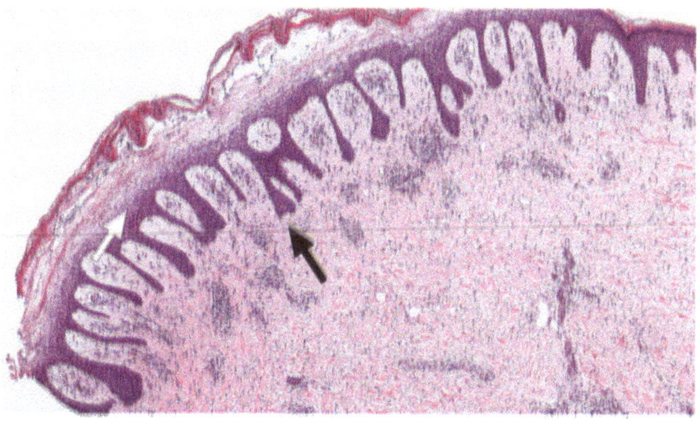

Fig. 22.4 Acrodermatitis enteropathica. Epidermal acanthosis (*black arrow*), with spongiosis, pallor, and ballooning degeneration of the upper epidermis (*white arrow*) (Image courtesy of Rajendra Singh, MD)

- Bullous form: intraepidermal vacuolar changes leading to intraepidermal blisters and vesiculation with prominent necrosis
- Candida and staph superinfection not uncommon

The diagnosis is made using a combination of [5]:

- Measuring zinc levels: need to draw in AM (diurnal variation with lower levels later in the day due to meals); watch for fluctuation with inflammation, increased with hemolysis
- Measuring zinc-dependent enzymes: alkaline phosphatase, which is low in zinc deficiency
- Hypoalbuminemia will decrease zinc levels

Treatment options include [8]:

- Zinc-sulfate: enteral supplementation; zinc-chloride: parenteral supplementation (need to monitor copper levels, which can be severely decreased with elevated Zn levels)
- Clinical improvement in 2–7 days and healing in 2–4 weeks

References

1. Ashok D, Kiely P. Bowel associated dermatosis-arthritis syndrome: a case report. J Med Case Rep. 2007;81:1.
2. Slater GH, Kerlin P, Georghiou PR, Fielding GA. Bowel associated dermatosis-arthritis syndrome after biliopancreatic diversion. Obes Surg. 2004;14:133–5.
3. Tu J, Chan JJ, Yu LL. Bowel bypass syndrome/bowel-associated dermatosis arthritis syndrome post laparoscopic gastric bypass surgery. Australas J Dermatol. 2011;52:e5–7.
4. Jen M, Yan AC. Syndromes associated with nutritional deficiency and excess. Clin Dermatol. 2010;28:669–85.
5. Maverakis E, Fung MA, Lynch PJ, et al. Acrodermatitis enteropathica and an overview of zinc metabolism. J Am Acad Dermatol. 2007;56:116–24.
6. Kim YJ, Kim MY, Kim H, et al. Acrodermatitis enteropathica-like eruption associated with combined nutritional deficiency. J Korean Med Sci. 2005;20:908–11.
7. Tabibian JH, Gerstenblith MR, Tedford RJ, et al. Necrolytic acral erythema as a cutaneous marker of hepatitis c: report of two cases and review. Dig Dis Sci. 2010;55:2735–43.
8. Fedeles F, Murphy M, Rothe MJ, Grant-Kels JM. Nutrition and bullous skin disease. Clin Dermatol. 2010;28:627–43.

Part III

Gastrointestinal Bleeding

23 Blue Rubber Bleb Nevus Syndrome: Gastrointestinal Features

Liam Zakko

Blue rubber bleb nevus syndrome is a rare condition that is estimated to affect fewer than 200,000 people in the United States.

Most patients with this syndrome are probably asymptomatic [1]. Gastrointestinal (GI) signs and symptoms [1–3] when present include:

- Bluish vascular nevi of the skin, hemangiomas of the GI tract, and GI hemorrhage
- GI lesions are typically found in the small intestine but can be found throughout the GI tract
- When viewed endoscopically the lesion characteristically appears as a discrete mucosal nodule with an overlying red cap (see Figs. 23.1, 23.2, and 23.3)
- Often present at birth or develops in early childhood
- GI bleed (hematemesis, melena, rectal bleeding) can be massive or occult
- Intussusception

The pathogenesis [1–3] of this condition is unclear:

- May be related to chromosome 9p mutation
- Appears to have autosomal dominant pattern of inheritance though there are sporadic cases

The typical pathology [1–3] reveals hemangiomas:

- Cavernous hemangiomas with clusters of dilated, irregular capillary spaces within the wall of the GI tract

The diagnosis [1–3] is based on visualizing the hemangiomas:

- Complete blood count/iron studies to check for anemia
- Endoscopic viewing is best technique for diagnosis
- Lesions will appear as filling defects on computed tomography and may be confused with polyps
- Magnetic resonance imaging can be used to screen asymptomatic family members

The differential diagnosis [1–3] includes other conditions associated with hemangiomas:

- Sturge-Weber disease
- Von-Hippel Lindau syndrome
- Cobb's disease
- Klippel-Trenaunay syndrome
- Parker-Weber disease
- Maffucci's syndrome

When treatment [1] is required, it is usually to manage GI bleeding:

- If occult bleeding is minimal, then symptomatic therapy with iron replacement and transfusions
- Life-threatening bleeds can be treated with surgical excision, but this is not a treatment of preference as lesions often recur
- Endoscopic management is preferred: electrocoagulation or laser photocoagulation

References

1. Dwivedi M, Misra SP. Blue rubber bleb nevus syndrome causing upper GI hemorrhage: a novel management approach and review. Gastrointest Endosc. 2002;55:943–6.
2. Gallo SH, McClave SA. Blue rubber bleb nevus syndrome: gastrointestinal involvement and its endoscopic presentation. Gastrointest Endosc. 1992;38:72–6.

L. Zakko (✉)
Yale Department of Internal Medicine, 20 York Street, Yale New Haven Hospital, New Haven, CT 06510, USA
e-mail: liam.zakko@yale.edu

G.Y. Wu et al. (eds.), *Atlas of Dermatological Manifestations of Gastrointestinal Disease*, DOI 10.1007/978-1-4614-6191-3_23, © Springer Science+Business Media New York 2013

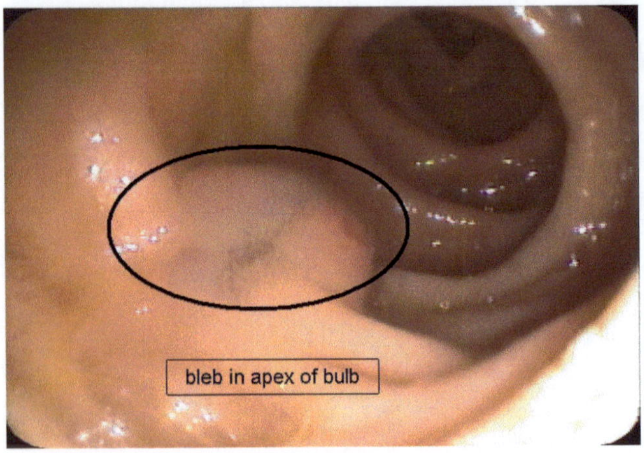

Fig. 23.1 An endoscopic view of a blue nevus in the duodenum (Image courtesy of Connecticut Gastroenterology Institute)

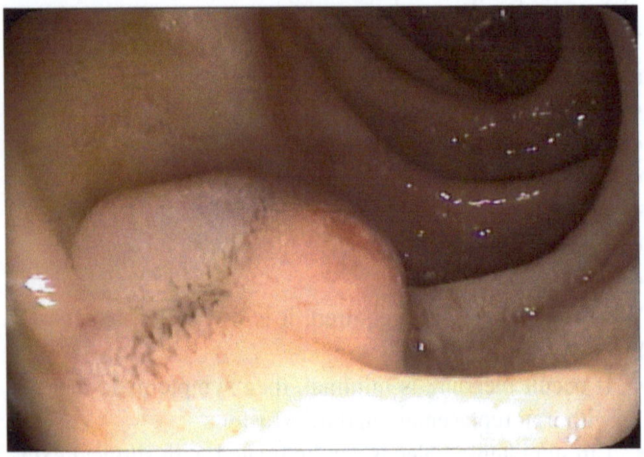

Fig. 23.2 A close-up endoscopic view of a blue nevus in the duodenum (Image courtesy of Connecticut Gastroenterology Institute)

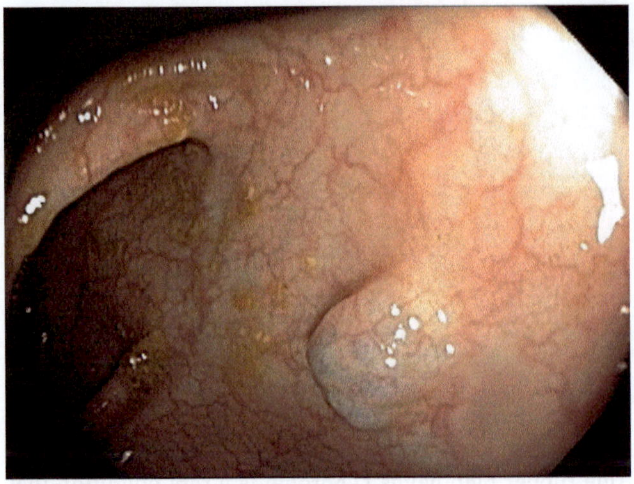

Fig. 23.3 An endoscopic view of a blue nevus in the colon (Image courtesy of Connecticut Gastroenterology Institute)

3. Wong CH, Tan YM, Chow WC, Tan PH, Wong WK. Blue rubber bleb nevus syndrome: a clinical spectrum with correlation between cutaneous and gastrointestinal manifestations. J Gastroenterol Hepatol. 2003;18:1000–2.

24 Blue Rubber Bleb Nevus Syndrome: Dermatological Features

Liam Zakko, Justin Finch, Marti J. Rothe, and Jane M. Grant-Kels

Clinical signs and features include [1]:

- Bluish venous hemangiomas (referred to as "vascular nevi" of the skin)
- Visceral hemangiomas involving most commonly the gastrointestinal (GI) tract
- GI hemorrhage
- Cutaneous lesions are compressible venous hemangiomas or malformations often on the trunk or upper extremities
- Often present at birth or develop in early childhood
  Three types of cutaneous lesions:
  - Large disfiguring lesions that can obstruct vital organs
  - Most commonly, crumpled blue rubber nipple-like lesions covered with skin (see Fig. 24.1)
  - Irregular blue-black macules or papules that may blanch with pressure
- Cutaneous lesions mostly asymptomatic
- Can cause increased sweating over lesion due to eccrine gland association with hemangiomas
- May be painful due to contraction of smooth muscle fibers within the vascular walls composing the hemangioma
- Large acral hemangiomas can cause angiomatous giantism and deformity that has lead to amputation or can cause chronic disseminated intravascular coagulation [2]
- There appears to be correlation between number of cutaneous hemangiomas and presence of visceral hemangiomas [3]

Pathogenesis of this disease involves:

- Unclear; may be related to chromosome 9p mutation [1]
- Appears to have autosomal dominant pattern of inheritance although there are sporadic cases

Histopathological features include:

- Venous hemangioma composed of clusters of dilated irregular capillary spaces lined by a thin layer of endothelial cells (see Fig. 24.2). Smooth muscle may be seen within some of the vascular walls.
- A varied amount of fibrous tissue will surround the vessel walls
- Eccrine sweat glands are frequently seen intimately related to vascular structures

The diagnosis is made using a combination of:

- Complete blood count/iron studies to check for anemia
- GI workup for occult bleeding

The differential diagnosis should include:

- Sturge-Weber syndrome
- von Hippel-Lindau syndrome
- Cobb's syndrome
- Klippel-Trenaunay syndrome
- Parkes-Weber disease
- Maffucci's syndrome

Treatment options include:

- Cutaneous lesions mostly treated for cosmetic effect
- Sclerosis with alcohol [1]
- Laser ablation with carbon dioxide laser irradiation
- Excision of disfiguring/functionally disabling lesions

L. Zakko (✉)
Yale Department of Internal Medicine, 20 York Street, Yale New Haven Hospital, New Haven, CT 06510, USA
e-mail: liam.zakko@yale.edu

J. Finch • M.J. Rothe • J.M. Grant-Kels
Department of Dermatology, University of Connecticut Health Center, 21 South Road, Farmington, CT 06030, USA
e-mail: finch@uchc.edu; rothe@uchc.edu; grant@uchc.edu

G.Y. Wu et al. (eds.), *Atlas of Dermatological Manifestations of Gastrointestinal Disease*, DOI 10.1007/978-1-4614-6191-3_24, © Springer Science+Business Media New York 2013

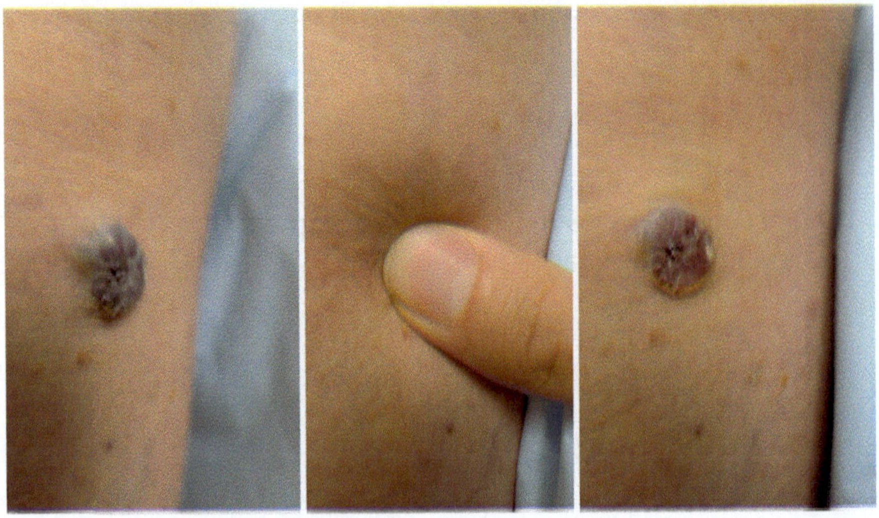

Fig. 24.1 Blue rubber bleb nevus. Rubbery blue nodule (*left*) that can be deflated with pressure (*center*), leaving a wrinkled sac (*right*) that slowly refills with venous blood (Image courtesy of Justin Finch, MD)

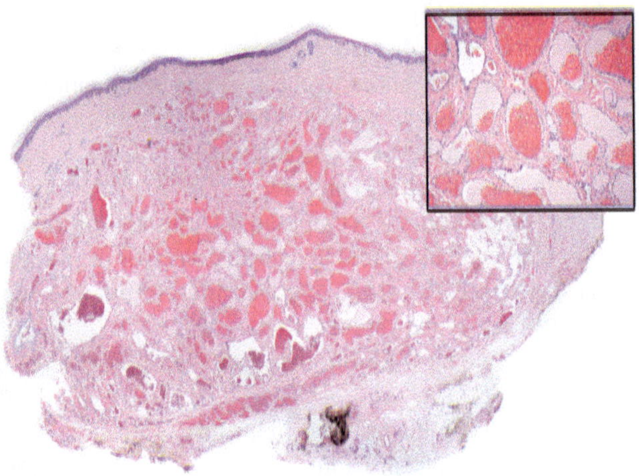

Fig. 24.2 Blue rubber bleb nevus. Poorly demarcated, nonlobular, proliferation of thin-walled blood vessels with flattened endothelium (10×; *inset* 100×)

References

1. Dwivedi M, Misra SP. Blue rubber bleb nevus syndrome causing upper gi hemorrhage: a novel management approach and review. Gastrointest Endosc. 2002;55:943–6.
2. Apak H, Celkan T, Ozkan A, et al. Blue rubber bleb nevus syndrome associated with consumption coagulopathy: treatment with interferon. Dermatology. 2004;208:345–8.
3. Wong CH, Tan YM, Chow WC, et al. Blue rubber bleb nevus syndrome: a clinical spectrum with correlation between cutaneous and gastrointestinal manifestations. J Gastroenterol Hepatol. 2003;18:1000–2.

Henoch–Schönlein Purpura: Gastrointestinal Features

25

Liam Zakko

Henoch–Schönlein purpura is a systemic vasculitis that is characterized by the deposition of IgA-containing immune complexes. The disease generally occurs in children, with 2:1 male to female predominance, and is usually preceded by a upper respiratory infection.

The gastrointestinal (GI) symptoms [1, 2] seen are:

- Abdominal pain (80% of patients): colicky, periumbilical, can be associated with vomiting and distension and may be severe enough to resemble a surgical abdomen
- GI bleeding: occult or symptomatic (see Figs. 25.1 and 25.2 [3]); occurs in 50% of patients, usually self-limited
- Intussusception: usually ileoileal

The clinical signs and findings [1, 2] include:

- Patients most often present with rash, GI symptoms, arthritis, and nephropathy
- Much more common in children (50% of cases in patients younger than 5 years old; 75% of cases in patients younger than 10 years old)
- Adults more likely to have more severe disease, though symptoms are still most often self limited, resolving in about 4 weeks
- Colonoscopy can show multiple hemorrhagic lesions (*see* Fig. 25.3) or ulcers

The pathogenesis of this condition is not entirely clear. There appear to be a number of potential triggering factors [1, 2, 4]:

- IgA1 is involved and found deposited in affected tissue; noted to have aberrant glycosylation of the hinge region
- B-hemolytic group A *Streptococcus* is most common preceding infection; also see with *Mycoplasma pneumoniae*, salmonella, parvovirus B, *Streptococcus pyogenes*, tuberculosis, *Toxocara canus*, *Campylobacter jejuni*, *Helicobacter pylori*, *Coxsackle B-1*, varicella, *Yersinia*, *Shigella*, *Entamoeba histolytica*, HIV, and *Bartonella henselae*
- Drug precipitants include chlorpromazine, ciprofloxacin, quinidine, ranitidine, clarithromycin, angiotensin-converting-enzyme inhibitors, aspirin, carbidopa/levodopa, ampicillin
- Environmental causes include insect bites

The pathology [1, 2, 4] typically features a vasculitis:

- Leukocytoclastic vasculitis of small vessels (dermal/post-capillary venules) with neutrophils and nuclear debris infiltration of the vessel wall

The diagnosis [1, 2, 4] involves consideration of several factors:

- Defined by two or more of the following: (1) palpable purpura not due to thrombocytopenia; (2) age ≤20 at onset; (3) abdominal pain with or without GI bleeding; and/or (4) biopsy showing a leukocytoclastic vasculitis
- Complete blood count; prothrombin time; partial thromboplastin time; C-reactive protein; erythrocyte-sedimentation rate; antinuclear antibody test; rheumatoid factor; anti-neutrophil cytoplasmic antibodies; complement 3; complement 4; immunoglobin A; urinalysis
- Biopsy: if needed per diagnostic criteria

The differential diagnosis [1, 2, 4] of Henoch–Schönlein purpura should include:

- Thrombocytopenic disease
- Other vasculitis

There is no cure for this condition but symptomatic treatment [1, 2, 4] involves:

- Supportive Care
- Prednisone will decrease abdominal pain/arthritis but will not shorten illness
- Severe/refractory disease consider cytotoxic agents/plasmapheresis

L. Zakko (✉)
Yale Department of Internal Medicine, Yale New Haven Hospital, 20 Yale Street New Haven, CT 06510, USA
e-mail: liam.zakko@yale.edu

G.Y. Wu et al. (eds.), *Atlas of Dermatological Manifestations of Gastrointestinal Disease*,
DOI 10.1007/978-1-4614-6191-3_25, © Springer Science+Business Media New York 2013

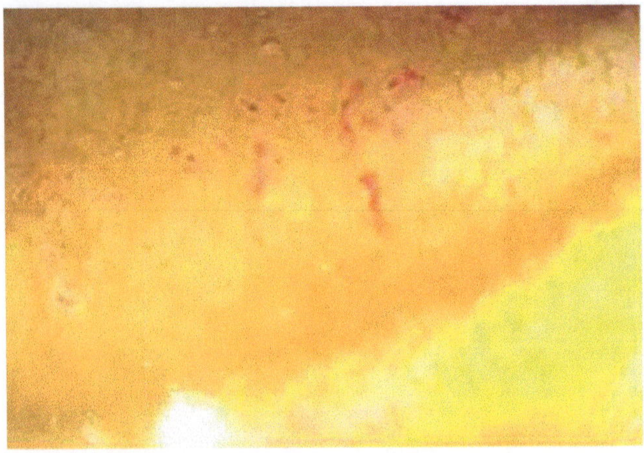

Fig. 25.1 Endoscopic findings from a patient with Henoch–Schönlein Purpura showing small nonbleeding vasculitic lesions in the ileum (Reprinted from Menon et al. [3]; with permission)

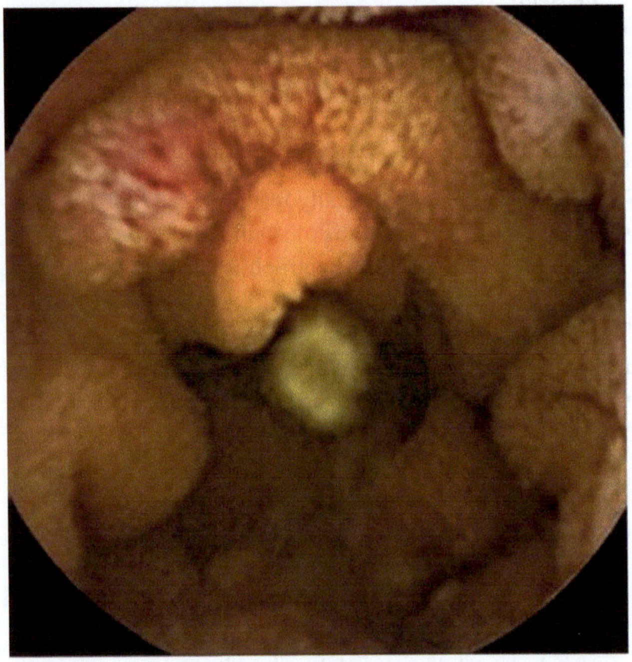

Fig. 25.2 Small bowel wireless capsule endoscopy image showing erythematous ulcerated mucosa in the jejunum (Reprinted from Menon et al. [3]; with permission)

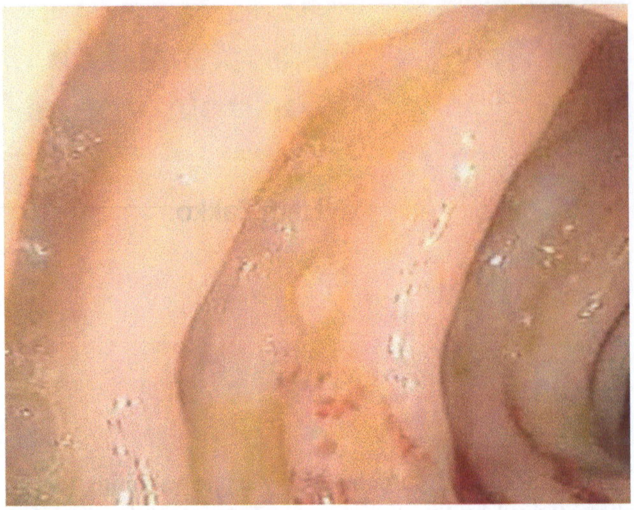

Fig. 25.3 An endoscopic view of vasculitic lesions in the sigmoid colon in a patient with Henoch–Schönlein Purpura (Reprinted from Menon et al. [3]; with permission)

References

1. Anh E, Luk A, Chetty R, Butany J. Vasculitis of the gastrointestinal tract. Semin Diagn Pathol. 2009;26:79–80.
2. Gedalia A. Henoch-Schönlein purpura. Curr Rheumatol Rep. 2004;6:195–202.
3. Menon P, Singh S, Ahuja N, Winter, TA. Gastrointestinal manifestations of Henoch-Schönlein purpura. Dig Dis Sci. 27 March 2012. (Epub ahead of print).
4. Salusbury FT. Henoch-Schönlein purpura. Curr Opin Rheumatol. 2010;22:598–602.

Henoch–Schönlein Purpura: Dermatological Features

26

Liam Zakko, Justin Finch, Marti J. Rothe, and Jane M. Grant-Kels

Clinical signs and features include:

- Besides dermatologic symptoms, patients most often present with gastrointestinal (GI) symptoms, arthritis, and nephropathy [1]
- Much more common in children (50% of cases in patients < 5 years old, 75% of cases in patients < 10 years old) [1]
- Adults more likely to have more severe disease [1], although symptoms are still most often self limited, resolving in about 4 weeks [2]
- Initially cutaneous manifestation is erythematous maculopapular rash with wheal-like spots [1]
- In 1–2 days characteristic nonblanching, palpable purpura develops usually starting symmetrically on the legs and buttock as lesions no larger than 1 cm in diameter (see Fig. 26.1) [1]
- Rash usually fades after 1–2 weeks but can reemerge in another 1–2 weeks and cycle through fading and reemerging over a year [1]
- Twenty percent to 46% (especially patients < age 3 years old) will develop an angioedema of the scalp, eyelids, lips, back, dorsal aspects of hands and feet, scrotum, and perineum not related to an underlying nephropathy [1]

L. Zakko (✉)
Yale Department of Internal Medicine,
Yale New Haven Hospital, 20 Yale Street New Haven, CT 06510, USA
e-mail: liam.zakko@yale.edu

J. Finch • M.J. Rothe • J.M. Grant-Kels
Department of Dermatology,
University of Connecticut Health Center,
21 South Road, Farmington, CT 06030, USA
e-mail: finch@uchc.edu; rothe@uchc.edu; grant@uchc.edu

Pathogenesis of this disease involves autoimmunity, including:

- IgA1 involved and found deposited in affected tissue; noted to have aberrant glycosylation of the hinge region [2]
- β-hemolytic Group A *Streptococcus* is most common preceding infection; also see with *Mycoplasma pneumoniae*, salmonella, parvovirus B, *Streptococcus pyogenes*, tuberculosis, *Toxocara canus*, *Campylobacter jejuni*, *Helicobacter pylori*, *Coxsackie B-1*, varicella, *Yersinia*, *Shigella*, *Entamoeba histolytica*, HIV, and *Bartonella henselae* [3]
- Drug precipitants include chlorpromazine, ciprofloxacin, quinidine, ranitidine, clarithromycin, angiotensin-converting enzyme inhibitors, aspirin, carbidopa/levodopa, ampicillin [3]
- Environmental causes include insect bites [3]
- Has been reported in association with malignancy (solid tumors more commonly than hematologic malignancy). In adults, consider malignancy workup if no other trigger is identified; should consider workup for metastatic disease in patients with prior history of malignancy [4]

Histopathological features include:

- Leukocytoclastic vasculitis of small vessels (dermal/post-capillary venules) demonstrating a perivascular and intravascular neutrophilic infiltration with leukocytoclasia, fibrinoid necrosis of the involved vessel wall, evidence of endothelial cell damage, and extravasated red blood cells (see Fig. 26.2) [1]
- Immunofluorescence shows IgA1 in vessel walls [1]; minor amounts of C3/C4 and fibrin also noted [3]

The diagnosis is made using a combination of:

- Defined by two or more of:
  1. Palpable purpura not due to thrombocytopenia
  2. Age ≤ 20 years at onset
  3. Abdominal pain with or without GI bleeding
  4. Biopsy showing a leukocytoclastic vasculitis [1, 3]
- Complete blood count; prothrombin time; partial thromboplastin time; C-reactive protein; erythrocyte-sedimentation

G.Y. Wu et al. (eds.), *Atlas of Dermatological Manifestations of Gastrointestinal Disease*,
DOI 10.1007/978-1-4614-6191-3_26, © Springer Science+Business Media New York 2013

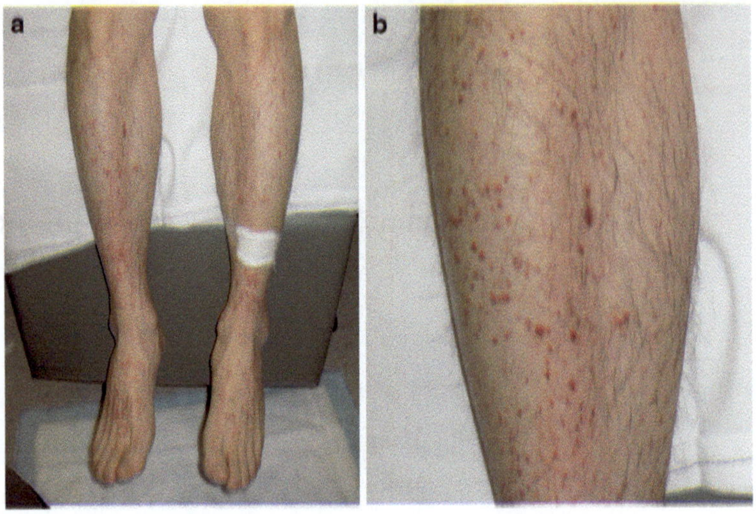

Fig. 26.1 (**a**) Henoch–Schönlein Purpura. (**b**) Palpable purpura on the lower legs

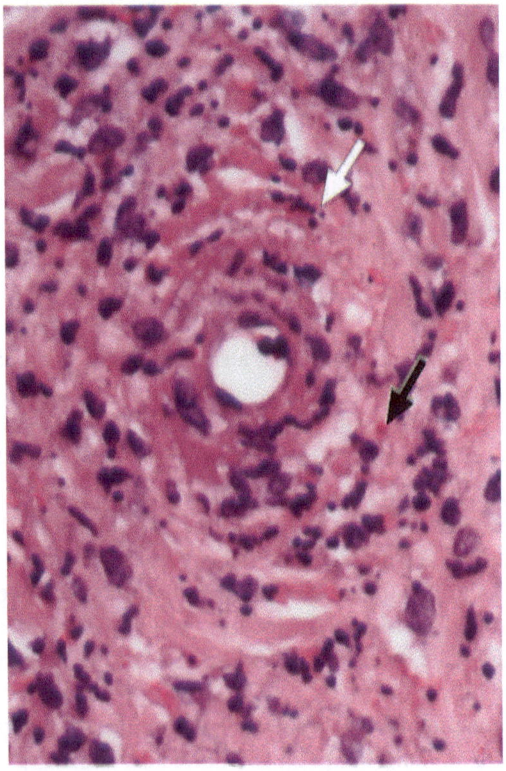

Fig. 26.2 Henoch–Schönlein Purpura. Vasculitis of small vessels, with neutrophils in the vessel wall, karyorrhexis (*white arrow*), and extravasated erythrocytes (*black arrow*) (400×)

rate; antinuclear antibody test; rheumatoid factor; anti-neutrophil cytoplasmic antibodies; C3;C4;IgA; urinalysis [1]

- Biopsy: if needed per diagnostic criteria [1]

The differential diagnosis should include:

- Thrombocytopenic disease
- Other causes of vasculitis

Treatment options include:

- supportive Care[1, 3]
- Prednisone will decrease abdominal pain/arthritis but will not shorten illness [1–3]
- Role of systemic steroids for preventing nephritis is controversial [2]
- Severe/refractory disease consider cytotoxic agents (as cyclophosphamide or azathioprine)/plasmapheresis [1, 3]

References

1. Gedalia A. Henoch-Schönlein purpura. Curr Rheumatol Rep. 2004;6:195–202.
2. Salusbury FT. Henoch-Schönlein purpura. Curr Opin Rheumatol. 2010;22:598–602.
3. Ahn E, Luk A, Chetty R, Butany J. Vasculitides of the gastrointestinal tract. Semin Diagn Pathol. 2009;26:79–80.
4. Misui H, Shibagaki N, Kawamura T, et al. A clinical study of Henoch-Schönlein purpura associated with malignancy. J Eur Acad Dermatol Venereol. 2009;23:394–401.

Pseudoxanthoma Elasticum: Gastrointestinal Features

27

Liam Zakko

Pseudoxanthoma elasticum is an autosomal recessive genetic disease. Those affected will have fragmentation of elastic fibers in various tissues throughout the body. The prevalence is thought to be about 1:25,000 with a 2:1 female to male predominance.

The most common gastrointestinal (GI) symptoms include [1, 2]:

- Recurrent acute gastrointestinal hemorrhages in about 13% of patients

The clinical signs and findings are [1, 2]:

- Disease in which elastic fibers become calcified and weak; manifests in the second and third decade
- Pseudoxanthoma elasticum also presents with eye lesions (angioid streaks and other degeneration of the retina) and vascular defects, calcification leading to GI bleeds.
- Imaging may show a nonspecific heterogeneous pattern (see Fig. 27.1).
- Myocardial infarction, cerebral vascular accidents, peripheral vascular disease, and hypertension have been reported.
- Macroscopically, the gastric mucosa may often have similar appearance to the skin with a yellow cobblestone appearance, with nodular, raised, yellow submucosal lesions. Often there are petechiae and erythema, as well.

The pathogenesis is based on a genetic defect [3]:

- Completely autosomal recessive although there may be some subclinical disease in carriers
- Hallmark of disease is mineralization of elastic fibers
- Mutation is on chromosome 16p in the *ABCC6* gene encoding a membrane transporter
- Affected gene is mainly expressed in the liver: how that causes disease is unclear
- There may be a mutation in the gene for γ-glutamyl carboxylase protein that leads to improper activation of matrix Gla protein, which prevents improper mineralization
- If the last aspect is true, it may explain coagulopathies seen in pseudoxanthoma elasticum-like disease

There are usually no pathological findings on mucosal biopsies. If present, the GI tract can rarely show [1]:

- Elastic tissue degeneration in the gastric arteries that is evident on biopsy

The diagnosis is made by a combination of [1, 2, 4]:

- Clinical: characteristic skin signs, characteristic ophthalmologic features, or characteristic histology on biopsy
- Genetic test is positive in 99% of cases: consider without clinical symptoms if there is a family history

The differential diagnosis of pseudoxanthoma elasticum should include [1, 2, 4, 5]:

- End-stage renal disease
- Ehlers–Danlos syndrome
- Anetoderma
- Focal cutaneous elastosis
- Elastosis perforans serpiginosa
- Buschke–Ollendorff syndrome

The treatment involves [1]:

- Medical management with proton-pump inhibitors and H2-blockers to try to prevent bleeding
- Esophagogastroduodenoscopy hemostasis and selective angiography with embolization of the bleeding vessel
- Surgical resections including total gastrectomy for severe bleeding

L. Zakko (✉)
Yale Department of Internal Medicine, Yale New Haven Hospital, 20 Yale Street New Haven, CT 06510, USA
e-mail: liam.zakko@yale.edu

G.Y. Wu et al. (eds.), *Atlas of Dermatological Manifestations of Gastrointestinal Disease*, DOI 10.1007/978-1-4614-6191-3_27, © Springer Science+Business Media New York 2013

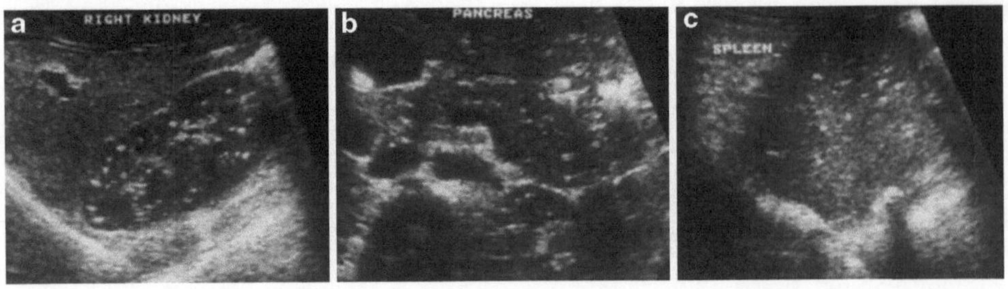

Fig. 27.1 Abdominal sonographic views of: kidneys (**a**), pancreas (**b**), and spleen (**c**) showing a hyperechogenic pattern in a patient with pseudoxanthoma elasticum

References

1. Finger RP, Issa PC, Ladewig MS, et al. Pseudoxathoma elasticum: genetics, clinical manifestations, and therapeutic approaches. Surv Ophthalmol. 2009;54:272–85.
2. Laube S, Moss C. Pseudoxanthoma elasticum. Arch Dis Child. 2005;90:754–6.
3. Li Q, Jiang Q, Pfender E, et al. Pseudoxanthoma elasticum: clinical phenotypes, molecular genetics, and putative pathomechanisms. Exp Dermatol. 2009;18:1–11.
4. Spinzi G, Strocchi E, Imperiali G, et al. Pseudoxanthoma elasticum: a rare cause of gastrointestinal bleeding. Am J Gastroenterol. 1996;91:1631–7.
5. Ward SK, Roenigk HH, Gordon KB. Dermatological manifestations of gastroenterological disorders. Gastroenterol Clin North Am. 1998;27:623–4.

Pseudoxanthoma Elasticum: Dermatological Features

28

Liam Zakko, Justin Finch, Marti J. Rothe, and Jane M. Grant-Kels

Clinical sign and symptoms include:

- Genetic disease in which elastic fibers become calcified and weak demonstrating skin manifestations in the second or third decade (but occasionally in childhood); serious ocular and vascular complications manifest in the third or fourth decade of life [1]
- Cutaneous lesions start as small (1–5 mm) yellowish papules in a reticular pattern at flexural areas (including the neck and axilla) associated with cutaneous laxity (see Fig. 28.1) [2]
- Cutaneous lesions coalesce into larger plaques of inelastic, leathery skin with a yellow hue; skin has a plucked chicken/cobblestone appearance [3]
- Also can have perforating pseudoxanthoma elasticum with calcified elastic fibers extruding from the skin; clinically, these lesions appear as keratotic papules [1]
- Pseudoxanthoma elasticum-like disorder also has symptoms of cutis laxa (laxity of face, neck, trunk) and may have a coagulation defect [4]
- Pseudoxanthoma elasticum also presents with eye lesions (angioid streaks due to alteration of the elastic fibers in the retina's Bruch membrane and subsequent retinal hemorrhages leading to central vision loss) and vascular calcification leading to GI bleeds, premature myocardial infarction, cerebral vascular accidents, peripheral vascular disease, and hypertension [1, 2]
- More common in women than in men [1, 2, 4]

Pathogenesis of this genetic disease involves:

- Autosomal recessive, although may be some subclinical disease in carriers [1, 2, 4]
- Hallmark of disease is ectopic mineralization of elastic fibers [4]
- Mutation is on chromosome 16p in the *ABCC6* gene for a membrane transporter [4]
- Affected protein is mainly expressed in the liver; how it causes disease is unclear
- There may be a mutation in the gene for γ-glutamyl carboxylase (GGCX) protein that leads to improper activation of matrix G1, a protein that prevents improper mineralization [4]; mutations in the *GGCS* gene also prevent normal γ-glutamyl carboxylation of vitamin K-dependent coagulation factors and may explain coagulopathies seen in association with PXE-like skin findings [4]

Histopathological features include:

- Hematoxylin and eosin stain shows within the mid to deep dermis an accumulation of basophilic material that represents fragmented and calcified elastic fibers [2] (see Fig. 28.2)
- Extracellular matrix components of fibronectin, vitronectin, and proteoglycans are associated with the altered elastic fibers [1, 2]
- Von Kossa stain reveals calcium on elastic fibers [2]
- Verhoeff–van Gieson stain reveals black clumped and irregular elastic fibers [2]

The diagnosis is made using a combination of:

- Clinical: characteristic skin signs, characteristic ophthalmologic features, or characteristic histology on biopsy [1, 4]

L. Zakko (✉)
Yale Department of Internal Medicine, Yale New Haven Hospital, 20 Yale Street New Haven, CT 06510, USA
e-mail: liam.zakko@yale.edu

J. Finch • M.J. Rothe • J.M. Grant-Kels
Department of Dermatology,
University of Connecticut Health Center,
21 South Road, Farmington, CT 06030, USA
e-mail: finch@uchc.edu; rothe@uchc.edu; grant@uchc.edu

G.Y. Wu et al. (eds.), *Atlas of Dermatological Manifestations of Gastrointestinal Disease*,
DOI 10.1007/978-1-4614-6191-3_28, © Springer Science+Business Media New York 2013

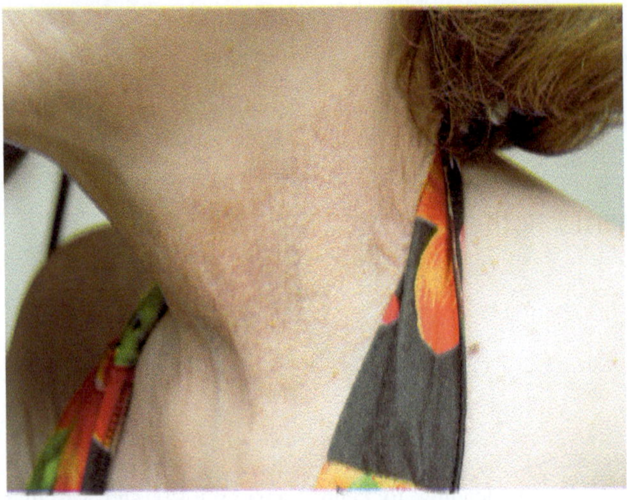

Fig. 28.1 Pseudothanthoma elasticum. Pseudothanthomatous yellowish papules on the lateral neck give the skin a "plucked chicken" appearance (Image courtesy of Steven Brett Sloan, MD)

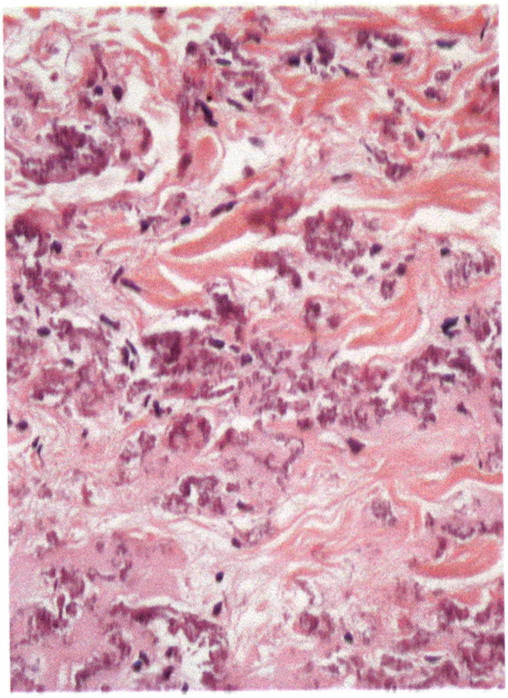

Fig. 28.2 Pseudothanthoma Elasticum. Clumped, calcified elastic fibers in the dermis (400×)

- Gene test is positive in 99% of cases: consider without clinical symptoms if there is a family history [4]

The differential diagnosis should include:

- End-stage renal disease
- B-thalassemia/sickle cell disease (PXE phenotype present in 20% of patients)
- Paget's disease (osteodystrophia deformans)
- Ehlers–Danlos syndrome
- Anetoderma
- Focal cutaneous elastosis
- Elastosis perforans serpiginosa
- Buschke–Ollendorff syndrome
- Aging skin

Treatment options include:

- Increased surveillance for vascular disease [1, 2]
- Low calcium diet may help slow progression [1]
- Avoidance of medications (e.g., nonsteroidal anti-inflammatory drugs and aspirin) that might increase bleeding risk [1, 2]
- Plastic surgery intervention for skin lesions can be performed [1]

References

1. Laube S, Moss C. Pseudoxanthoma elasticum. Arch Dis Child. 2005;90:754–6.
2. Finger RP, Issa PC, Ladewig MS, et al. Pseudoxathoma elasticum: genetics, clinical manifestations and therapeutic approaches. Surv Ophthalmol. 2009;54:272–85.
3. Ward SK, Roenigk HH, Gordon KB. Dermatological manifestations of gastroenterological disorders. Gastroenterol Clin North Am. 1998;27:623–4.
4. Li Q, Jiang Q, Pfender E, et al. Pseudoxanthoma elasticum: clinical phenotypes, molecular genetics, and putative pathomechanisms. Exp Dermatol. 2009;18:1–11.

29 Ehlers–Danlos Syndrome Type IV (Vascular): Gastrointestinal Features

Liam Zakko

Ehlers–Danlos syndrome is a group of inherited connective tissue disorders caused by a defect in the synthesis of collagen. Severity of the disease depends on the mutation inherited. The disorder occurs in approximately one in 5,000 births [1].

Gastrointestinal (GI) signs and findings include [2, 3]:

- Epigastric discomfort, hematemesis, melena, abdominal pain, constipation, peritoneal signs
- In general, Ehlers–Danlos Syndrome is characterized by skin hyperextensibility, joint hypermobility, and wound-healing abnormalities
- Type IV (vascular) Ehlers–Danlos is most often associated with GI pathology
- Type IV has less skin hyperextensibility; major skin finding is very translucent skin with easily visible veins (particularly on the chest); thin faces, pinched nose, and large eyes
- Common GI pathology includes:
  - Esophagus: hiatal hernia, esophageal diverticula, macroesophagus, esophageal rupture with forceful vomiting
  - Gastric: volvulus from adhesions, severe peptic ulcer disease due to mucosal fragility
  - Small intestine: perforation due to studded diverticula on the mesentery border, megaduodenum leading to bacterial overgrowth, intramural hematoma, and bleeding
  - Colon (see Fig. 29.1) [4]: perforation (particularly type IV disease); rectal prolapse

The pathogenesis lies in the specific collagen formation defect [3, 5]:

- Type IV: autosomal dominant disease with mutation in *COL3A1* gene, which codes for type III procollagen; patients have quantitative and/or qualitative defects in type III collagen (*see* Fig. 29.2) [4].
- Type I, II: abnormalities of type V and type I collagen inherited in an autosomal dominant pattern; worse clinical disease with type I
- Type III; mutation in *COL3A1* and/or *TNXB* genes leading to small joint hyperextensibility (usually mild clinical disease) in an autosomal dominant or autosomal recessive pattern

The pathology may show typical features [3, 5]:

- Decreased dermal thickness with increased lamellae around dermal blood vessels
- Increased elastic fibers; finer (decreased diameter) and more loosely organized collagen
- Fibroblasts have dilated endoplasmic reticulum

The diagnosis is made by considering [1–3, 5, 6]:

- Family history of Type IV Ehlers–Danlos
- Four main clinical findings: rupture of blood vessels or internal organs (arterial rupture, intestinal rupture, uterine rupture during pregnancy); striking facial appearance (thin lips/philtrum, small chin, thin nose, large eyes); easy bruising; translucent skin
- Also see: acrogeria, hypermobility of small joints, early onset varicose veins, tendon/muscle rupture, arteriovenous carotid/cavernous sinus fistula, pneumothorax, chronic joint dislocations, congenital dislocation of the hips, talipes equinovarum, gingival recession
- Cultures of fibroblasts show abnormal type III collagen production
- Genetic testing can reveal *COL3A1* mutation
- Type I–III Ehlers–Danlos based on clinical findings of skin hyperextensibility, joint hypermobility, and wound healing abnormalities

Differential diagnosis of Ehlers–Danlos should include [1–3]:

- Neoplasm
- Diverticulitis
- Inflammatory bowel disease
- Colitis
- Steroid use

L. Zakko (✉)
Yale Department of Internal Medicine, Yale New Haven Hospital, 20 Yale Street New Haven, CT 06510, USA
e-mail: liam.zakko@yale.edu

G.Y. Wu et al. (eds.), *Atlas of Dermatological Manifestations of Gastrointestinal Disease*, DOI 10.1007/978-1-4614-6191-3_29, © Springer Science+Business Media New York 2013

There is no cure for this disease but treatment includes [1–3]:

- Symptomatic treatment for GI conditions: H2-antagonists/proton pump inhibitors and antibiotics for those with *Helicobacter pylori* to prevent gastric ulcers; laxatives to prevent constipation that often leads to perforations requiring surgical treatments; anastomosis can lead to recurrent perforation and breakdown due to weak fibrous tissue (therefore, perforation may require colectomy); surgery is also often complicated by wound dehiscence and infection.

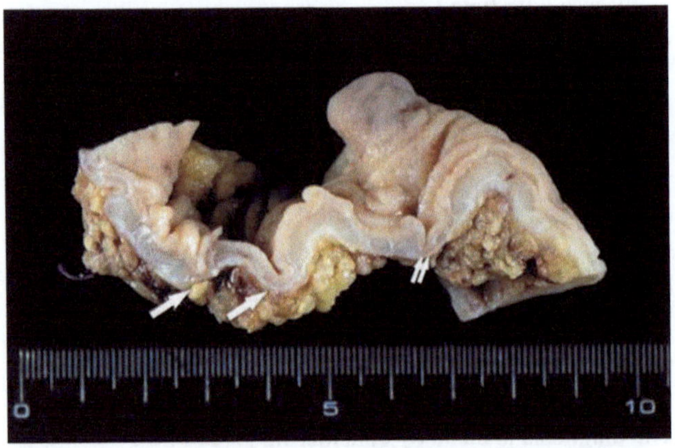

Fig. 29.1 Gross appearance of the resected colon from a patient with Ehlers–Danlos syndrome. The muscularis propria has abrupt changes in thickness, and in some areas, it is practically absent (*large arrows*). In some areas, diverticula penetrating through the muscularis propria can be seen (*small arrows*) (Reprinted from Bläker et al. [4]; with permission)

Fig. 29.2 A photomicrograph of colon sections from a patient with Ehlers–Danlos syndrome Type IV (**a**). Immunohistochemical staining for collagen type III is markedly decreased compared to a normal control specimen (**b**) (Reprinted from Bläker et al. [4]; with permission)

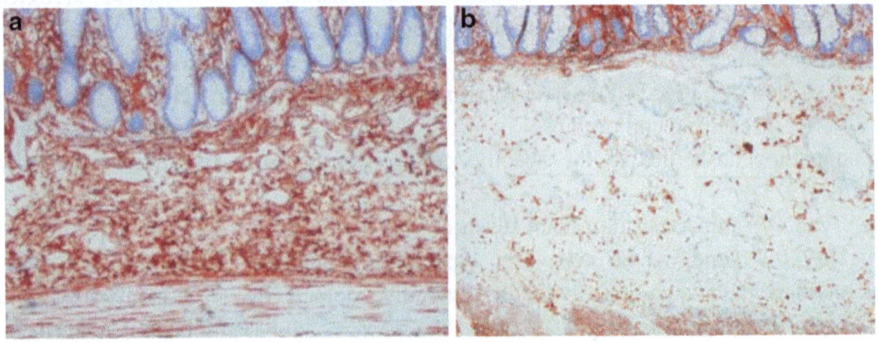

References

1. Malfait F, Wenstrup RJ, Paepe AD. Clinical and genetic aspects of Ehlers–Danlos syndrome, classic type. Genet Med. 2010;12:597–605.
2. Solomon JA, Abrams L, Lichtenstein GR. GI manifestations of Ehlers–Danlos syndrome. Am J Gastroenterol. 1996;91:2282–8.
3. Pepin M, Schwarze U, Superti-Furga A, Byers PH. Clinical and genetic features of Ehlers–Danlos syndrome type IV, the vascular type. N Eng J Med. 2000;342:673–80.
4. Bläker H, Funke B, Hausser I, et al. Pathology of the large intestine in patients with vascular type Ehlers-Danlos syndrome. Virchows Arch. 2007;450:713–7.
5. Smith LT, Schwarze U, Goldstein J, Byers PH. Mutations in the COL3A1 gene results in Ehlers–Danlos syndrome type IV and alterations in the size and distribution of the major collage fibrils of the dermis. J Invest Dermatol. 1997;108:241–7.
6. Ward SK, Roenigk HH, Gordon KB. Dermatological manifestations of gastroenterological disorders. Gastroenterol Clin North Am. 1998;27:624–5.
7. Watanabe A, Shimada T. The vascular type of Ehlers–Danlos syndrome. J Nippon Med Sch. 2008;75:254–61.

Ehlers–Danlos Syndrome Type IV (Vascular): Dermatological Features

30

Liam Zakko, Justin Finch, Marti J. Rothe, and Jane M. Grant-Kels

Clinical signs and features include:

- In general, Ehlers–Danlos syndrome is characterized by skin hyperextensibility (see Fig. 30.1), joint hypermobility, and wound healing abnormalities (see Fig. 30.2)
- Type IV (vascular) Ehlers-Danlos is the type most commonly associated with gastrointestinal (GI) pathology
- Type IV has less skin hyperextensibility. The major cutaneous finding is very translucent skin with easily visible veins particularly on the chest, abdomen, and extremities. The most common, and often the first sign of the disease, is pronounced bruising [1].
- Series of patients show that 7–25% of patients experience the first major complication by age 20 years and more than 75% by age 40 years [1, 2].

Pathogenesis of this disease involves a genetic mutation [3]:

- Autosomal dominant disease with mutation in *COL3A1* gene, which codes for type III procollagen
- Patients have quantitative and/or qualitative defects in type III collagen

Histopathological features include:

- Reticular dermal thickness decreased by one half to three quarters of normal thickness
- Reticular dermis with loosely organized thin collagen and a relative increase in elastic fibers that are shortened and fragmented
- Collagen bundles in subcutaneous septae are thin and decreased
- In areas of trauma where pseudotumor formation is noted clinically there can be evidence of fibrosis, with increased but finer (decreased in diameter) elastic fibers, numerous capillaries, and occasional foreign body giant cells
- Markedly decreased factor XIIIa dermal dendrocytes in the reticular dermis
- Ultrastructural anomalies of blood vessels have been described including replication of the lamina densa, altered dermal arteriolar wall morphology, and dissociation of vascular smooth muscle cells
- Fibroblasts have dilated endoplasmic reticulum

The diagnosis is made using a combination of [4, 5]:

- Family history of type IV Ehlers–Danlos
- Four main clinical findings:
  1. Rupture of blood vessels or internal organs (arterial rupture, intestinal rupture, uterine rupture during pregnancy)
  2. Striking facial appearance (thin lips/philtrum, small chin, thin nose, large eyes, lobeless ears)
  3. Easy bruising
  4. Translucent skin
- Also see: acrogeria (extreme wrinkling and thinness of skin of the dorsal hands and feet), hypermobility of small joints, early-onset varicose veins, tendon/muscle rupture, arteriovenous carotid/cavernous sinus fistula, pneumothorax, chronic joint dislocations, congenital dislocation of the hips, talipes equinovarum, gingival recession
- Cultures of fibroblasts show abnormal type III collagen production
- Genetic testing can reveal *COL3A1* mutation

The differential diagnosis should include:

- Marfan syndrome

L. Zakko (✉)
Yale Department of Internal Medicine, Yale New Haven Hospital, 20 Yale street New Haven, CT 06510, USA
e-mail: liam.zakko@yale.edu

J. Finch • M.J. Rothe • J.M. Grant-Kels
Department of Dermatology, University of Connecticut Health Center, 21 South Road, Farmington, CT 06030, USA
e-mail: finch@uchc.edu; rothe@uchc.edu; grant@uchc.edu

G.Y. Wu et al. (eds.), *Atlas of Dermatological Manifestations of Gastrointestinal Disease*, DOI 10.1007/978-1-4614-6191-3_30, © Springer Science+Business Media New York 2013

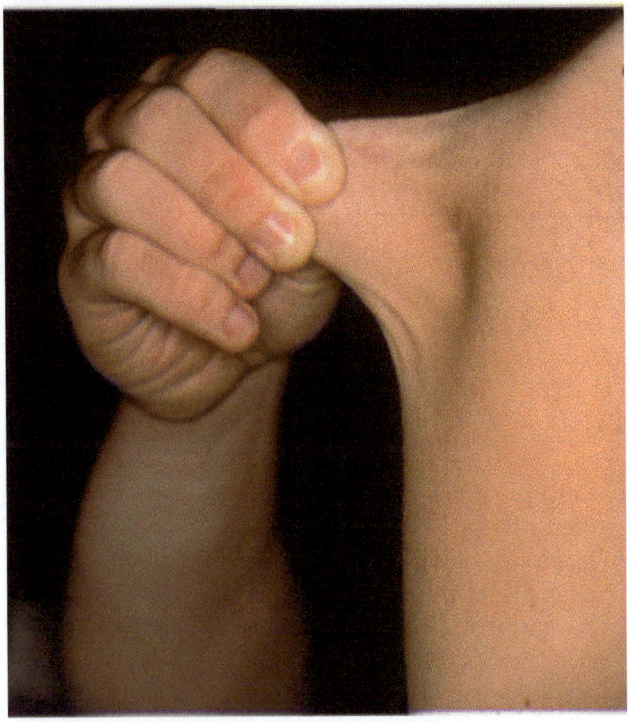

Fig. 30.1 Ehlers–Danlos syndrome. Hyperplastic skin

- Loeys–Dietz syndrome
- Cutis laxa syndromes
- Other types of Ehlers–Danlos

Treatment options include:

- No specific treatment for cutaneous manifestations but preventive measures should be taken including avoidance of trauma, contact sports, and heavy exercise; wearing protective padding; supplementation with oral vitamin C and desamino-D-arginine-vasopressin, which may help to decrease bruising [6].

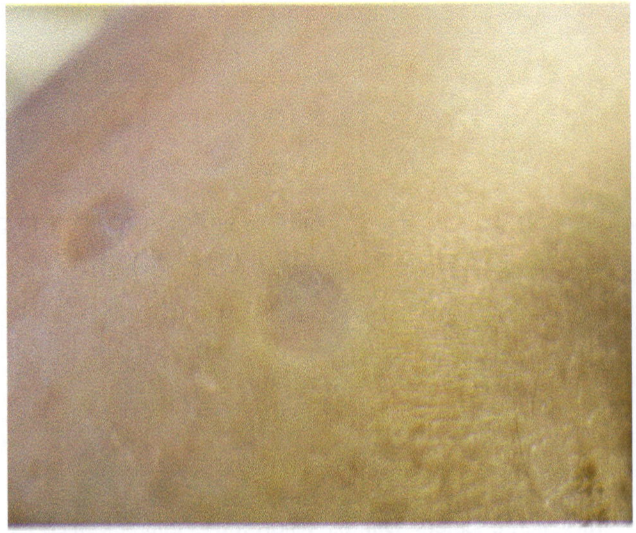

Fig. 30.2 Ehlers–Danlos syndrome. Atrophic scars

References

1. De Paepe A, Malfait F. The Ehlers-Danlos syndrome, a disorder with many faces. Clin Genet. 2012;82:1–11.
2. Pepin M, Schwarze U, Superti-Furga A, Byers PH. Clinical and genetic features of Ehlers-Danlos syndrome type IV, the vascular type. N Eng J Med. 2000;342:673–80.
3. Smith LT, Schwarze U, Goldstein J, Byers PH. Mutations in the COL3A1 gene results in Ehlers-Danlos syndrome type IV and alterations in the size and distribution of the major collage fibrils of the dermis. J Invest Dermatol. 1997;108:241–7.
4. Watanabe A, Shimada T. The vascular type of Ehlers-Danlos syndrome. J Nippon Med Sch. 2008;75:254–61.
5. Beighton P, De Paepe A, Steinmann B, et al. Ehlers-Danlos syndromes: revised nosology, Villefrance, 1997. Ehlers-Danlos National Foundation (USA) and Ehlers-Danlos Support Group (UK). Am J Med Genet. 1998;77:31–7.
6. Malfait F, Wenstrup RJ, De Paepe AD. Clinical and genetic aspects of Ehlers-Danlos syndrome, classic type. Genet Med. 2010;12:597–605.

31 Gastric Cancer: Gastrointestinal Features

Michael Tadros

Gastric cancer consists of primary malignant lesions in any part of the stomach. This group is thought to cause about 800,000 deaths per year worldwide. Unfortunately, this disease often causes no or nonspecific symptoms in early stages and does not manifest itself until late stages are reached.

Gastrointestinal (GI) symptoms include [1, 2]:

- Asymptomatic in early cancers
- Advanced cancer may present with:
  - Weight loss
  - Abdominal pain
  - Nausea, vomiting, anorexia, and early satiety
  - Upper GI bleeding
  - Gastric outlet obstruction if the tumors obstruct the pylorus
  - Pseudoachalasia and dysphagia if the tumor involves the cardia

Typical clinical signs and findings are [1, 3]:

- Gastric cancer can be localized to the stomach (see Fig. 31.1) or present with regional spread or metastatic disease
- Cachexia and malnutrition
- Epigastric mass, hepatomegaly, and ascites in advanced cases
- Sister Mary Joseph's nodule (spread to the periumbilical area)
- Virchow's node (left supraclavicular lymph node involvement)
- Krukenberg's tumor (involvement of the ovaries)
- Intestinal obstruction
  - Paraneoplastic syndromes may occur in the form of skin involvement: acanthosis nigricans, seborrheic dermatosis, and pruritus

M. Tadros (✉)
Department of Internal Medicine, University of Connecticut Health Center, Farmington, CT, USA

560 Hudson Street, Apt 750, Hartford, CT 06106, USA
e-mail: MTadros@resident.uchc.edu

Pathogenesis is likely multifactorial but includes [1, 2]:

- Several factors increase the risk of gastric cancer such as:
  - *Helicobacter pylori* infection
  - Chronic atrophic gastritis, intestinal metaplasia, and dysplasia
  - Genetic factors such as DNA aneuploidy
  - Family history of gastric cancer
  - Environmental factors such as high salt intake, salt-preserved food, smoking
  - Prior gastric surgery

Typical pathological findings are [1, 2]:

- Gross appearance:
  - Gastric cancer can be polypoid, fungating, ulcerated, depressed, and infiltrating lesions (linitis plastica)
- Microscopic appearance:
  - Adenocarcinoma is the most common. It can be subclassified into intestinal, diffuse, papillary, tubular, mucinous, signet ring cells (see Fig. 31.2).
  - Squamous cell
  - Undifferentiated
  - Others

The diagnosis is made by considering [1, 2]:

- Laboratory studies: complete blood count for anemia, abnormal liver function tests, hepatic involvement, nutritional laboratory tests, and tumor markers such as CEA, CA19.7, and CA 72.4
- Esophagogastroduodenoscopy to establish the diagnosis and obtain tissue biopsy
- Endoscopic ultrasound helps in detecting the depth and extent of the tumor especially, if neoadjuvant treatment is planned.
- Chest radiograph, computed tomography, or magnetic resonance imaging of the chest, abdomen, and pelvis for staging

The differential diagnosis of gastric cancer should include [1, 2]:

- Esophagitis and esophageal cancer
- Peptic ulcer disease

G.Y. Wu et al. (eds.), *Atlas of Dermatological Manifestations of Gastrointestinal Disease*,
DOI 10.1007/978-1-4614-6191-3_31, © Springer Science+Business Media New York 2013

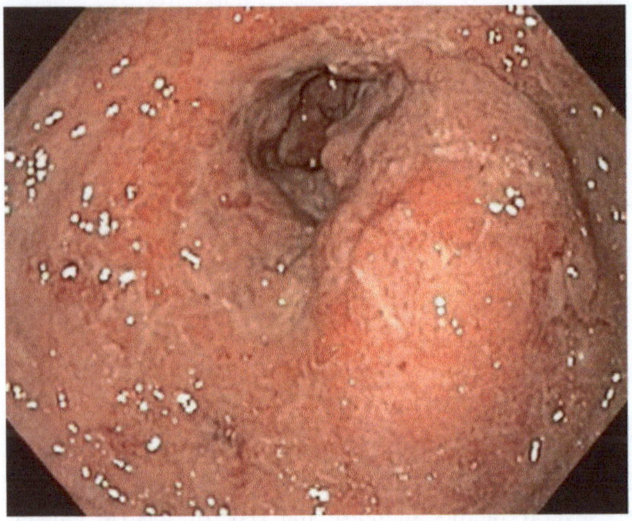

Fig. 31.1 An endoscopic view of a large, exophytic malignancy in the distal stomach. The mass is friable and contains shallow ulcers on the surface

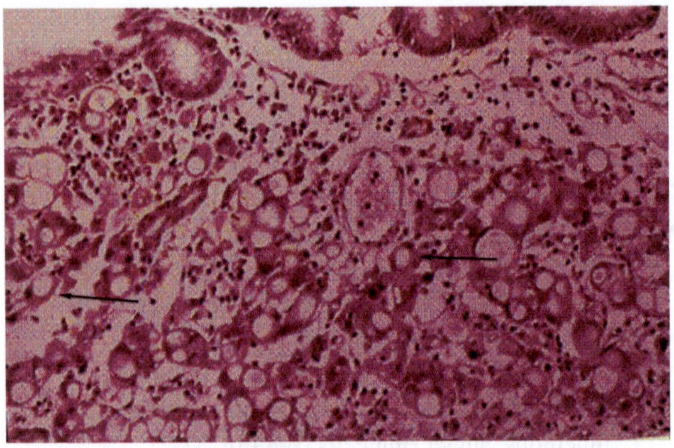

Fig. 31.2 A photomicrograph of a gastric adenocarcinoma specimen showing typical "signet ring" cells (*arrows*). Hematoxylin and eosin stain, high power (Image courtesy of Dr. Qian Wu, University of Connecticut Health Center, Farmington, CT)

- Gastritis
- Gastric lymphoma
- Gastrointestinal stromal tumor

Treatment involves multiple modalities [1, 2]:

- Endoscopic mucosal resection and submucosal dissection: advanced endoscopic techniques for early cancers
- Surgical therapy: depends on tumor location (total gastrectomy, subtotal gastrectomy, esophagogastrectomy); some centers perform lymph node dissection, distal pancreatectomy, splenectomy
- Chemotherapy/radiation therapy/immunotherapy [3]
- Specific regimens are given depending on the extent of the cancer
- Some regimens are used as neoadjuvant therapy to downstage the cancer before surgery

References

1. Feldman M, Friedman LS, Brandt LJ, editors. Sleisenger and Fordtran's gastrointestinal and liver disease. 9th ed. Philadelphia: Saunders; 2010.
2. Fuchs CS, Mayer RJ. Gastric carcinoma. N Engl J Med. 1995;333:32–41.
3. Kim HK, Choi IJ, Kim CG, et al. Gene expression signatures to predict the response of gastric cancer to cisplatin and fluorouracil. J Clin Oncol. 2009;05:27.

32 Malignant Acanthosis Nigricans, Sign of Leser–Trélat, and Tripe Palms

Liam Zakko, Justin Finch, Marti J. Rothe, and Jane M. Grant-Kels

Clinical signs and features include:

- Malignant acanthosis nigricans, sign of Leser–Trélat, and tripe palms are often found together
- Malignant acanthosis nigricans is rare: in total, worldwide, only 1,000 reported cases [1]
  - Involves symmetric hyperpigmented plaques with variable amounts of epidermal hypertrophy, creating a velvety texture; ranges in color from yellow to gray/black; often has overlying scaling/papillomas (if extensive then cutaneous papillomatosis)
  - Progressive—generally advances with cancer, begins with increased pigmentation and advances to hypertrophy with accentuation of the skin lines; maybe associated with pruritus
  - Most commonly found on flexural areas, posterior neck, or mucosally (particularly the mouth) (*see* Fig. 32.1)
- Tripe palms: <100 cases reported, men affected more commonly than women [1]
  - Condition involves hypertrophy of the palms and soles with papillations creating a velvety, rugose appearance often with a yellow hue and exaggeration of the skin lines (they can become distorted with extensive epidermal hyperkeratosis), associated with clubbing and pruritus
- Leser-Trélat: rare, <100 cases reported worldwide [1]
  - Numerous eruptive seborrheic keratoses on trunk and extremities, possible in Christmas tree like pattern, often with pruritus
  - Controversial whether this is a valid sign as both malignancies and seborrheic keratoses are common in the elderly (see Fig. 32.1)
- In general about 60% of the time these conditions precede diagnosis of cancer, 10% are with diagnosis, and 30% follow diagnosis [1]
- Associated with gastric, intestinal, pulmonary, uterine, liver, ovarian, renal, and lymphoproliferative neoplasms; malignancies are often aggressive with poor prognosis

The differential diagnosis should include:

- Benign acanthosis nigricans
- Nonmalignant causes of seborrheic keratosis: HIV, transplants, erythroderma, acromegaly, age
- Keratoderma

Pathogenesis of this disease is unclear but hypotheses include:

- May be related to release of growth factors (e.g., growth factors tumor necrosis factor alpha [TNF-α] and epidermal growth factor [EGF]) from the neoplasm that act on receptors, particularly EGF receptor [1]

Histopathological features include:

- Malignant acanthosis nigricans: hyperkeratosis and papillomatosis with minimal or slight and irregular acanthosis; often alternating acanthosis with atrophy; none or occasionally only slightly increased basal layer hyperpigmentation (see Fig. 32.2)
- Tripe palms: hyperkeratosis, acanthosis, and papillomatosis; increased dermal mucin with an increased number of mast cells can be seen
- Leser–Trélat, seborrheic keratosis: varying hyperkeratosis, papillomatosis, acanthosis often with horn pseudocysts (see Fig. 32.3)

L. Zakko (✉)
Yale Department of Internal Medicine, Yale New Haven Hospital, 20 Yale StreetNew Haven, CT 06510, USA
e-mail: liam.zakko@yale.edu

J. Finch • M.J. Rothe • J.M. Grant-Kels
Department of Dermatology,
University of Connecticut Health Center,
21 South Road, Farmington, CT 06030, USA
e-mail: finch@uchc.edu; rothe@uchc.edu; grant@uchc.edu

G.Y. Wu et al. (eds.), *Atlas of Dermatological Manifestations of Gastrointestinal Disease*,
DOI 10.1007/978-1-4614-6191-3_32,

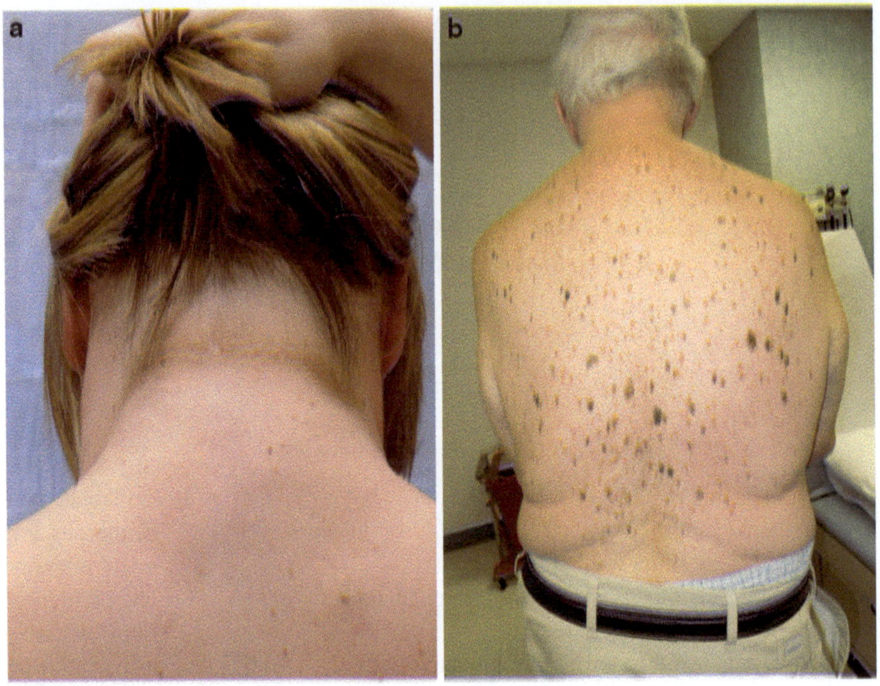

Fig. 32.1 (**a**) Acanthosis nigricans. (**b**) Seborrheic keratoses (Leser-Trélat)

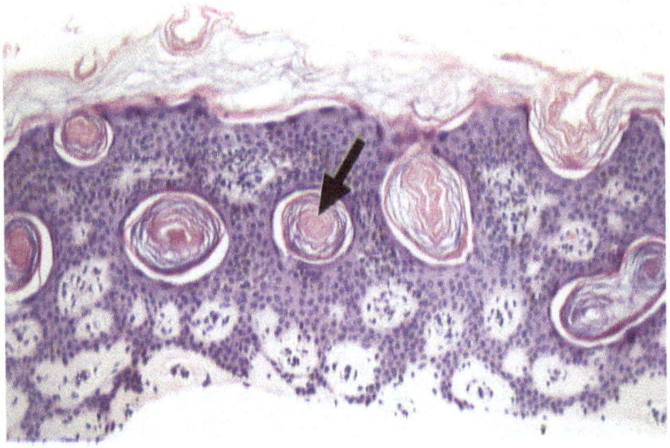

Fig. 32.2 Acanthosis nigricans. Hyperkeratosis and basal layer hyperpigmentation (*arrow*) (100×)

The diagnosis is based on:

- History of malignancy and timing/progression of cutaneous lesions

Treatment options include [1]:

- Treat underlying malignancy as disease parallels tumor growth
- Also treat symptoms, particularly pruritus

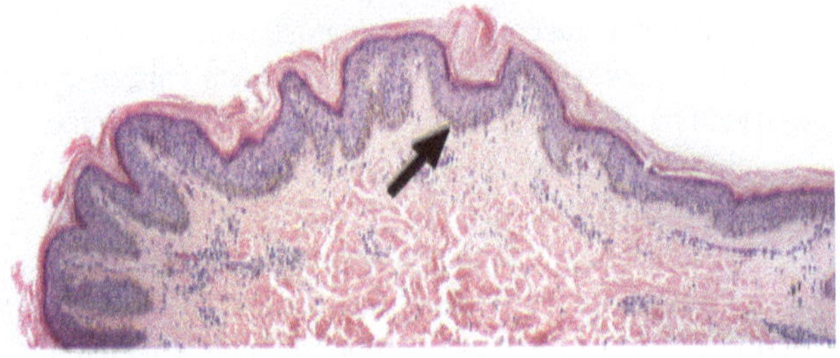

Fig. 32.3 Seborrheic keratosis. Acanthosis and horn pseudocysts (*arrow*) (200×)

- Malignant acanthosis nigricans: acitretin and PUVA (psoralen and ultraviolet A)
- Tripe palms: methotrexate, keratolytics, topical steroids
- Leser-Trélat: cryotherapy or local excision of irritating seborrheic keratosis

Reference

1. Moore RL, Devere TS. Epidermal manifestations of internal malignancy. Dermatol Clin. 2006;26:17–29.

Hereditary Hemorrhagic Telangiectasia: Gastrointestinal Features

33

Liam Zakko

Hereditary hemorrhagic telangiectasia (HHT), also known as Osler–Weber–Rendu disease, is an autosomal dominant disorder characterized by abnormal blood vessel formation. The incidence is one in 5,000, with five genetic variants currently recognized.

The gastrointestinal symptoms include [1]:

- Occult bleeding with iron deficiency
- Symptomatic bleeding with melena, hematemesis, rectal bleeding (25% of patients >60 Yo)
- Rarely portal hypertension, biliary disease, hepatic encephalopathy

The most common clinical signs and findings are [1, 2]:

- 80% present as spontaneous epistaxis
- Arteriovenous malformations (AVMs) occur throughout the body including the GI tract (see Figs. 33.1 and 33.2), lungs, liver, brain/spinal cord
- Telangiectasia appears in the stomach, small bowel (see Fig. 33.3), and colon (see Fig. 33.4) in 10–33% of patients and can lead to GI bleeding
- Liver AVMs occur in up to 75% of patients and are mostly asymptomatic; large lesions, however, can present with high output heart failure, portal hypertension, biliary disease, and hepatic encephalopathy

The pathogenesis involves a genetic disorder caused by a specific mutation [1, 2]:

- Autosomal dominant mutations: HHT1, mutation in *ENG* on chromosome 9; HHT2, mutation in *ACRVL1/ALK1* on chromosome 12; HHT3, mutation on chromosome 5q; HHT4, mutation on chromosome 7p; HHT with juvenile polyposis, mutation of *SMAD4*
- Mutations lead to aberrant response to transforming growth factor beta (TGF-β) family signals for angiogenesis
- Ultimately signal errors cause blood vessels to mature inappropriately

Typical pathology seen includes [1, 2]:

- Initially see dilation of post-capillary venules
- Ultimately dilated post-capillary venules enlarge and connect with arterioles eliminating capillary bed
- Vessels are often thin-walled and surrounded by fibrosis
- Changes are in the setting of a perivascular lymphocytic infiltrate

The diagnosis is made by considering the following [2, 3]:

- Curaçao criteria: (1) epistaxis; (2) telangiectasias at characteristic sites; (3) visceral AVMs in GI tract/liver/lungs/brain/spinal cord; (4) family history: de novo mutation is rare and the disease has a nearly 100% penetrance by age 40
- If ≤3 of the above, HHT can be diagnosed; if ≤2, HHT can be suspected; if only one, HHT is unlikely
- In children with a parent who has HHT, cannot rule out HHT until genetic tests confirm no mutation
- Genetic testing reveals mutation in 80–90% of cases

The differential diagnosis of hereditary hemorrhagic telangiectasia should include [2, 3]:

- Von Willebrand disease

There is no cure but treatment generally involves hemostasis [2, 3]:

- Esophagogastroduodenoscopy with photocoagulation or laser coagulation to control bleeding
- Estrogen/progesterone may reduce the incidence of bleeding
- Only treat symptomatic liver AVM; embolization is not used due to high incidence of liver infarct. Therefore the mainstay treatment is liver transplantation

L. Zakko (✉)
Yale Department of Internal Medicine,
Yale New Haven Hospital, 20 Yale Street New Haven, CT 06510, USA
e-mail: liam.zakko@yale.edu

G.Y. Wu et al. (eds.), *Atlas of Dermatological Manifestations of Gastrointestinal Disease*,
DOI 10.1007/978-1-4614-6191-3_33, © Springer Science+Business Media New York 2013

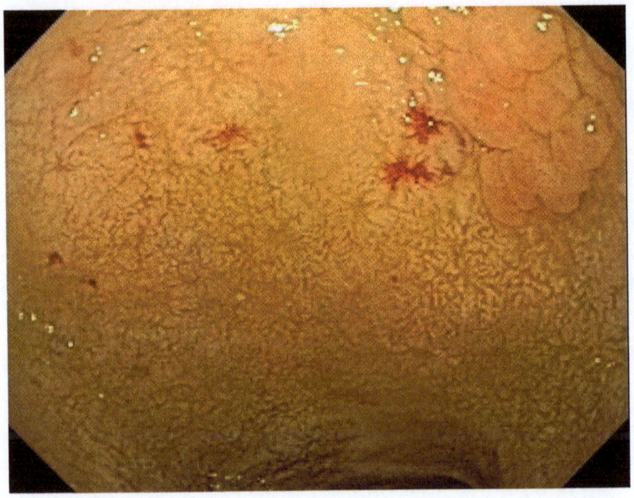

Fig. 33.1 An endoscopic view of telangiectasias in the duodenum of a patient with HHT. Rupture of, or trauma to, these structures can lead to hemorrhage, the most common GI complication associated with this disorder

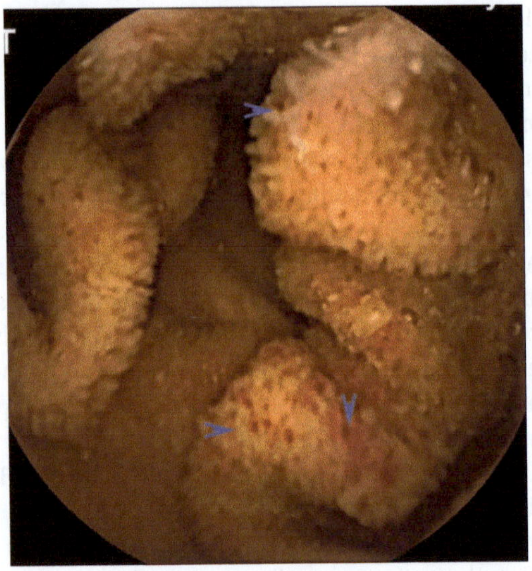

Fig. 33.2 A PillCam view of minute telangiectasias (*arrowheads*) in the small bowel of a patient with HHT

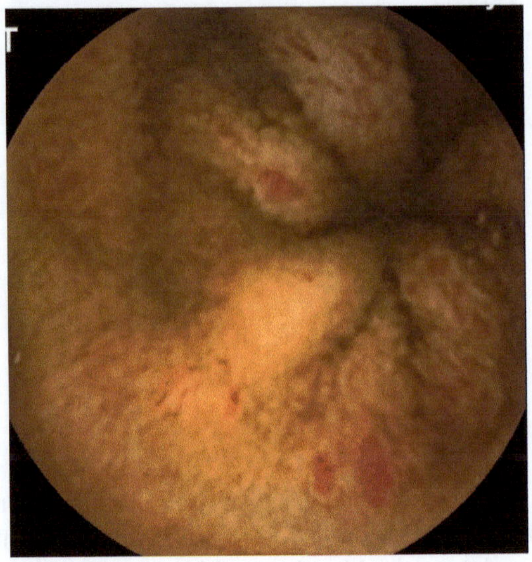

Fig. 33.3 A PillCam view of multiple telangiectasias in the small bowel of a patient with HHT

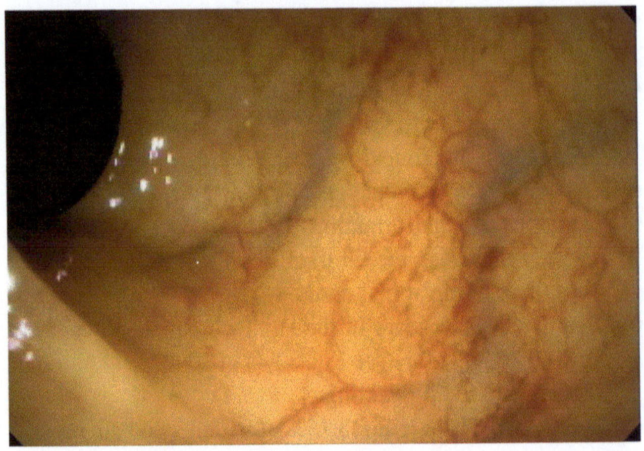

Fig. 33.4 An endoscopic view of telangiectasias of varying sizes scattered in the colon of a patient with HHT

References

1. Dupis-Girod S, Bailly S, Plauchu H. Hereditary hemorrhagic telangiectasia: from molecular biology to patient care. J Thromb Haemost. 2010;8:1447–56.
2. Shlovin CL. Hereditary haemorrhagic telangiectasia: pathophysiology, diagnosis, and treatment. Blood Rev. 2010;24:203–19.
3. Ward SK, Roenigk HH, Gordon KB. Dermatological manifestations of gastroenterological disorders. Gastroenterol Clin North Am. 1998;27:621–2.

Hereditary Hemorrhagic Telangiectasia: Dermatological Features

34

Liam Zakko, Justin Finch, Marti J. Rothe, and Jane M. Grant-Kels

Clinical signs and features include:

- Also known as Osler-Weber-Rendu disease
- Eighty percent present as spontaneous epistaxis [1]
- Arteriovenous malformations (AVMs) occur throughout the body including the gastrointestinal (GI) tract, lungs, liver, brain/spinal cord
- Cutaneous lesions start to appear in adulthood and increase with age [1]
- Lesions appear as small macular telangiectasia that are 1–2 mm in diameter and blanch [1]
- Telangiectasia commonly occur on lips, tongue, palate, face (sun-exposed areas), nares, ears, conjunctiva, chest, hands, and feet (see Fig. 34.1) [1]
- Fingertips can develop painful ulcers from the telangiectasia

Pathogenesis of this disease involves:

- Autosomal dominant mutations: hereditary hemorrhagic telangiectasia (HHT)1, mutation in *ENG* on chromosome 9; HHT2, mutation in *ACRVL1/ALK1* on chromosome 12; HHT3, mutation on chromosome 5q; HHT4, mutation on chromosome 7p; HHT with juvenile polyposis, mutation of *SMAD4*; HHT2 with primary pulmonary hypertension, mutation of *BMPRII* on chromosome 2 [2, 3]
- Mutations lead to aberrant response to transforming growth factor beta (TGF-β) family signals for angiogenesis
- Ultimately signal errors cause blood vessels to mature inappropriately

Histopathological features include:

- Initially see dilatation post-capillary venules
- Ultimately dilated post-capillary venules enlarge and connect with arterioles eliminating capillary bed
- Vessels are often thin walled and surrounded by fibrosis
- A perivascular lymphocytic infiltrate may also be noted around involved vessels

The diagnosis is made using a combination of:

- Curaçao criteria: (1) epistaxis; (2) telangiectasias at characteristic sites; (3) visceral AVMs in GI tract/liver/lungs/brain/spinal cord; (4) family history: de novo mutation is rare and the disease has a nearly 100% penetrance by age 40 [4]
- If ≤3 of above, HHT can be diagnosed; if ≤2, HHT is suspected; if only 1, HHT is unlikely
- In children with a parent who has HHT, cannot rule out HHT until genetic tests confirm no mutation [2]
- Genetic testing reveals mutation in 80–90% of cases

The differential diagnosis should include:

- Von Willebrand disease

Treatment options include [4]:

- Mostly cosmetic for cutaneous lesions
- Long-pulsed Nd: YAG (neodymium-doped yttrium aluminum garnet) laser is effective
- Skin grafts effective for painful ulcerations on fingertips

L. Zakko (✉)
Yale Department of Internal Medicine, Yale New Haven Hospital, New Haven, CT 06510, USA
e-mail: liam.zakko@yale.edu

J. Finch • M.J. Rothe • J.M. Grant-Kels
Department of Dermatology, University of Connecticut Health Center, 21 South Road, Farmington, CT 06030, USA
e-mail: finch@uchc.edu; rothe@uchc.edu; grant@uchc.edu

G.Y. Wu et al. (eds.), *Atlas of Dermatological Manifestations of Gastrointestinal Disease*, DOI 10.1007/978-1-4614-6191-3_34, © Springer Science+Business Media New York 2013

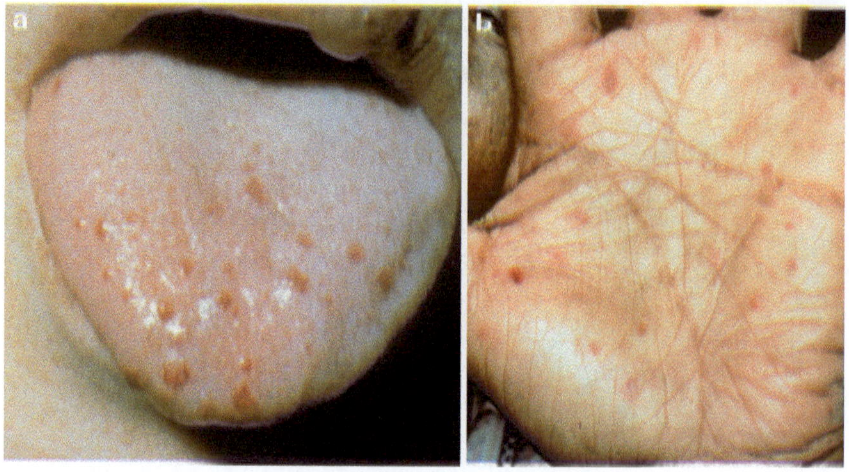

Fig. 34.1 Hereditary hemorrhagic telangiectasia. (**a**) Telangiectasia of the oral mucosa. (Image courtesy of Jeff Shornick, MD.) (**b**) Telangiectasia of the palms (Image courtesy of the New York University Image Collection)

References

1. Ward SK, Roenigk HH, Gordon KB. Dermatological manifestations of gastroenterological disorders. Gastroenterol Clin N Am. 1998;27:615–36.
2. Sharathkumar AA, Shapiro A. Hereditary haemorrhagic telangiectasia. Haemophilia. 2008;14:1269–80.
3. Shlovin CL. Hereditary haemorrhagic telangiectasia: pathophysiology, diagnosis, and treatment. Blood Rev. 2010;24:203–19.
4. Dupis-Girod S, Bailly S, Plauchu H. Hereditary hemorrhagic telangiectasia: from molecular biology to patient care. J Thromb Haemost. 2010;8:1447–56.

Peutz–Jeghers Syndrome: Gastrointestinal Features

35

Liam Zakko

Peutz–Jeghers syndrome is a genetic disease characterized by the development of benign hamartomatous polyps in the gastrointestinal (GI) tract and macules on the lips and oral mucosa. The incidence rate is not clear.

GI symptoms include [1, 2]:

- Bleeding, anemia, abdominal pain
- More severe: intussusception, obstruction, infarct

Clinical signs and findings should include [1, 2]:

- Characteristic "hamartoma" polyps found in the small bowel (90%) and colon (50%) (*see* Fig. 35.1) [3]
- Symptoms from polyps arise in 33% of patients by age 10 years and 50% by age 20 years
- Mucocutaneous hyperpigmented macules that develop in early childhood
- Extent of cutaneous lesions is not associated with the extent of polyps
- It is not clear if polyps increase risk of cancer or if instability in the mucosa does
- Patients with Peutz–Jeghers syndrome do appear to be at higher risk for esophageal, gastric, small bowel, colorectal, pancreatic, lung, prostate, breast, and female reproduction carcinomas

The pathogenesis is based on a genetic defect [1, 2]:

- Autosomal dominant mutation in the *STK11* gene at chromosome 19p13.3
- *STK11* is a tumor suppressor gene that acts during G1 cell-cycle and with p53 in apoptosis
- *STK11* is also involved in Wnt signaling for cell polarization and cell metabolism/energy homeostasis

The pathology includes [1, 2]:

- Polyps: frond-like epithelial component with cystic gland dilation extending into the submucosa/muscularis propria. Smooth muscles extend into the polyp fronds (*see* Fig. 35.2)
- Small bowel polyps may demonstrate "pseudoinvasion" but lack cytological atypia seen in truly invasive lesions

Diagnosis is made by considering the following [1, 2, 4]:

- Clinical diagnosis if ≤ one of the following true: (1) ≥ three histologically confirmed Peutz–Jeghers polyps; (2) any Peutz–Jeghers polyps in an individual with a family history of Peutz–Jeghers; (3) characteristic mucocutaneous pigmentation in an individual with a family history of Peutz–Jeghers; (4) any Peutz–Jeghers polyps in an individual with the characteristic mucocutaneous pigmentation
- Genetic testing reveals *STK11* mutation in 94% of those with a clinical diagnosis

The differential diagnosis should include [1–3]:

- Canada-Cronkite
- Carney complex
- Cowden's
- Laugier-Hunziker
- Leopard syndrome

There is no cure for this disease but treatment should include [1, 2]:

- Mainstay of GI treatment is surveillance
- Colonoscopy recommended at age eight, then every 3 years if significant polyps are found, and at age 18, and then every 3 years if no polyps, and then after age 50 every 1–2 years due to a rapidly increasing risk for colon cancer after this age
- Video capsule endoscopy starting at age 8 (or earlier if symptoms). If polyps are found, repeat every 3 years; if not, can repeat again at age 18 and then every 3 years
- No proven benefit to screening for other malignancies beyond routine health screening

L. Zakko (✉)
Yale Department of Internal Medicine, Yale New Haven Hospital, 20 Yale street, New Haven, CT 06510, USA
e-mail: liam.zakko@yale.edu

G.Y. Wu et al. (eds.), *Atlas of Dermatological Manifestations of Gastrointestinal Disease*,
DOI 10.1007/978-1-4614-6191-3_35, © Springer Science+Business Media New York 2013

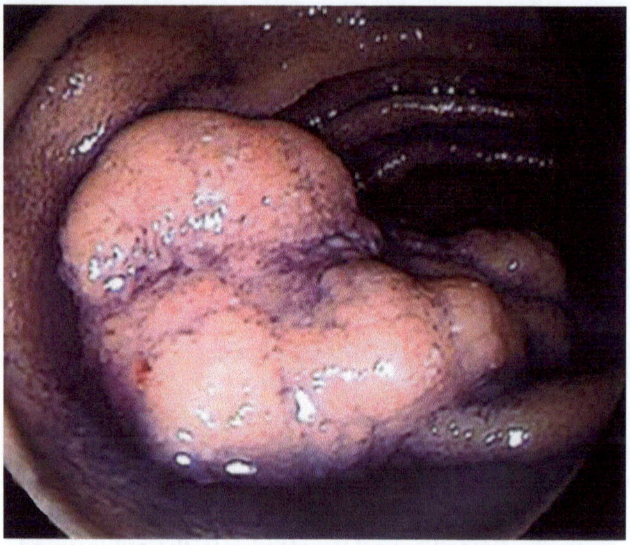

Fig. 35.1 An endoscopic view of a sessile polyp, stained with indigo carmine, 20 mm in diameter in the ileum of a patient with Peutz–Jeghers syndrome (Reprinted from Hosogi et al. [3]; with permission)

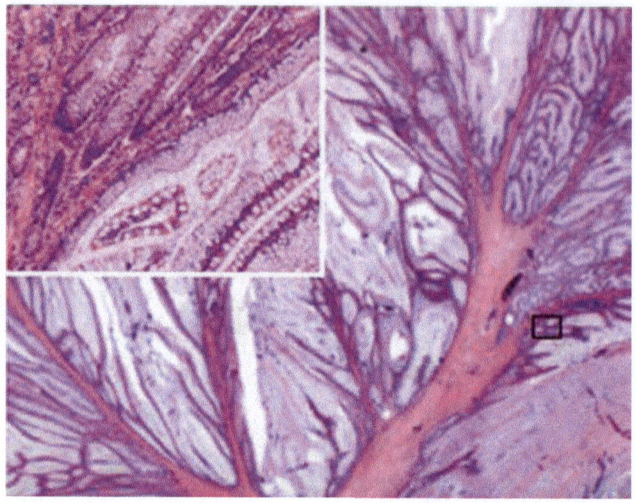

Fig. 35.2 A photomicrograph of a section of a resected ileal polyp showing a mixture of hyperplastic glandular epithelium with prominent branching of the thick smooth muscle bundles characteristic of Peutz–Jeghers polyps. *Inset* shows a higher magnification. Hematoxylin and eosin staining (Reprinted from Hosogi et al. [3]; with permission)

- Clean sweep polypectomy should be performed if patient has had severe symptoms from a polyp requiring surgical intervention

References

1. Begs AD, Latchford AR, Vasen HFA, et al. Peutz–Jeghers syndrome: a systematic review and recommendations for management. Gut. 2010;59:975–86.
2. Higham P, Alawi F, Stoopler ET. Medical management update: Peutz–Jeghers syndrome. Oral Surg Oral Med Oral Pathol Oral Radiol Endod. 2010;109:5–11.
3. Hosogi H, Nagayama S, Kawamura J, et al. Molecular insights into Peutz-Jeghers syndrome: two probands with a germline mutation of LKB1. J Gastroenterol. 2008;43:492–7.
4. Ward SK, Roenigk HH, Gordon KB. Dermatological manifestations of gastroenterological disorders. Gastroenterol Clin N Am. 1998;27:626–7.

Peutz–Jeghers Syndrome: Dermatological Features

36

Liam Zakko, Justin Finch, Marti J. Rothe, and Jane M. Grant-Kels

Clinical signs and features include:

- Mucocutaneous hyperpigmented macules that develop in early childhood [1]
- Melanocytic pigmented macules 1–5 mm in size ("freckles") on vermillion border of lips (see Fig. 36.1), buccal mucosa, labial mucosa, palate, tongue, distal fingers, toes, nostrils, perianal area, dorsal and volar hands and feet [2]
- Some will diminish with age but those around mouth in particular will persist [2, 3]
- Other significant clinical finding is numerous small intestine hamartomatous polyps
- Extent of cutaneous lesions is not associated with the extent of polyps [3]

Pathogenesis of this disease involves:

- Autosomal dominant mutation in the *STK11* gene at chromosome 19p13.3 [2]
- *STK11* is a tumor suppressor gene that acts during G1 cell cycle and with p53 in apoptosis [2]
- *STK11* is also involved in cell metabolism/energy homeostasis and in Wnt signaling for cell polarization [2]
- Cutaneous pigment may be caused by an inflammatory block to melanin migration from melanocyte to keratinocyte [2]

Histopathological features include:

- Increased melanin predominantly in basal cell layer [2]
- Slight melanocytic hyperplasia at the dermoepidermal junction [1]
- Melanophages in the superficial dermis [1]

The diagnosis is made using a combination of:

- Clinical diagnosis if greater than one of the following present [1, 2]:
  - ≥3 histologically confirmed Peutz-Jeghers gastrointestinal (GI) hamartomatous polyps
  - ≥1 Peutz-Jeghers GI polyps in an individual with a family history of Peutz-Jeghers
  - Characteristic mucocutaneous pigmentation in an individual with a family history of Peutz-Jeghers
  - ≥1 Peutz-Jeghers GI polyps in an individual with the characteristic mucocutaneous pigmentation
- Genetic testing reveals *STK11* mutation in 94% of those with a clinical diagnosis [2]

The differential diagnosis should include:

- Canada-Cronkite
- Carney complex
- Cowden's
- Laugier-Hunziker
- Leopard syndrome

Treatment options include:

- Cosmetic interactions for cutaneous lesions, often without good results [1]
- Q-switched ruby laser and filtered intense pulse light laser may offer best results [1]

L. Zakko (✉)
Yale Department of Internal Medicine, Yale New Haven Hospital, 20 York Street, New Haven, CT 06510, USA
e-mail: liam.zakko@yale.edu

J. Finch • M.J. Rothe • J.M. Grant-Kels
Department of Dermatology,
University of Connecticut Health Center,
21 South Road, Farmington, CT 06030, USA
e-mail: finch@uchc.edu; rothe@uchc.edu; grant@uchc.edu

G.Y. Wu et al. (eds.), *Atlas of Dermatological Manifestations of Gastrointestinal Disease*,
DOI 10.1007/978-1-4614-6191-3_36, © Springer Science+Business Media New York 2013

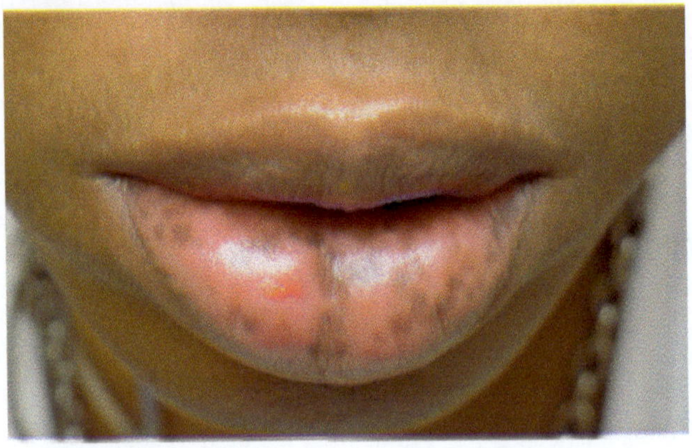

Fig. 36.1 Peutz-Jeghers syndrome. Melanotic macules of the oral mucosa

References

1. Higham P, Alawi F, Stoopler ET. Medical management update: Peutz-Jeghers syndrome. Oral Surg Oral Med Oral Pathol Oral Radiol Endod. 2010;109:5–11.
2. Begs AD, Latchford AR, Vasen HFA, et al. Peutz-Jeghers syndrome: a systematic review and recommendations for management. Gut. 2010;59:975–86.
3. Ward SK, Roenigk HH, Gordon KB. Dermatological manifestations of gastroenterological disorders. Gastroenterol Clin N Am. 1998;27:626–7.

Cowden's Syndrome: Gastrointestinal Features

37

Liam Zakko

Cowden's syndrome is a rare hereditary condition affecting about one per 200,000 people in the United States [1].

In terms of gastrointestinal (GI) symptoms, most individuals are asymptomatic and pathology is found incidentally when present, the most common GI signs and findings are [1]:

- Polyps, predominantly in the colon (see Fig. 37.1), but also in the stomach (see Fig. 37.2), small bowel, and esophagus (see Fig. 37.3) [2]
- Forty percent of individuals have GI findings, but this is likely an underestimate as asymptomatic individuals rarely get a full work up. Some studies have estimated up to 85% of individuals have GI involvement
- A possible pathognomonic lesion for the disease is glycogen acanthosis of the esophagus
- Syndrome also includes increased risk of breast/thyroid/endometrial cancer

From genetic studies, the pathogenesis of Cowden's syndrome is based on [3]:

- Autosomal dominant disease with mutation of *PTEN* gene on chromosome 10q23.3
- *PTEN* codes for a tumor suppressor gene that regulates the P13K/AKT/mTDR pathway
- After a second hit to the function, *PTEN* gene protein in cells undergo increased phosphorylation leading to changes in the cell cycle, metabolism, translation, growth, migration, invasion, angiogenesis, and apoptosis

The characteristic pathologic features are benign but the condition is associated with the development of malignancies [3]:

- Glycogen acanthosis of the esophagus: epidermal hyperplasia with increased glycogen deposits [3]
- Polyps: mostly hamartomatous but can also have hyperplastic, inflammatory, juvenile, leiomyomatous, lipomatous, lymphoid, and neuromatous

To make a diagnosis, certain criteria need be fulfilled [4, 5]:

- Three-generation family history of malignancy can be helpful
- Clinical criteria: any pathognomonic lesions; 2+ major lesions, with one being macrocephaly; 1+ major and 3+ minor, or 4+ minor
- Pathognomonic lesions: Lhermitte-Duclos disease (LDD), a cerebellar tumor; 6+ facial papules with 3+ being trichilemmomas; cutaneous facial papules with oral mucosal papillomatous lesions; oral mucosal papillomatosis and acral keratosis; 6+ palmoplantar keratosis
- Major criteria: breast carcinoma; nonmedullary thyroid carcinoma; endometrial carcinoma; macrocephaly
- Minor criteria: thyroid lesions, mental retardation, GI hamartomas, fibrocystic disease of the breast, lipomas, fibromas, genitourinary (GU) tumors (especially renal cell carcinoma), GU structural abnormalities, uterine fibroids
- If a direct relative has Cowden's syndrome, then a diagnosis can be made with: 1+ major criteria, 2+ minor criteria, history of Bannayan-Riley-Ruvalcaba syndrome
- More than 80% of patients will have a detectable *PTEN* mutation

Other conditions associated with the development of GI polyps should be considered in the differential diagnosis [4, 5]:

- Juvenile polyposis syndrome
- Viral warts
- Darier's disease
- Tuberous sclerosis
- Neurofibromatosis

L. Zakko (✉)
Yale Department of Internal Medicine, Yale New Haven Hospital, 20 York Street, New Haven, CT 06510, USA
e-mail: liam.zakko@yale.edu

G.Y. Wu et al. (eds.), *Atlas of Dermatological Manifestations of Gastrointestinal Disease*,
DOI 10.1007/978-1-4614-6191-3_37, © Springer Science+Business Media New York 2013

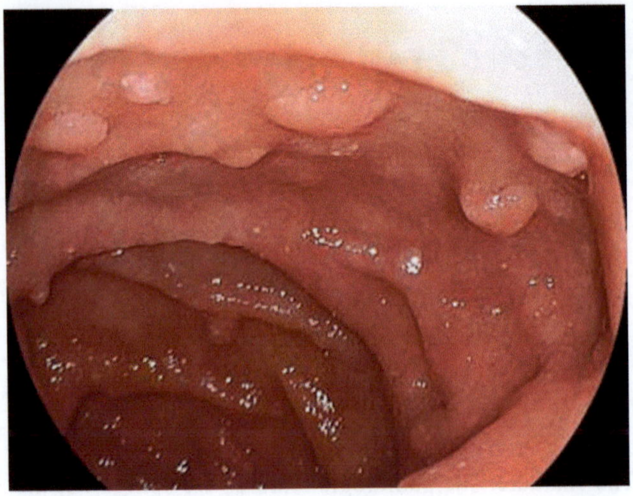

Fig. 37.1 An endoscopic view of hamartomatous polyps of the colon (Reprinted from Coriat et al. [2]; with permission)

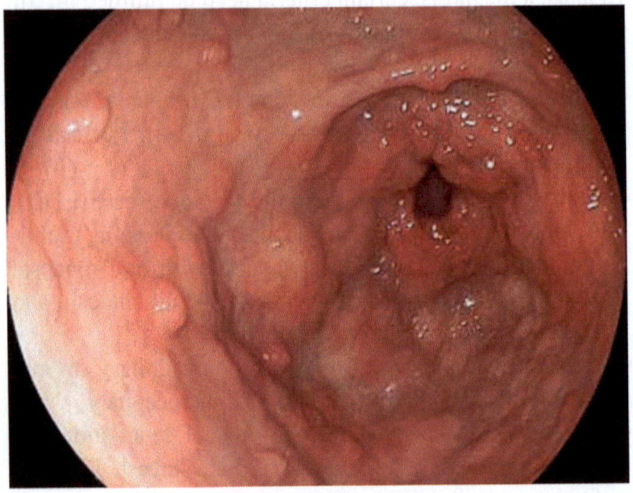

Fig. 37.2 An endoscopic view of hamartomatous polyps of the stomach (Reprinted from Coriat et al. [2]; with permission)

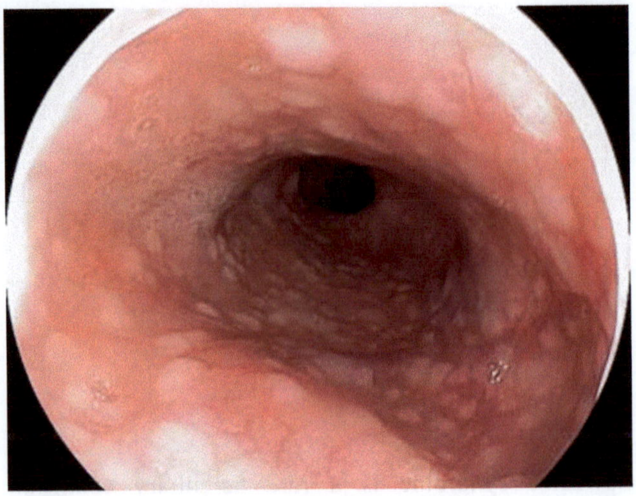

Fig. 37.3 An endoscopic view of acanthosis of the esophagus, scattered white papules on the esophageal mucosa (Reprinted from Coriat et al. [2]; with permission)

There is no treatment for the condition:

- Screening for malignancy is the most important treatment
- GI lesions are noteworthy for helping make the diagnosis so that appropriate screening can occur

References

1. Farooq A, Walker LJ, Bowling J, Audisio RA. Cowden syndrome. Cancer Treat Rev. 2010;36:577–83.
2. Coriat R, Mozer M, Caux F, et al. Endoscopic findings in Cowden syndrome. Endoscopy. 2011;43:723–6.
3. McGarrity TJ, Baker MJW, Ruggerio FM, et al. GI polyposis and glycogenic acanthosis of the esophagus associated with PTEN mutation positive Cowden syndrome in absence of cutaneous manifestations. Am J Gastroenterol. 2003;98:1429–34.
4. Pilarski R. Cowden syndrome: a critical review of the literature. J Genet Counsel. 2009;18:13–27.
5. Ward SK, Roenigk HH, Gordon KB. Dermatological manifestations of gastroenterological disorders. Gastroenterol Clin N Am. 1998;27:628–9.

38 Cowden's Syndrome: Dermatological Features

Liam Zakko, Justin Finch, Marti J. Rothe, and Jane M. Grant-Kels

The skin manifestations of Cowden's syndrome include three common lesions (see Fig. 38.1) [1, 2]:

1. Facial trichilemmomas: 1–5 mm diameter, flesh-colored, flat-topped or elongated verrucous papules in periorofacial and centrofacial distribution
2. Papillomatous papules: small, smooth, flesh-colored papules on labial, gingival, palatal surfaces leading to a cobblestone appearance; also occur on face and pressure-points (palmar/plantar surfaces) where they tend to be more translucent, hard papules
3. Acral keratoses: flesh-colored, flat-topped, rough papules on the dorsum of the hands or feet that resemble common warts; can be pits if small or microplaques/papules if larger
   - Less common skin manifestations include lipomas, hemangiomas (associated with related Bannayan-Riley-Ruvalcaba syndrome), scrotal tongue, neuromas [2]
   - Syndrome also includes increased risk of breast/thyroid/endometrial cancer and gastrointestinal (GI) hamartomatous polyps [1–4]

The pathogenesis of this genetic disease involves:

- Autosomal dominant disease with mutation of *PTEN* gene that codes for a tumor-suppressor gene that regulates the P13K/AKT/mTOR pathway [3, 4]
- Mutations of the *PTEN* gene causes increased phosphorylation leading to changes in the cell cycle, metabolism, translation, growth, migration, invasion, angiogenesis, and apoptosis [4]

The histopathological features of Cowden's syndrome include [2]:

- Trichilemmomas: benign hamartomatous lesions of the outer root sheath of hair follicles [3]; demonstrates papillated and endophytic epithelial hyperplasia with clear cell differentiation and overlying hyperkeratosis (see Fig. 38.2)
- Acral keratosis: discrete foci of epidermal hyperplasia with orthokeratosis [1]
- Papillomatous papules: papillomatous epidermal hyperplasia with hyperkeratosis or dermal fibromas [1]

Because there are several similar syndromes, it has been recommended that the diagnosis be made using a combination of [1, 3, 4]:

- Three-generation family history of malignancy
- Clinical criteria:
  - Pathognomonic mucocutaneous lesions; or
    - ≥2 major criteria, with one being macrocephaly or adult Lhermitte-Duclos disease (LDD); or
    - 1 major and ≥3 minor; or
    - ≥4 minor
- Pathognomonic lesions:
  - LDD: a dysplastic gangliocytoma of the cerebellum
  - Skin changes including
    - o ≥6 facial papules with ≥3 being trichilemmomas, or
    - o Cutaneous facial papules with oral mucosal papillomatous lesions, or
    - o Oral mucosal papillomatosis and acral keratosis, or
    - o ≥6 palmoplantar keratosis
- Major criteria: breast carcinoma; nonmedullary thyroid carcinoma; endometrial carcinoma; macrocephaly; LDD

L. Zakko (✉)
Yale Department of Internal Medicine, Yale New Haven Hospital, 20 York Street, New Haven, CT 06510, USA
e-mail: liam.zakko@yale.edu

J. Finch • M.J. Rothe • J.M. Grant-Kels
Department of Dermatology, University of Connecticut Health Center, 21 South Road, Farmington, CT 06030, USA
e-mail: finch@uchc.edu; rothe@uchc.edu; grant@uchc.edu

G.Y. Wu et al. (eds.), *Atlas of Dermatological Manifestations of Gastrointestinal Disease*, DOI 10.1007/978-1-4614-6191-3_38, © Springer Science+Business Media New York 2013

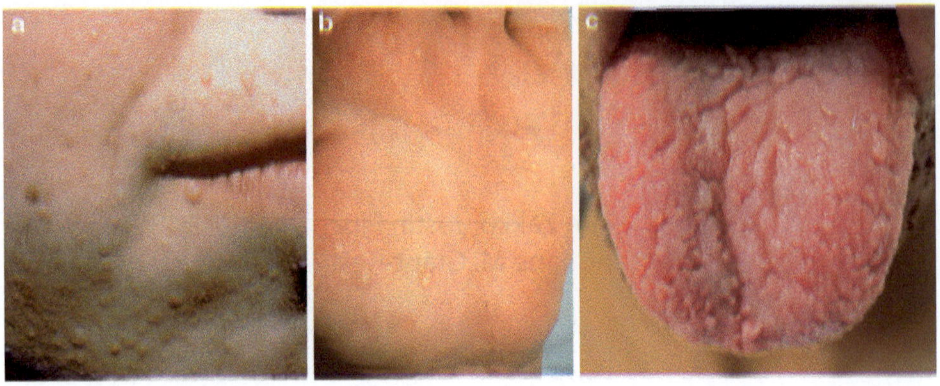

Fig. 38.1 (**a**) Skin-colored warty facial papules (Image courtesy of Yale Residency Collection). (**b**) Acral keratoses. (**c**) Cobblestone tongue

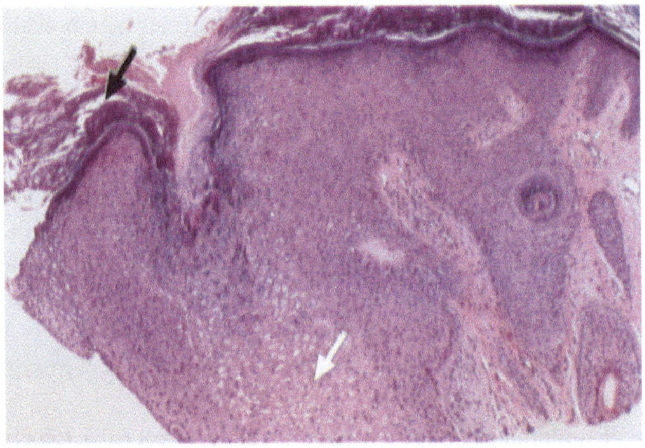

Fig. 38.2 Trichilemmoma, displaying downward lobular growth of epidermis, comprising clear glycogen-filled keratinocytes (*white arrow*) with overlying hyperkeratosis (*black arrow*) (20×). Hematoxylin and eosin

- Minor criteria: thyroid lesions, mental retardation, GI hamartomas, fibrocystic disease of the breast, lipomas, fibromas, genitourinary (GU) tumors (especially renal cell carcinoma), GU structural abnormalities, uterine fibroids
- If a direct relative has Cowden's syndrome, make diagnosis with: ≥1 major criteria, ≥2 minor criteria, history of Bannayan-Riley-Ruvalcaba Syndrome
- >80% of patients will have a detectable *PTEN* mutation

The differential diagnosis should include other entities associated with polyposis:

- Juvenile polyposis syndrome
- Viral warts
- Darier's disease
- Tuberous sclerosis
- Neurofibromatosis

Treatment options include a variety of ablative measures:

- Cutaneous lesions can be treated with carbon dioxide laser ablation, surgical excision, electrosurgery, cryotherapy, dermabrasion, or topical 5-fluorouracil for cosmetic reasons [1]
- Rapamycin may have a role in preventing progression of lesions [1]
- Screening for malignancy is the most important treatment [1, 3, 4]

References

1. Farooq A, Walker LJ, Bowling J, Audisio RA. Cowden syndrome. Cancer Treat Rev. 2010;36:577–83.
2. Ward SK, Roenigk HH, Gordon KB. Dermatological manifestations of gastroenterological disorders. Gastroenterol Clin N Am. 1998;27:628–9.
3. Jornayvaz FR, Philippe J. Mucocutaneous papillomatous papules in Cowden's syndrome. Clin Exp Dermatol. 2007;33:151–3.
4. Pilarski R. Cowden syndrome: a critical review of the literature. J Genet Counsel. 2009;18:13–27.

Behçet's Syndrome: Gastrointestinal Features

39

Liam Zakko

Behçet's syndrome causes gastrointestinal (GI) manifestations in 3–26% of patients and is more common in patients from Asia than from the Middle East or the Mediterranean region [1].

GI features include:

- Anorexia, diarrhea, abdominal pain, bloody stools, abdominal masses, small bowel obstructive symptoms
- More severe: intestinal stenosis, perforation, persistent bleeding

Clinical signs and findings in Behçet's Syndrome include [2]:

- Punched-out ulcers are the most common GI finding, found most often in the ileum, then the cecum (*see* Fig. 39.1a) [3], then the rest of colon (*see* Fig. 39.1b) [4]; ileocecal ulcers have a tendency to perforate
- Hallmark is recurrent aphthous ulcers; also skin findings of genital ulcers, papulopustular acne-like rash, nodular rashes (erythema nodosum-like and superficial thrombosis)
- Also manifestations in the eyes, musculoskeletal system, joints, pulmonary vessels, heart, and central nervous system

The mechanism of pathogenesis of this condition are not well understood, but there is evidence for an immune-mediated vasculitis [1, 2]:

- Vasculitis of all-sized vessels, although some lesions appear to lack vasculitis (especially papulopustular rash)
- Associated with human leukocyte antigen (HLA)-B51 and with populations along the Old Silk Road
- Immune complex-mediated reaction in the endothelium is suggested by some pathology
- Possible role of streptococci or herpes simplex virus 1 with protein homolog leading to autoimmune reaction

The pathological features are not specific and include [1, 2]:

- Ulcers with inflammatory cell infiltrate consisting of neutrophils, lymphocytes, plasma cells, and eosinophils (*see* Fig. 39.2)
- Blood vessels with fibrinoid necrosis and perivascular infiltrates

The diagnosis is made by endoscopic and pathologic findings [1, 2]:

- Complete blood count may show increased white blood count; C-reactive protein and erythrocyte sedimentation rate may be slightly elevated
- May have increased serum immunoglobulins and complement
- Negative rheumatoid factor/antineutrophil cytoplasmic antibodies /antinuclear antibodies/anti-cardiolipin
- Colonoscopy/endoscopy to identify and biopsy gastrointestinal lesions
- Clinical diagnosis (91% sensitive; 96% specific): recurrent oral ulceration (3 times/12 months) with two or more of (1) recurrent genital ulcers; (2) eye lesions; (3) skin lesions; (4) pathergy

The differential diagnosis should include [1, 2]:

- Reactive arthritis/seronegative arthropathy/inflammatory arthropathy
- Inflammatory bowel disease/sarcoidosis/multiple sclerosis
- Venereal disease/HIV/enteroviruses
- Steven Johnson syndrome
- Vogt-Koyanagi-Harada syndrome
- Other vasculitides

There is no cure for this condition but treatment can alleviate symptoms [1, 2]:

- Treatment similar to Crohn's disease with 5-aminosalicylic acid, 6-mercaptopurine, corticosteroids, methotrexate, azathioprine, thalidomide, interferon-α, tumor necrosis factor-α inhibitors [3].

L. Zakko (✉)
Yale Department of Internal Medicine, Yale New Haven Hospital, 20 York Street, New Haven, CT 06510, USA
e-mail: liam.zakko@yale.edu

G.Y. Wu et al. (eds.), *Atlas of Dermatological Manifestations of Gastrointestinal Disease*, DOI 10.1007/978-1-4614-6191-3_39, © Springer Science+Business Media New York 2013

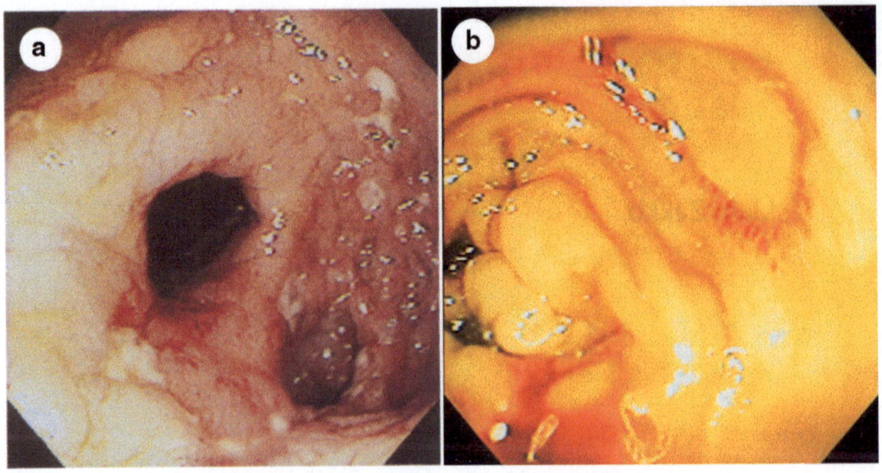

Fig. 39.1 (**a**) An endoscopic view of an ulcer in Behçet's syndrome involving the cecum (Reprinted with permission from Hassard et al. [3]). (**b**) An endoscopic view of a deep punched-out ulcer due to Behçet's syndrome in the transverse colon (Reprinted with permission from Kram et al. [4])

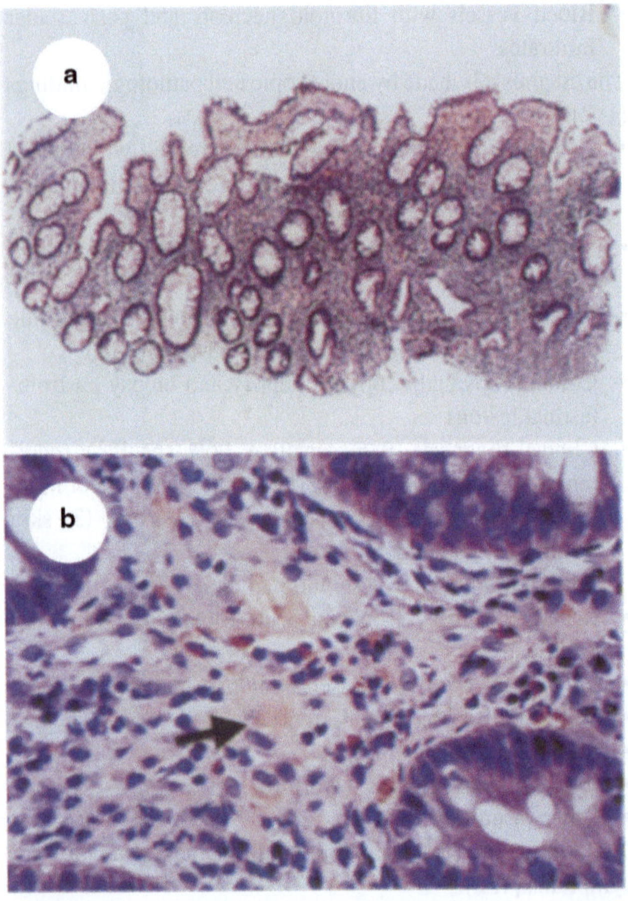

Fig. 39.2 (**a**) Low-power photomicrograph of a colonic biopsy showing distorted crypt architecture and mixed inflammatory infiltrate in Behçet's syndrome involving the colon (Reprinted with permission from Hassard et al. [3]). (**b**) High-power photomicrograph of a colonic biopsy showing an inflammatory infiltrate consisting of neutrophils, lymphocytes, and eosinophils. *Arrow* indicates fibrinoid necrosis and perivascular infiltrates (Reprinted with permission from Hassard et al. [3])

References

1. Mendes D, Correia M, Barbedo M, et al. Behçets disease: a contemporary review. J Autoimmunity. 2009;32:178–88.
2. Yaziei Y, Yurdakul S, Yaziei H. Behçets syndrome. Curr Rheumatol Rep. 2010;12:429–35.
3. Hassard PV, Binder SW, Nelson V, Vasiliauskas EA. Anti-tumor necrosis factor monoclonal antibody therapy for gastrointestinal Behçet's disease: a case report. Gastroenterology. 2001;120:995–9.
4. Kram MT, May LD, Goodman S, et al. Behçet's ileocolitis: successful treatment with tumor necrosis factor-alpha antibody (infliximab) therapy: report of a case. Dis Colon Rectum. 2003;46:118–21.

40 Behçet's Syndrome: Dermatological Features

Liam Zakko, Justin Finch, Marti J. Rothe, and Jane M. Grant-Kels

Clinical signs and features include:

- Hallmark is recurrent aphthous ulcers: three types: minor (<10 mm) (see Fig. 40.1), major (>10 mm; more painful and more likely to scar), herpetiform [1]
- Oral ulcers are usually the earliest manifestation of disease and may be the only symptom for many years
- The disease usually first presents during the third decade of life and affects males and females equally [2]
- Genital ulcers occur in 57–93% of patients (see Fig. 40.1) and subside after weeks and recur in days to months [1]
- Ulcers affect the scrotum rather than the glans penis and the labia minora and majora [2]
- Large genital ulcers may scar while small ulcers usually do not
- Extragenital cutaneous ulcerations occur in 3% of patients, recur, and resemble aphthous ulcers [1]
- Nodular eruptions are present in 50%of patients and manifest as erythema nodosum (EN)-like and superficial thrombosis [2]
- Superficial thrombosis differs from the EN-like rash in that it appears to move from day to day along the vein; it is also associated with deep vein thrombosis
- Pathergy is also commonly present (papulopustular formation 24–48 h after a needle is inserted into the dermis)
- Also there maybe manifestations in the eyes, musculoskeletal system, joints, pulmonary vessels, heart, central nervous system, and gastrointestinal tract

Pathogenesis of this disease involves:

- Vasculitis of all sized vessels, although some lesions appear to lack vasculitis (especially papulopustular rash)
- Associated with human leukocyte antigen (HLA)-B51 and with populations along the Old Silk Road in the Middle East and Central Asia
- Immune complex-mediated reaction in the endothelium is suggested by some pathology
- Possible role of streptococci or herpes simplex virus-1 with protein homolog leading to autoimmune reaction
- T helper-17 and interleukin-17 pathways are active [3]

Histopathological features include:

- Early skin lesions: leukocytoclastic vasculitis or neutrophilic vascular reaction ± fibrinoid necrosis/thrombosis of postcapillary venules
- Older lesions: lymphocytic vasculitis
- Aphthous lesions demonstrate exuberant granulation tissue (see Fig. 40.2)
- Papulopustular rash: resembles acne; need to look for vasculitis
- Erythema nodosum (EN)-like lesions have vasculitis/vascular reaction unlike classic EN plus evidence of septal panniculitis
- Pathergy-induced lesions demonstrate leukocytoclastic vasculitis

The diagnosis is made using a combination of:

- Complete blood count may show increased white blood count; C-reactive protein and erythrocyte sedimentation rate may be slightly elevated
- May have increased serum immunoglobulin and complement
- Negative rheumatoid factor/antineutrophil cytoplasmic antibodies/antinuclear antibodies/anti-cardiolipin

L. Zakko (✉)
Yale Department of Internal Medicine, Yale New Haven Hospital, 20 York Street, New Haven, CT 06510, USA
e-mail: liam.zakko@yale.edu

J. Finch • M.J. Rothe • J.M. Grant-Kels
Department of Dermatology, University of Connecticut Health Center, 21 South Road, Farmington, CT 06030, USA
e-mail: finch@uchc.edu; rothe@uchc.edu; grant@uchc.edu

G.Y. Wu et al. (eds.), *Atlas of Dermatological Manifestations of Gastrointestinal Disease*, DOI 10.1007/978-1-4614-6191-3_40, © Springer Science+Business Media New York 2013

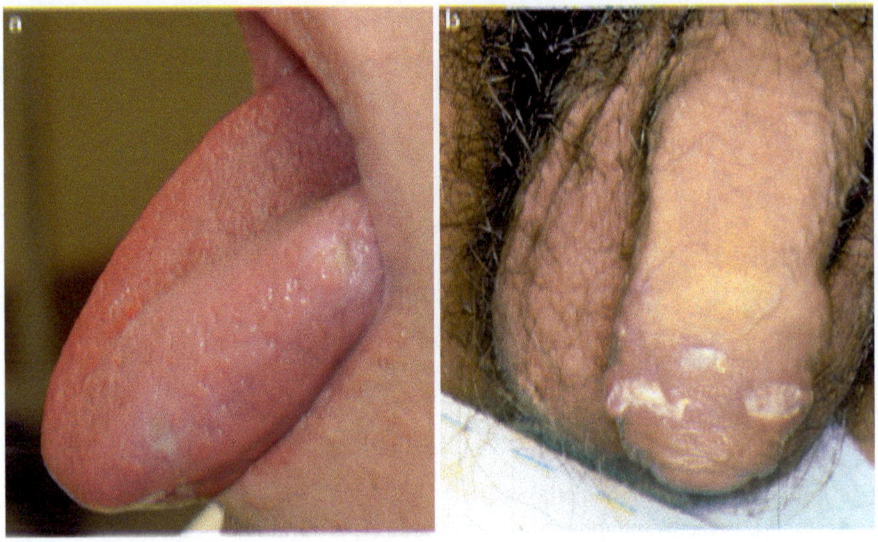

Fig. 40.1 Behçet's syndrome. (**a**) Aphthous ulcer. (**b**) Genital ulcer

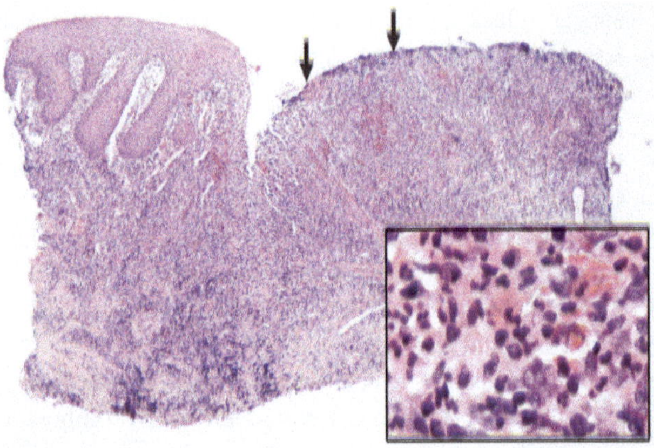

Fig. 40.2 A photomicrograph of a skin biopsy of an aphthous ulcer. Mucosal ulceration (*black arrows*) with a predominantly neutrophilic infiltrate visible on high power. Hematoxylin and eosin stain (*white arrow*; *inset*) (40×; *inset* 400×)

- Clinical diagnosis (91% sensitive; 96% specific): recurrent oral ulceration (at least three episodes in a single year) with two or more of (1) recurrent genital ulcers; (2) eye lesions; (3) skin lesions; (4) pathergy [4]

Treatment options include [5]:

- Topical antimicrobial agents, sucralfate, corticosteroids, pimecrolimus or tacrolimus
- Moderate genital ulcers/nodular lesions: systemic corticosteroids in combination with colchicine ± benzathine penicillin
- Severe disease: azathioprine, thalidomide (but can exacerbate nodular disease), dapsone, pentoxifylline, methotrexate, cyclosporine, interferon-α, tumor necrosis factor-α inhibitors, rituximab

The differential diagnosis should include:

- Reactive arthritis/seronegative arthropathy/inflammatory arthropathy
- Inflammatory bladder disease/sarcoidosis/multiple sclerosis
- Venereal disease/HIV/enteroviruses
- Herpes simplex
- Stevens Johnson syndrome
- Vogt-Koyanagi-Harada syndrome
- Other vasculitis

References

1. Mendes D, Correia M, Barbedo M, et al. Behçets disease: a contemporary review. J Autoimmun. 2009;32:178–88.
2. Yazici Y, Yurdakul S, Yazici H. Behçet's syndrome. Curr Rheumatol Rep. 2010;12:429–35.
3. Ekinci NS, Alpsoy E, Karakas AA, et al. IL-17A has an important role in the acute attacks of Behcet's disease. J Invest Dermatol. 2010;130:2136–8.
4. O'Neill TW, Rigby AS, Silman AJ, et al. Validation of the international study group criteria for Behcet's disease. Br J Rheumatol. 1994;33:115–7.
5. Alpsoy E. New evidence-based treatment approach in Behçet's disease. Patholog Res Int. 2012;2012:11, 871019.

Gardner's Syndrome: Gastrointestinal Features

41

Liam Zakko

Gardner's syndrome is genetic disease characterized by adenomatous polyps of the gastrointestinal (GI) tract associated with tumors outside of the colon. Failure to remove the colon results in a very high risk of cancer.

- GI symptoms include [1]:
- Rectal bleeding, anemia
- Change in bowel habits (constipation or diarrhea)
- Abdominal pain
- Palpable abdominal masses
- Weight loss

Clinical signs and findings include [1]:

- Variant of familial adenomatous polyposis
- Classically, hundreds to thousands of polyps throughout the colon. Polyps begin to develop as intramucosal nodules in early childhood in the rectosigmoid colon. By adolescence, they have spread throughout the colon. Fifty percent develop adenomas by age 15, 95% by age 35
- 70% to 80% of tumors occur on the left side of the colon
- 26% percent to 61% develop gastric fundic polyps and 25% show dysplasia, a few of which progress to cancer
- 90% develop adenomatous polyps in the duodenum (see Figs. 41.1, 41.2 and 41.3) and periampullary region by the age of 70. These can progress to bowel cancer, which is the third leading cause of death in these patients
- Polyps in the gastrointestinal tract, skull/mandible osteomas, dental abnormalities (multiple unerupted teeth), desmoids tumors, and congenital hypertrophy of the retinal epithelium bilaterally
- Skin manifestations include epidermoid cysts, lipomas, sebaceous cysts, and fibromas which may be the first clinical signs

L. Zakko (✉)
Yale Department of Internal Medicine, Yale New Haven Hospital, 20 York Street, New Haven, CT 06510, USA
e-mail: liam.zakko@yale.edu

Pathogenesis is due to [2]:

- Mutation of *APC* gene on chromosome 5q21
- *APC* codes for a tumor suppressor protein that regulates β-catenin, thus playing a role in Wnt signaling. Unregulated β-catenin leads to differences in cell proliferation, migration, differentiation, and apoptosis

The pathology associated with the disease is [1, 3]:

- Adenomatous polyps are essential to differentiating the disorder from other polyposis syndromes

The diagnosis is made by considering a combination of factors [1, 3]:

- Family history of colon cancer in 70–75% of patients
- Physical examination revealing extracolonic manifestations
- GI symptoms of pain and occult/chronic lower GI bleeding
- If above are present, then confirm with colonoscopy and genetic testing
- Classify duodenal lesions by Spigelman criteria

The differential diagnosis of Gardner's syndrome should include [1–4]:

- Peutz-Jeghers syndrome
- Familial juvenile polyposis
- Lynch syndrome
- Hereditary mixed polyposis syndrome
- Lymphoid disease
- Turcot's syndrome

Treatment is not curative but should include [1–4]:

- Proctocolectomy with an ileal pouch—anal anastomosis—in children can defer with screening to adulthood; avoid subtotal colectomy because of colorectal cancer risk in remaining rectal tissue; if subtotal colectomy is obtained, should get screening of remaining rectal mucosa every 6 months
- Duodenal adenomatosis is challenging as the number of lesions leads to a high risk of scarring and structuring of the ampulla. Surgical options should be considered though appropriate timing and technique are unclear. Definite consideration should be made in patients with

G.Y. Wu et al. (eds.), *Atlas of Dermatological Manifestations of Gastrointestinal Disease*,
DOI 10.1007/978-1-4614-6191-3_41, © Springer Science+Business Media New York 2013

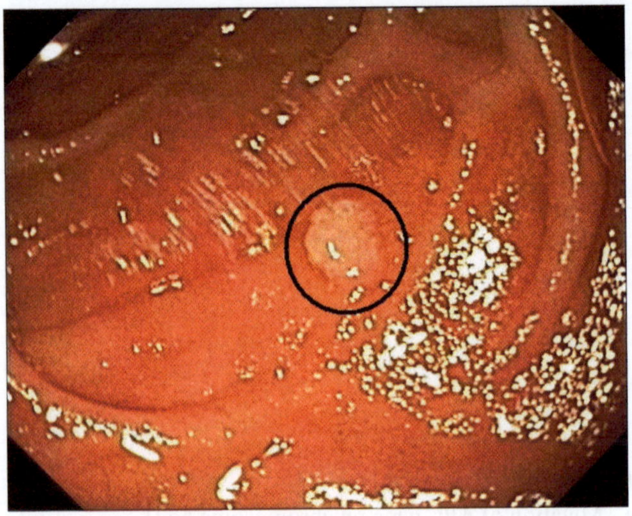

Fig. 41.1 Endoscopic view of a duodenal polyp in a patient with Gardner's syndrome. A small polyp is circled (Image courtesy of Connecticut Gastroenterology Institute)

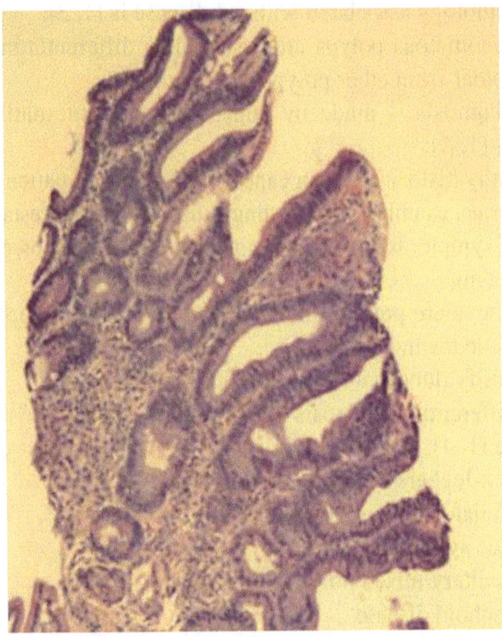

Fig. 41.2 Duodenal adenoma. A photomicrograph of the biopsy of a polyp from a patient with Gardner's syndrome. Dysplastic features of crowded, hyperchromatic nuclei of a tubular adenoma can be appreciated. Hematoxylin and eosin stain; low-power magnification (Image courtesy of Connecticut Gastroenterology Institute)

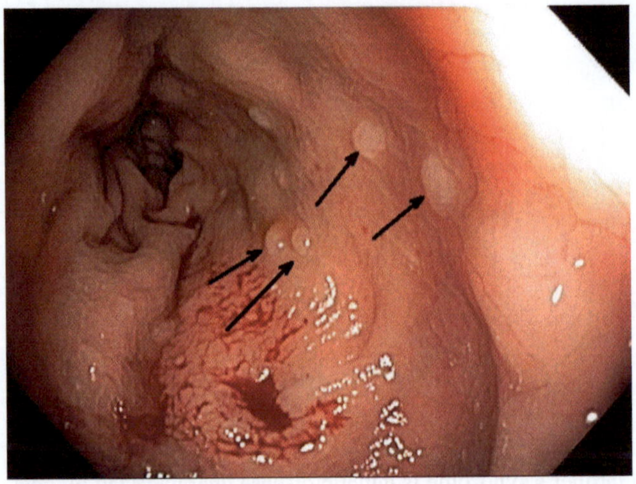

Fig. 41.3 Typical endoscopic view of multiple duodenal polyps (*arrows*), one of which has been biopsied where there is a small amount of hemorrhage (Image courtesy of Connecticut Gastroenterology Institute)

Spigelman stage III and IV lesions or a family history of duodenal cancer

References

1. Galiatsatos P, Foulkes WD. Familial adenomatous polyposis. Am J Gastroenterol. 2006;101:385–98.
2. García EBG, Knoers NVAM. Gardner's syndrome (familial adenomatous polyposis): a cilia related disorder. Lancet Oncol. 2009;10:727–35.
3. Half E, Bercovich D, Rozen P. Familial adenomatous polyposis. Orphanet J Rare Dis. 2009;4:1–23.
4. Ward SK, Roenigk HH, Gordon KB. Dermatological manifestations of gastroenterological disorders. Gastroenterol Clin N Am. 1998;27:615–36.

Gardner Syndrome: Dermatological Features

42

Liam Zakko, Justin Finch, Marti J. Rothe, and Jane M. Grant-Kels

Clinical signs and features include:

- Variant of familial adenomatous polyposis
- Clinically presents with polyps in the gastrointestinal tract (GI), skull/mandible osteomas, dental abnormalities (multiple impacted or unerupted teeth), fibromas, desmoid tumors, and congenital hypertrophy of the retinal epithelium bilaterally [1]
- First sign is often epidermoid cysts, which can present about 10 years before the polyps (see Fig. 42.1) [2]
- Cysts appear just before puberty on the face, extremities, and scalp
- Cysts are usually asymptomatic but can present with pruritus, inflammation, and rupture
- Other skin manifestations include lipomas and leiomyomas
- Colonic polyps are associated with increased risk of colon cancer

Pathogenesis of this disease involves a genetic mutation:

- Autosomal dominant; usually one parent involved
- Mutation of *APC* (adenomatous polyposis coli) gene on chromosome 5q21
- *APC* codes for a tumor suppressor protein that regulates β-catenin, thus playing a role in Wnt signaling [2]
- Cutaneous manifestations may be due to increased β-catenin causing cilia dysfunction leading to cyst formation [3]

Histopathological features include:

- Epidermoid cyst is a cyst lined by squamous epithelium with a granular layer and filled with lamellated keratinous material (see Fig. 42.2)
- Dermoid cyst can also show hair follicles and sebaceous glands as well as eccrine and/or apocrine glands in the wall of the cyst and fragments of hairs within the contents of the cyst
- Pilomatricoma (see Fig. 42.3) is a benign follicular tumor composed of well-circumscribed islands of basophilic cells and shadow cells (anucleate epithelial cells) within the lower dermis; granulomatous inflammation and focal calcification are often identified

The diagnosis is made using a combination of:

- Family history of colon cancer in 70–75% of patients
- Physical examination revealing extracolonic manifestations
- GI symptoms of pain and occult/chronic lower GI bleeding
- If above, then confirm with colonoscopy and genetic testing

The differential diagnosis should include:

- Peutz-Jeghers syndrome
- Familial juvenile polyposis
- Lynch syndrome
- Hereditary mixed polyposis syndrome
- Lymphoid disease
- Turcot syndrome

Treatment options include [4]:

- Epidermoid cysts, if not infected, can be treated with intralesional triamcinolone injections

L. Zakko (✉)
Yale Department of Internal Medicine, Yale New Haven Hospital, 20 York Street, New Haven, CT 06510, USA
e-mail: liam.zakko@yale.edu

J. Finch • M.J. Rothe • J.M. Grant-Kels
Department of Dermatology, University of Connecticut Health Center, 21 South Road, Farmington, CT 06030, USA
e-mail: finch@uchc.edu; rothe@uchc.edu; grant@uchc.edu

G.Y. Wu et al. (eds.), *Atlas of Dermatological Manifestations of Gastrointestinal Disease*, DOI 10.1007/978-1-4614-6191-3_42, © Springer Science+Business Media New York 2013

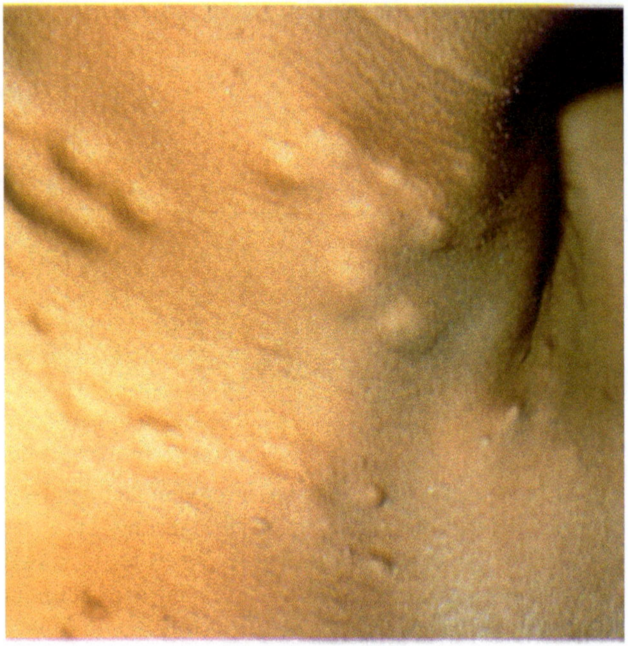

Fig. 42.1 Gardner syndrome. Multiple epidermal inclusion cysts (Image courtesy of Yale Residency Collection)

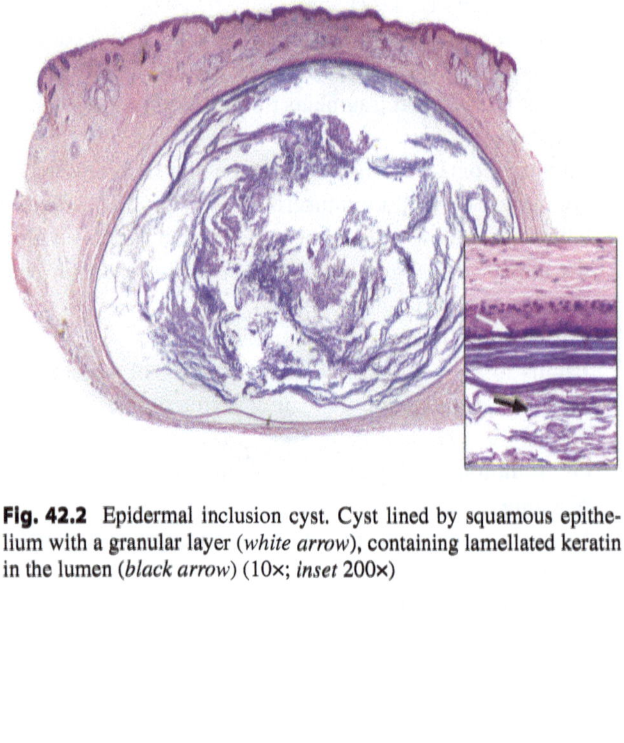

Fig. 42.2 Epidermal inclusion cyst. Cyst lined by squamous epithelium with a granular layer (*white arrow*), containing lamellated keratin in the lumen (*black arrow*) (10×; *inset* 200×)

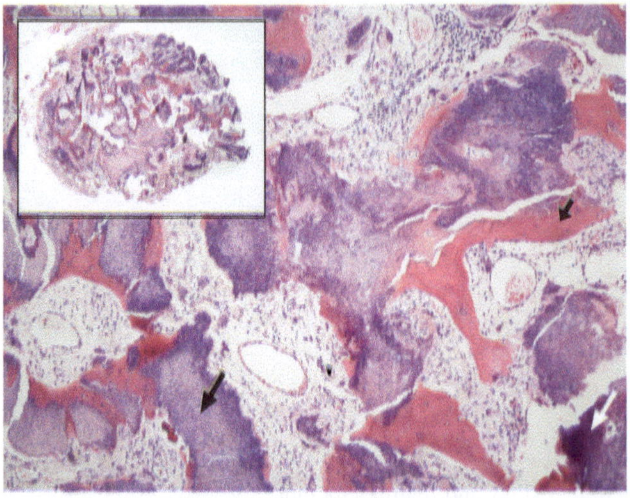

Fig. 42.3 Pilomatricoma. Circumscribed nodule (*inset*, 20×) comprising islands of shadow cells devoid of nuclei (*long black arrow*), calcification (*white arrow*), keratinous debris, and shards of ossification (*short black arrow*) (200×)

- Infected epidermoid cysts can be treated with surgical incision and drainage followed by antistaphylococcal antibiotics

References

1. Juhn E, Khachemoune A. Gardner syndrome: skin manifestations, differential diagnosis, and management. Am J Clin Dermatol. 2010;11:117–22.
2. Ward SK, Roenigk HH, Gordon KB. Dermatological manifestations of gastroenterological disorders. Gastroenterol Clin N Am. 1998;27:615–36.
3. Half E, Bercovich D, Rozen P. Familial adenomatous polyposis. Orphanet J Rare Dis. 2009;4:1–23.
4. Gomez-García EB, Knoers NVA. Gardner's syndrome (familial adenomatous polyposis): a cilia related disorder. Lancet Oncol. 2009;10:727–35.

Klippel–Trenaunay–Weber Syndrome: Gastrointestinal Features

43

Michael Tadros

Klippel–Trenaunay–Weber syndrome is a congenital condition characterized by a failure of blood or lymph vessels to form properly. There is ongoing discussion about the classification of this disease as it has clinical overlap with several other diseases.

Gastrointestinal (GI) symptoms include [1, 2]:

- Hematochezia: the most common GI complaint
- Occult to severe and fatal bleeding; recurrent episodes
- Visceral organ involvement can occur
- Splenic hemangioma can spontaneously rupture, leading to internal bleeding

GI clinical signs and findings are [1, 2, 4]:

- Klippel–Trenaunay–Weber syndrome consists of a triad of
  - Varicose veins
  - Port-wine stain
  - Bony and soft tissue hypertrophy all tissues of the involved limb
- Parkes–Weber syndrome variant includes arteriovenous fistulas
- GI involvement up to 20% of patients (see Fig. 43.1)
- Rectum and colon are the most common sites followed by the jejunum and the esophagus
- Hematochezia from arteriovenous malformations, varices due to internal iliac system obstruction, or portal hypertension
- Hematuria from genitourinary involvement
- Visceral organ involvement

The pathogenesis is not completely clear but appear to involve [3]:

- A congenital syndrome
- Most are sporadic but recent reports exist of autosomal dominant inheritance
- Genetic defects in angiogenic factors regulation

The pathology will show [1, 3]:

- Arteriovenous malformations
- Mucosal polypoid nodules and masses with abundant vasculature

The diagnosis is made by [4–6]:

- Physical diagnosis of the affected limb can be sufficient
- Multiple imaging modalities to confirm diagnosis and evaluate anatomy of the vasculature; computed tomography, magnetic resonance imaging, venography, and arteriography
- For GI involvement, endoscopy
- Interventional angiography

The differential diagnosis should include [1, 4, 5]:

- Osler–Weber–Rendu disease
- Portal colopathy and enteropathy
- Blue Rubber Bleb nevus syndrome
- Kasabach–Merritt syndrome

Treatment should involve [4]:

- Endoscopic therapeutic intervention (thermal)
- Angiographic (embolization)
- Surgical exploration and correction of the vascular malformation
- Surgical resection if the involved bowel segment (rectum)

References

1. Feldman M, Friedman LS, Brandt LJ, editors. Sleisenger and Fordtran's gastrointestinal and liver disease. 9th ed. Philadelphia: Saunders; 2010.
2. Servelle M, Bastin R, Loygue J, et al. Hematuria and rectal bleeding in the child with Klippel and Trenaunay syndrome. Ann Surg. 1976;183:418–28.

M. Tadros (✉)
Department of Internal Medicine, University of Connecticut Health Center, Farmington, CT, USA

560 Hudson Street, Apt 750, Hartford, CT 06106, USA
e-mail: mtadros@resident.uchc.edu

G.Y. Wu et al. (eds.), *Atlas of Dermatological Manifestations of Gastrointestinal Disease*,
DOI 10.1007/978-1-4614-6191-3_43, © Springer Science+Business Media New York 2013

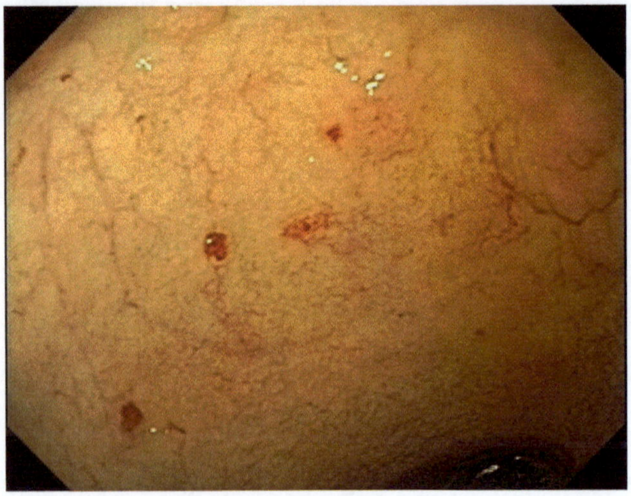

Fig. 43.1 Hemangiomas in the duodenum in a patient with Klippel-Trenaunay-Weber syndrome

3. Ceballos-Quintal JM, Pinto-Escalante D, Castillo-Zapata I. A new case of Klippel-Trenaunay-Weber (KTW) syndrome: evidence of autosomal dominant inheritance. Am J Med Genet. 1996;63:426–7.
4. Jacob AG, Driscoll DJ, Shaughnessy WJ, et al. Klippel-Trénaunay syndrome: spectrum and management. Mayo Clin Proc. 1998;73:28–36.
5. Wilson CL, Song LM, Chua H, et al. Bleeding from cavernous angiomatosis of the rectum in Klippel-Trenaunay syndrome: report of three cases and literature review. Am J Gastroenterol. 2001;96:2783–8.
6. Wang ZK, Wang FY. Klippel-Trénaunay syndrome with gastrointestinal bleeding, splenic hemangiomas and left inferior vena cava. World J Gastroentero. 2010;16:1548.

Klippel–Trenaunay–Weber Syndrome: Dermatological Features

44

Liam Zakko, Justin Finch, Marti J. Rothe, and Jane M. Grant-Kels

Clinical signs and features include:

- Classic triad:
  - Boney/soft tissue hypertrophy: increased length and/or girth of limb, affecting at least one extremity; presents with slight findings at birth but becomes much more evident with continually imbalanced growth during first few years of life [1]
  - Cutaneous capillary malformations: usually port wine stains, red to purple plaques, which may or may not blanch, in a dermatomal distribution limited by the midline (see Fig. 44.1); usually on the same side as the affected limb but on other areas of the skin as well, and rarely occur in the bone, pleura, spleen, bladder [1]
  - Varicosities/venous malformations: often with persistent lateral embryologic veins; 60–80% have large lateral incompetent vein on affected leg (vein of Servelle [2]); these may develop cellulitis, hemorrhage, thrombus leading to pulmonary embolism, stasis dermatitis, stasis ulcerations, thrombophlebitis [1]
- Associated with hip dislocation, scoliosis, syndactyly, hypoplasia of lymph system resulting in lymphedema [1]
- Parkes–Weber syndrome: classic triad with clinically apparent arteriovenous fistula [1]
- No sex or ethnic predilection [3]

Pathogenesis of this disease is unclear but hypotheses include:

- No clear chromosomal or gene linkage, all cases appearing to be sporadic [2]
- Some hypotheses [2]:
  - Congenital spinal cord anomaly with autonomic dysfunction of growth control
  - Disturbed vasculogenesis
  - Generalized mesodermal defects
  - Genetic mosaicisms

Histopathological features include:

- Vascular malformations: tortuous vascular channels of varying size and shape, lined by a continuous endothelium, and surrounded by an abnormal complement of mural cells [2]
- Cutaneous capillary malformations (port wine stains): dilated capillary blood vessels in superficial dermis of the skin; when the lesions become nodular, deeper vessels in the dermis and subcutis are also dilated; cavernous hemangioma or arteriovenous malformation may also be associated with deeper lesions. [2, 3]

The diagnosis is made using a combination of:

- Two major features (one from group A and at least one from group B) [2]
  - Group A: congenital vascular malformations: cutaneous malformations (including port wine stains); venous malformations: hypoplasia or aplasia of veins, persistence of fetal veins, varicosities, hypertrophy, tortuosity, and valvular malformations; arteriovenous malformations; lymphatic malformations
  - Group B: disturbed growth of bone length or girth; disturbed growth of soft tissue in length or girth (hypertrophy [frequent] or hypotrophy [rare])

The differential diagnosis should include:

- Parkes–Weber Syndrome
- Chuvash polycythemia Proteus syndrome

L. Zakko (✉)
Yale Department of Internal Medicine, Yale New Haven Hospital, 20 York Street, New Haven, CT 06510, USA
e-mail: liam.zakko@yale.edu

J. Finch • M.J. Rothe • J.M. Grant-Kels
Department of Dermatology, University of Connecticut Health Center, 21 South Road, Farmington, CT 06030, USA
e-mail: finch@uchc.edu; rothe@uchc.edu; grant@uchc.edu

G.Y. Wu et al. (eds.), *Atlas of Dermatological Manifestations of Gastrointestinal Disease*,
DOI 10.1007/978-1-4614-6191-3_44, © Springer Science+Business Media New York 2013

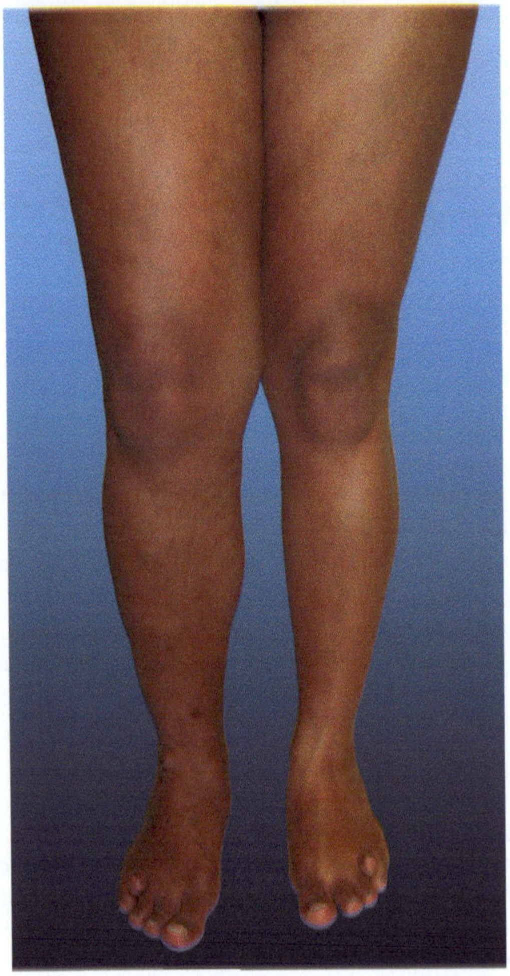

Fig. 44.1 Klippel-Trenaunay-Weber syndrome. Geographic-patterned vascular malformation with ipsilateral limb hypertrophy

- Bannayan–Riley–Ruvalcaba syndrome
- Maffucci syndrome
- Stewart–Bluefarb syndrome

Treatment options include:

- Capillary malformations: if symptomatic lesions or if port wine stains on face and neck, then use pulse dye lasers [1]
- Varicose veins: compression stockings [1]
- When lower limb discrepancy is >2 cm, stapling epiphysiodesis of knee cartilage can be performed to delay growth of the longer limb [4]

References

1. Meier S. Kippel-Trenaunay syndrome. Adv Neonatal Care. 2009;9:120–4.
2. Oduber CE, van der Horst CM, Hennekam RC. Klippel-Trenaunay syndrome: diagnostic criteria and hypothesis etiology. Ann Plast Surg. 2008;60:217–23.
3. Redondo P, Aguado L, Martinez-Cuestra A. Diagnosis and management of extensive vascular malformations of the lower limb. Part I. Clinical diagnosis. J Am Acad Dermatol. 2011;65:893–906.
4. Redondo P, Aguado L, Martinez-Cuestra A. Diagnosis and management of extensive vascular malformations of the lower limb. Part II. Systemic repercussions, diagnosis, and treatment. J Am Acad Dermatol. 2011;65:909–23.

Tuberous Sclerosis: Gastrointestinal Features

45

Jameel Uddeen

Tuberous sclerosis is a genetic disease characterized by nonmalignant tumor growth in all organs due to the inactivation of tumor growth suppressors. The current prevalence is thought to be one in 12,500 [1]. Gastrointestinal (GI) symptoms [2, 3] include:

- Usually asymptomatic
- Rectal bleeding
- Constipation

Typical clinical signs and findings [2, 3] are:

- Rectal bleeding
- Hamartomatous polyps, most commonly in colon (see Fig. 45.1) and rectum, can also be found in the stomach (see Fig. 45.2) [4]
- Papillomas in GI tract
- Oral and gingival fibromas
- Esophageal mucosal protrusions
- Hepatic angiomyolipomas
- Epilepsy
- Mental retardation

The pathogenesis is based on a genetic defect [5]:

- Mutations that inactivate *TSC1* (hamartin) gene on chromosome 9 or *TSC2* (tuberin) gene on chromosome 16, resulting in impaired tumor suppression

The pathology [5, 6] of polyp biopsies shows:

- Gross: semispherical, whitish polyps (see Fig. 45.2)
- Histological: hyperplastic mucosa with an excess of smooth muscle fibers in the stroma (see Figs. 45.3 and 45.4)

The diagnosis [5, 6] is made by considering a number of criteria:

- Laboratory tests: complete blood count, electrolytes, liver enzymes, DNA testing to identify mutations in *TSC1* and *TSC2* genes
- Studies: colonoscopy, flexible sigmoidoscopy, barium enema, computed tomography/magnetic resonance imaging brain, renal ultrasound, echocardiogram
- Clinical diagnosis
  - Definite: two major features or one major feature plus two minor features
  - Probable: one major feature plus one minor feature
  - Possible: one major feature or two or more minor features
  - Major features
    - Facial angiofibromas or forehead plaque
    - Nontraumatic ungual or periungual fibromas
    - ≥3 hypomelanotic macules (ash leaf spots)
    - Shagreen patch (connective tissue nevus)
    - Multiple retinal nodular hamartomas
    - Cortical tuber
    - Subependymal nodule
    - Subependymal giant cell astrocytoma
    - Cardiac rhabdomyoma, single or multiple
    - Lymphangiomyomatosis
    - Renal angiomyolipoma
  - Minor features
    - Multiple dental enamel pits
    - Hamartomatous rectal polyps
    - Bone cysts
    - Cerebral white matter radial migration lines
    - Gingival fibromas
    - Nonrenal hamartoma
    - Retinal achromic patch
    - "Confetti" skin lesions
    - Multiple renal cysts

J. Uddeen (✉)
Department of Internal Medicine,
University of Connecticut Health Center, Farmington, CT, USA

University of Connecticut, 2 Earls Court Unit E,
Farmington, CT 06032, USA
e-mail: uddeen@resident.uchc.edu

G.Y. Wu et al. (eds.), *Atlas of Dermatological Manifestations of Gastrointestinal Disease*,
DOI 10.1007/978-1-4614-6191-3_45, © Springer Science+Business Media New York 2013

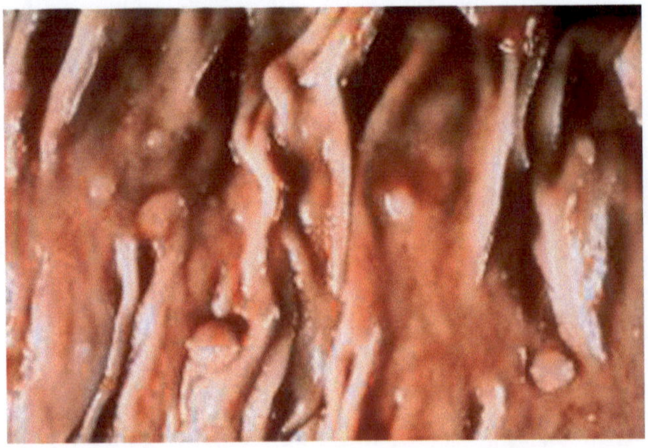

Fig. 45.1 A colonoscopic view of multiple hamartomatous polyps seen in tuberous sclerosis

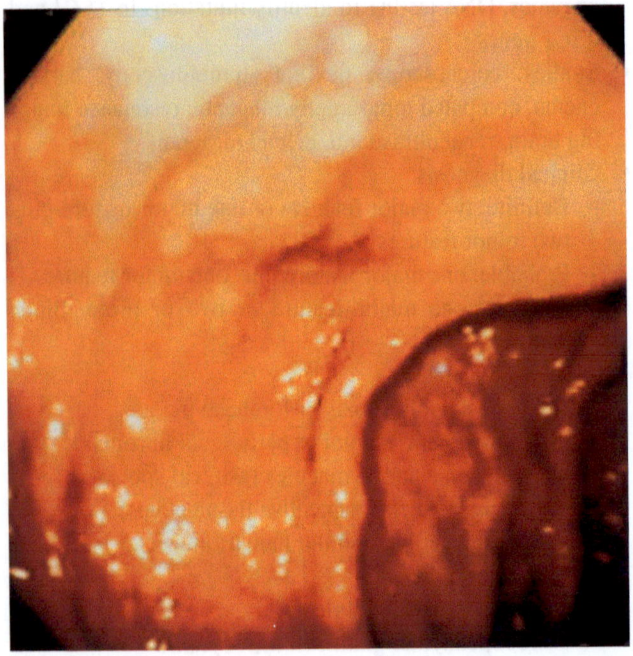

Fig. 45.2 Endoscopic findings in a patient with tuberous sclerosis. Diffusely scattered whitish polyps on the fundic mucosa representing hamartomatous gastric polyps (From Kim et al. [4]; with permission)

The differential diagnosis of tuberous sclerosis should include other polyposis syndromes [4, 5]:

- Familial adenomatous polyposis
- Gardner syndrome
- Inflammatory bowel disease
- Peutz–Jeghers syndrome
- Cowden disease

The treatment involves [5, 6]:

- Symptomatic (i.e., stool softener for constipation)
- Polypectomy
- Rapamycin

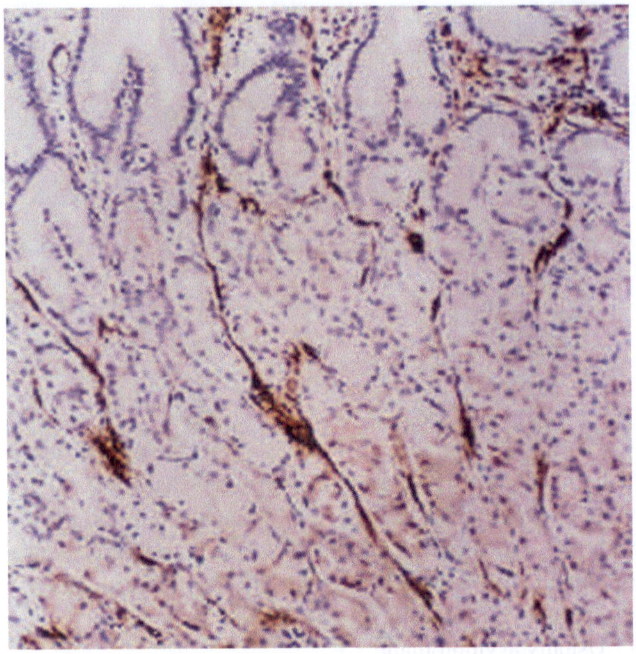

Fig. 45.3 A photomicrograph showing immunochemical staining of smooth muscle actin. Smooth muscle fibers are prominent in the lamina propria extending up to the surface epithelium. (100×) (From Kim et al. [4]; with permission)

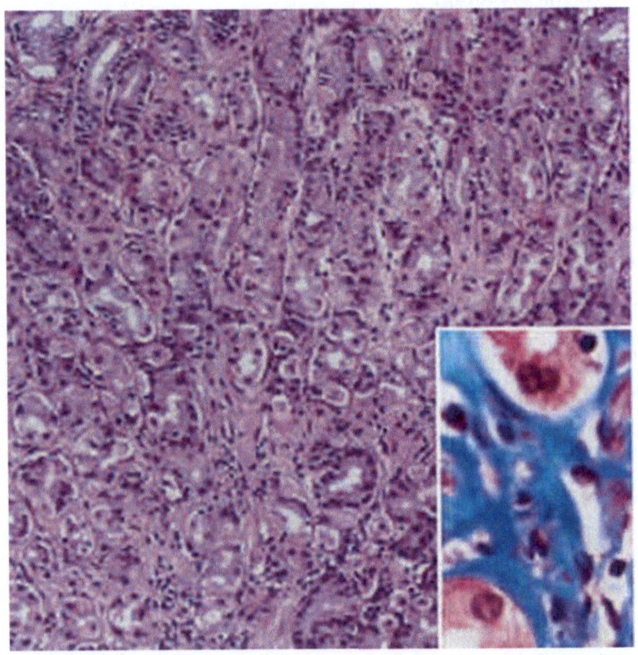

Fig. 45.4 Smooth muscle bundles between fundic glands in the lamina propria (H and E stain, 100×) (From Kim et al. [4]; with permission)

References

1. Goldman L. Tuberous sclerosis. Goldman's Cecil medicine. 24th ed. Philadelphia: Saunders; 2012.
2. Kliegman RM. Clinical manifestations of tuberous sclerosis. In: Kliegman RM, Stanton B, St Geme J, editors. Nelson textbook of pediatrics. 19th ed. Saunders: Philadelphia; 2011.
3. Sarigol-Blanchard S, et al. Unusual endoscopic and histologic findings in teenagers presenting with constipation and rectal bleeding. Am J Gastroenterol. 2001;96:S240–1.
4. Kim BK, Kim YI, Kim WH. Hamartomatous gastric polyposis in a patient with tuberous sclerosis. J Korean Med Sci. 2000;15:467–70.
5. Schwartz RA, Fernández G, Kotulska K, Jóźwiak S. Tuberous sclerosis complex: advances in diagnosis, genetics, and management. J Am Academy Dermatol. 2007;57:189–202.
6. Hizawa K, Iida M, Matsumoto T, et al. Gastrointestinal involvement in tuberous sclerosis. J Clin Gastroenterol. 1994;19:46–9.

Tuberous Sclerosis: Dermatological Features

46

Liam Zakko, Justin Finch, Marti J. Rothe, and Jane M. Grant-Kels

Clinical signs and features include:

- Neurocutaneous syndrome: variable phenotype characterized by the development of multiple hamartomas throughout the body [1]
- Classically presents with seizures, mental retardation, facial angiofibromas (this triad is found in only 29% of cases) [1]
- Incidence is about 1:6,000–1:10,000, although it is hard to calculate as individuals with mild or asymptomatic disease may never be diagnosed [1]
- Manifests in the brain (cortical tubers, subendymal nodules, and giant cell astrocytomas leading to seizures and mental retardation), kidney (angiomyolipoma), lung (lymphangiomyomatosis), heart (rhabdomyoma), and eyes (retinal hamartomas) [1]
- Cutaneous features are present in nearly 100% of patients and include [1]:
  - Facial angiofibromas: red to pink papules/nodules with a smooth, glistening surface, symmetrically and bilaterally distributed over the centrofacial areas sparing the central upper lip and appearing at 2–5 years of age in 75–85% of patients and may grow rapidly during puberty (*see* Fig. 46.1)
  - Large hypomelanotic macules (ash leaf spot): 1–2 cm in diameter lesions that occasionally are more round or polygonal than "leaf" shaped; these are often the earliest visible signs of the condition as usually present at birth; they are present on 97% of affected persons
  - Confetti-like lesions: 1–3 mm white macules, symmetrically distributed over the extremities and appear in adulthood in about 3% of cases; Shagreen patches and plaques present in 50% of cases, increase in number and size with age, and are found on the dorsal body, especially the lumbosacral area. These have a rough texture resembling an orange peel
  - Ungual/periungual fibromas: first develop at puberty, affect 15% of cases, and appear as red/skin-colored papules that arise from the lateral nail grove, plate, and folds; forehead fibrous plaques: yellow to brown to skin-colored large, soft, doughy plaques with variable size and shape that may appear at any age and affect nearly 20% of patients (*see* Fig. 46.1)

Pathogenesis of this genetic disease involves:

- Autosomal dominant inheritance, although two thirds of cases are from sporadic mutation [1]
- Two tuberous sclerosis genes: *TSC2*: 16p13.3 (more severe phenotype); *TSC1*: 9q34
- Two proteins—tuberin and hamartin—form a tight binding relationship that regulates cell growth and tumor genesis by inhibiting mTOR, a cell cycle regulating protein, GAP portion of *TSC1*/*TSC2* protein is the site of mutations that results in tuberous sclerosis (TS) [1]

L. Zakko (✉)
Yale Department of Internal Medicine, Yale New Haven Hospital, 20 York Street, New Haven, CT 06510, USA
e-mail: liam.zakko@yale.edu

J. Finch • M.J. Rothe • J.M. Grant-Kels
Department of Dermatology, University of Connecticut Health Center, 21 South Road, Farmington, CT 06030, USA
e-mail: finch@uchc.edu; rothe@uchc.edu; grant@uchc.edu

G.Y. Wu et al. (eds.), *Atlas of Dermatological Manifestations of Gastrointestinal Disease*, DOI 10.1007/978-1-4614-6191-3_46,

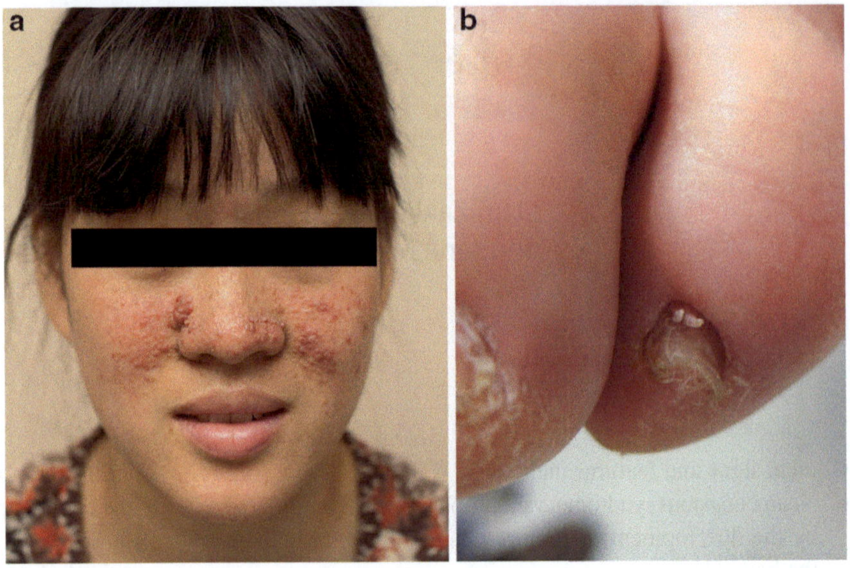

Fig. 46.1 Tuberous sclerosis. (**a**) Adenoma sebaceum, presenting clinically as red papules clustered on the central face; (**b**) Koenen tumors appear as a periungual skin-colored papule on the fingers or toes

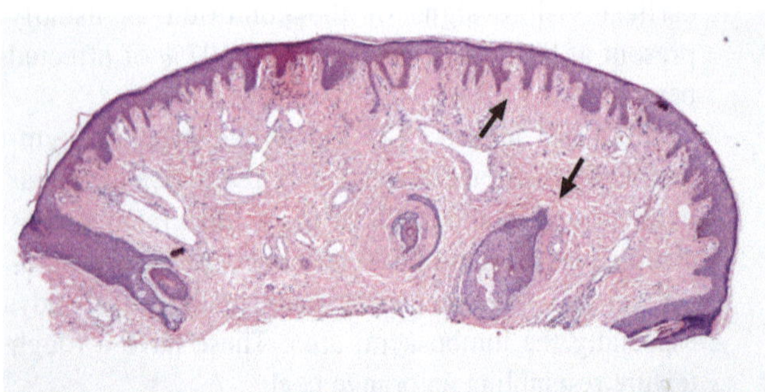

Fig. 46.2 Tuberous sclerosis. Histologically, both adenoma sebaceum and Koenen tumors are angiofibromas. Note the dome-shaped papule with dilated vessels (*white arrow*) and collagen fibers oriented concentrically around follicles and vertically near the epidermis (*black arrows*) (20×)

Histopathological features include:

- Ash leaf spots: melanocytes normal in number but decreased pigmentation (decrease in dopamine response); melanosomes in both melanocytes and keratinocytes are decreased in size and associated with less melanization [1]
- Angiofibromas: atrophic sebaceous glands with dermal fibrosis and capillary dilation with large stellate fibroblasts and occasional multinucleated giant cells; elastic fibers reduced or absent (*see* Fig. 46.2) [1]
- Forehead fibrous plaque similar to angiofibromas with more sclerotic collagen in concentric layers around atrophic pilosebaceous follicles [1]
- Ungual/periungual fibromas: similar to angiofibromas [1]
- Shagreen patch: connective tissue hamartoma with dense bands of collagen and variable adipose tissue, smooth muscle, cutaneous appendages without increased vascularity; elastic tissue usually fragmented, clumped, and reduced [1]

The diagnosis is made using a combination of:

- Clinical: definite TS, two majors features or one major and two minor; probable TS, one major and one minor; possible TS, one major or more than two minor [1]
- Major criteria: facial angiofibromas or forehead plaques; nontraumatic ungual/periungual fibroma; hypomelanotic macule (3+); shagreen patch; multiple retinal nodular hamartomas; cortical tubers; subependymal nodule; subependymal giant cell astrocytoma; cardiac rhabdomyoma; lymphangiomatosis; renal angiomyolipoma
- Minor criteria: multiple randomly distributed pits in dental enamel; hamartomatous rectal polyps; bone cysts; cerebral white matter radial migration lines; gingival fibromas; nonrenal hamartomas; retinal achromic patch; "confetti" skin lesions; multiple renal cysts
- Molecular genetic testing will be positive in 75–80% of cases; can help rule out parents as having disease when children have a spontaneous mutation [1]

The differential diagnosis should include:

- Sporadic skin tumors (e.g., angiofibroma, collagenoma)
- Multiple endocrine neoplasia, type 1 [1]
- Vitiligo
- Nevus anemicus
- Nevus depigmentosus

Treatment options include:

- Neuroimaging, electroencephalography (EEG), renal ultrasound, chest computed tomography followed by surgical intervention if indicated [1]

- Facial angiofibromas that disfigure: cryosurgery, curettage, dermabrasion, chemical peeling, excision, laser therapy [1]
- Rapamycin orally may have a role in decreasing lesions by stabilizing mTOR [1]

Reference

1. Schwartz RA, Fernandez G, Kotulska K, Jozwiak S. Tuberous sclerosis complex: advances in diagnosis, genetics, and management. J Am Acad Dermatol. 2007;57:189–202.

47 Churg-Strauss Syndrome: Gastrointestinal Features

Liam Zakko

Churg-Strauss syndrome (CSS) is characterized by small- and medium-vessel vasculitis frequently associated with asthma. This autoimmune disease affects the lungs, gastrointestinal (GI) system, peripheral nerves, heart, skin, and kidneys.

GI symptoms include [1, 2]:

- Abdominal pain (59%), diarrhea (33%), bloody stools (18%), ileus, nausea, anorexia, odynophagia, ischemic bowel disease

Clinical signs and findings include [1, 2]:

- Systemic and pulmonary small and medium vessel vasculitis, tissue and peripheral hypereosinophilia, and extravascular granulomas, which occur in the presence of severe asthma
- Diagnosis usually made at about age 50 with an incidence of 1.3–6.8 per million of the general population and an incidence of 34.6–67 per million in asthmatics
- Stage I (prodromal) begins in the second or third decade of life with allergic rhinitis, nasal polyposis, sinusitis, and asthma
- Stage II (eosinophilic phase) increased peripheral eosinophils that infiltrate the organs (lungs, GI tract)
- Stage III (vasculitic) systemic vasculitis
- GI symptoms occur in 33% of patients (fourth most common site of involvement after lungs, skin, and peripheral nervous system)
- GI disease most commonly involves ulcers in the small intestine [3] or colon [4] with rare perforating ulcers (see Fig. 47.1) [5] in either (perforation is more common in the small intestine); endoscopy often shows acute serosal inflammation, hemorrhage, and marked adhesions with deep ulcers intervening with edematous areas
- Congestive esophagitis [6], liver abscesses [7], cholecystitis [8], serosal disease with eosinophilic ascites
- GI (like cardiac involvement) is a poor prognostic indicator

The pathogenesis is not entirely clear but there are several hypotheses [1, 9]:

- Strong association with asthma, atopy, increased eosinophilia, heightened T-cell immunity, and antineutrophil cytoplasmic antibodies (ANCA) increase suggests an autoimmune mechanism is likely
- Appears possible infectious, foreign, or autoantigen initiates the Th-2 response leading to rhinosinusitis, asthma, then eosinophilic infiltration of vessels and organs
- Strong association with anti-asthma medications particularly antileukotriene receptor antagonists
- Forty percent are ANCA-positive and 90% of those with positive ANCA have perinuclear ANCA; those with positive ANCA are more likely to have a vasculitis pattern with increased renal involvement, neuropathy, alveolar hemorrhage, increased heart and lung disease, and increased fibrinoid degeneration/necrosis
- It is controversial whether asthma medications cause CSS or whether these medications make it possible to taper steroid doses, thus unmasking CSS; steroids may lead to fibrinoid changes in vessels that lead to acute ulcers and perforation
- Ischemic ulcers may also be caused by eosinophilic infiltration of GI mucosa

The pathology often shows [1, 9]:

- Leukocytoclastic vasculitis involving small- and medium-sized arteries and veins
- Necrotizing granulomas in the interstitium and perivascular regions (see Fig. 47.2)
- Prominent regions of necrosis
- Eosinophilic infiltration

The diagnosis is made based on [1, 9]:

- New onset of four of the following: asthma, peripheral blood eosinophilia (>10% of total leukocyte count), mono- or polyneuropathy, paranasal sinus abnormalities,

L. Zakko (✉)
Yale Department of Internal Medicine, Yale New Haven Hospital, 20 York Street, New Haven, CT 06510, USA
e-mail: liam.zakko@yale.edu

G.Y. Wu et al. (eds.), *Atlas of Dermatological Manifestations of Gastrointestinal Disease*, DOI 10.1007/978-1-4614-6191-3_47, © Springer Science+Business Media New York 2013

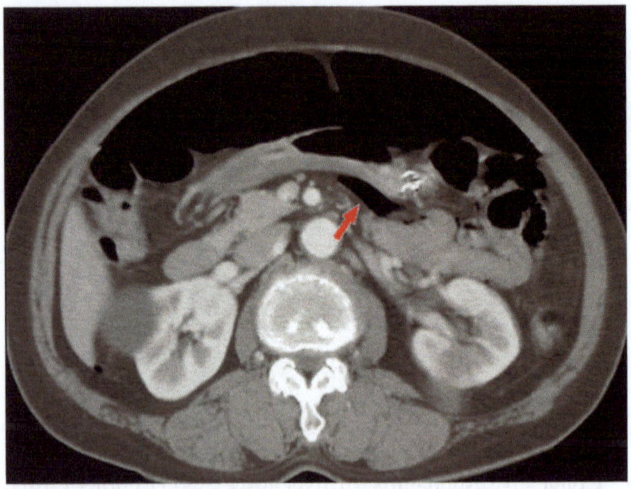

Fig. 47.1 Computed tomography image showing pneumoperitoneum (*arrow*) due to colonic perforation in a patient with Churg-Strauss syndrome treated with corticosteroids (From Venditti et al. [5]; with permission)

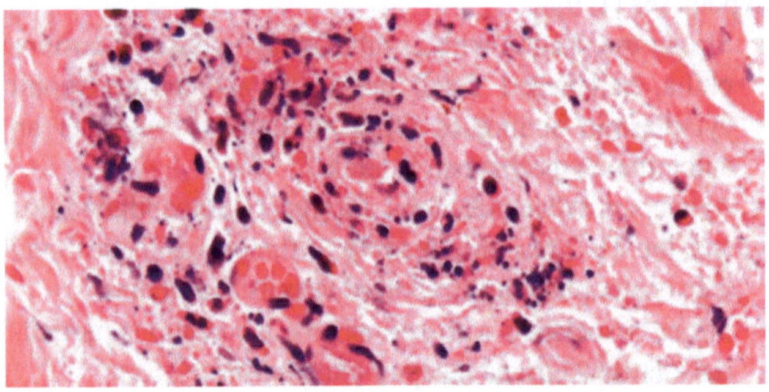

Fig. 47.2 A photomicrograph showing extravascular granulomas in a specimen of resected colon from a patient with Churg-Strauss syndrome. Hematoxylin and eosin stain, high power (From Venditti et al. [5]; with permission)

eosinophilia in tissues on biopsy, migratory pulmonary infiltrates

- Chapel Hill criteria: "eosinophil-rich and granulomatous inflammation involving the respiratory tract and necrotizing vasculitis affecting small to medium sized vessels associated with asthma and eosinophilia" [9]; the problem with this criteria is that it relies on biopsy characteristics that rarely exist at the same time
- For GI involvement, abdominal films may show gaseous distension of the small intestine
- Angiography may show irregularities of vessel walls and disruption of arteries, suggesting vasculitis

The differential diagnosis of CSS should include [1, 9]:

- Asthma
- Hypereosinophilia syndromes (eosinophilic gastroenteritis)
- Other causes of vasculitis (polyarteritis nodosa, Wegner's granulomatosis)

There is no cure for this disease. However, treatment may include [1, 9]:

- Corticosteroids and cyclophosphamide to induce remission
- Use corticosteroids with azathioprine or methotrexate for maintenance
- Refractory disease-consider mycophenolate, infliximab, etanercept, rituximab, intravenous immunoglobin, interferon-α, mepolizumab, omalizumab

References

1. Ahn E, Luk A, Chetty R, Butany J. Vasculitis of the gastrointestinal tract. Semin Diagn Pathol. 2009;26:81–2.
2. Baldini C, Jalarico R, Della Rossa A, Bobardieri S. Clinical manifestations and treatment of Churg-Strauss syndrome. Rheum Dis Clin North Am. 2010;36:527–43.
3. Murakami S, Misumi M, Sakata H, et al. Churg-Strauss syndrome manifesting as perforation of the small intestine: report of a case. Surg Today. 2004;34:788–92.
4. Kim YB, Choi SW, Park IS, et al. Churg-Strauss syndrome with perforating ulcers of the colon. J Korean Med. 2000;15:585–8.
5. Venditti D, Balassone V, Ielpo B, et al. Bowel perforations in a patient affected by Churg-Strauss syndrome under high-dose steroid treatment: will alternative drugs reduce risk of surgery? Rheumatol Int. 2011;31:1239–41.
6. Mir O, Nazal EM, Cohen P, et al. Esophageal involvement as an initial manifestation of Churg-Strauss syndrome. Presse Med. 2007;36:57–60.
7. Sinico RA, Bottero P. Churg-Strauss angiitis. Best Pract Clin Rheumatol. 2009;23:355–66.
8. Suzuki M, Nabeshima K, Miyazaki M, et al. Churg-Strauss syndrome complicated by colon erosion, acalculous cholecystitis, and liver abscesses. World J Gastroenterol. 2005;11:5248–50.
9. Szczeklik W, Jakiela B, Adamek D, Musial J. Cutting edge issues in Churg-Strauss syndrome. Clin Rev Allerg Immunol. 2013;44:39–50.

Churg–Strauss Syndrome: Dermatological Features

48

Liam Zakko, Justin Finch, Marti J. Rothe, and Jane M. Grant-Kels

Clinical signs and features include:

- Systemic and pulmonary small and medium vessel vasculitis, tissue and peripheral hypereosinophilia, and extravascular granulomas, which occur in the presence of severe asthma
- Diagnosis usually made at about age 50 with an incidence of 1.3–6.8 per million of the general population [1] and an incidence of 34.6–67 per million in asthmatics [2]
- Stage I (prodromal) begins in the second or third decade of life with allergic rhinitis, nasal polyposis, sinusitis, and asthma
- Stage II (eosinophilic phase) increased peripheral eosinophils that infiltrate the organs (eosinophilic pneumonia, eosinophilic gastroenteritis)
- Stage III (vasculitic) systemic vasculitis
- Most frequently involved systems involve peripheral nervous system in 65–76%, lungs in 51–65%, and skin in 52–57% [1]
- Skin changes occur in one half to two thirds of patients and include nonthrombocytopenic palpable purpura (most common), occasional nodules, papules, petechiae, urticaria, and livedo of the extremities/trunk [2] (see Fig. 48.1)
- Peripheral nervous system disease is usually mononeuritis multiplex but symmetrical peripheral neuropathy can develop

Pathogenesis of this disease involves:

- Unknown although strong association with asthma, atopy, eosinophilia, heightened T-cell immunity, and positive antineutrophil cytoplasmic antibodies (ANCA) suggests autoimmune disorder is likely [3]
- Appears as though infectious, foreign, or autoantigen initiates the Th-2 response, leading to rhinosinusitis, asthma, then eosinophilic infiltration of vessels and organs [2]
- Strong association with anti-asthma medications particularly anti-leukotriene receptor antagonists [2]
- Controversial whether asthma medications cause Churg–Strauss syndrome (CSS) or whether these medications make it possible to taper steroid doses, thus unmasking CSS [3]
- Forty percent are positive ANCA and 90% of those with positive ANCA are perinuclear ANCA; those with positive ANCA are more likely to have a vasculitis pattern with greater incidence of renal involvement, neuropathy, alveolar hemorrhage, and fibrinoid degeneration/necrosis; heart and lung disease (excluding alveolar hemorrhage) are more likely in ANCA-negative patients [2]

Histopathological features include:

- Eosinophilic infiltrates within the dermis
- Extravascular granulomas (see Fig. 48.2)
- Leukocytoclastic vasculitis involving small and medium sized vessels (see Fig. 48.2)

The diagnosis is made using a combination of [2]:

- New onset of four of the following: asthma, peripheral blood eosinophilia (>10% of total leukocyte count), mono- or polyneuropathy, paranasal sinus abnormalities, eosinophilia in tissues on biopsy, migratory pulmonary infiltrates

L. Zakko (✉)
Yale Department of Internal Medicine, 20 York Street, Yale New Haven Hospital, New Haven, CT 06510, USA
e-mail: liam.zakko@yale.edu

J. Finch • M.J. Rothe • J.M. Grant-Kels
Department of Dermatology, University of Connecticut Health Center, 21 South Road, Farmington, CT 06030, USA
e-mail: finch@uchc.edu; rothe@uchc.edu; grant@uchc.edu

G.Y. Wu et al. (eds.), *Atlas of Dermatological Manifestations of Gastrointestinal Disease*, DOI 10.1007/978-1-4614-6191-3_48, © Springer Science+Business Media New York 2013

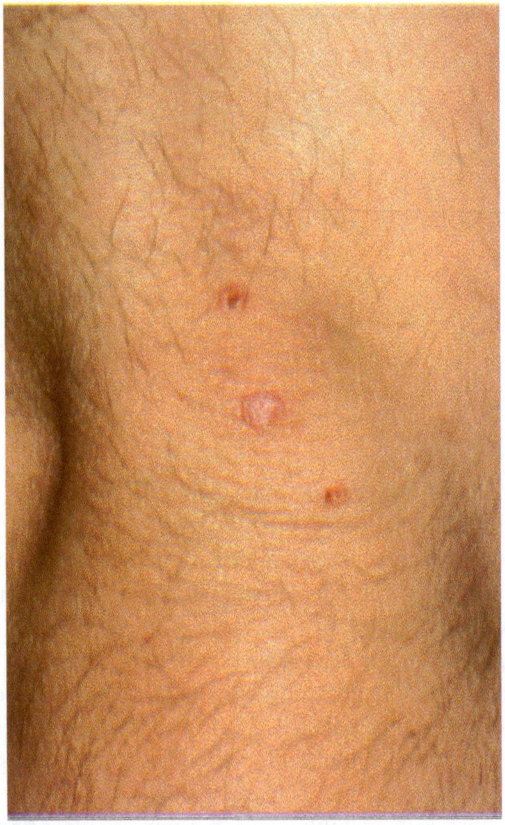

Fig. 48.1 Churg–Strauss syndrome. Necrotic papules on the elbow (Image courtesy of Yale Residency Collection)

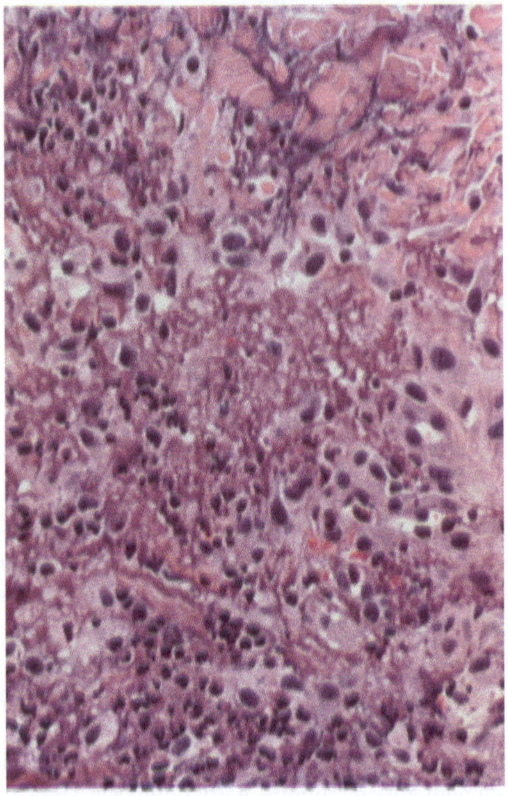

Fig. 48.2 Churg–Strauss syndrome. Extravascular necrotizing granuloma (400×) (Image courtesy of Yale Residency Collection)

- Chapel Hill criteria: "eosinophil-rich and granulomatous inflammation involving the respiratory tract and necrotizing vasculitis affecting small to medium sized vessels associated with asthma and eosinophilia" [2]; a problem with this criteria, however, is that it relies on biopsy characteristics that rarely exist at the same time

The differential diagnosis should include:

- Asthma
- Hypereosinophilia syndromes
- Other causes of vasculitis

Treatment options include [2, 4]:

- Corticosteroids and pulse cyclophosphamide to induce remission
- Use corticosteroids with azathioprine or methotrexate or cyclosporine for maintenance
- Refractory disease consider mycophenolate, infliximab, etanercept, rituximab, intravenous immunoglobin, interferon-alpha, mepolizumab, omalizumab, plasma exchange

References

1. Sinico RA, Bottero P. Churg-Strauss angiitis. Best Pract Clin Rheumatol. 2009;23:355–66.
2. Szczeklik W, Jakiela B, Adamek D, et al. Cutting edge issues in Churg-Strauss syndrome. Clin Rev Allerg Immunol. Clin Rev Allergy Immunol. 2013;44:39–50.
3. Ahn E, Luk A, Chetty R, et al. Vasculitides of the gastrointestinal tract. Semin Diagn Pathol. 2009;26:81–2.
4. Baldini C, Talarico R, Della Rossa A, et al. Clinical manifestations and treatment of Churg-Strauss syndrome. Rheum Dis Clin North Am. 2010;36:527–43.

Ulcerative Colitis: Gastrointestinal Features

49

Nathan Selsky

Ulcerative colitis is an inflammatory bowel disease likely due to an autoimmune process. In North America, the prevalence of this disease is 1 per 1000, with a bimodal distribution of age of onset in the second and sixth decade of life [1].

The gastrointestinal (GI) symptoms include [1, 2]:

- Intermittent diarrhea mixed with blood and mucous, more than ten episodes per day in severe disease
- Intermittent rectal bleeding
- Tenesmus
- Abdominal cramping

The most common clinical signs and findings are [1, 2]:

- Initially limited to rectum/distal colon in 33%, extending proximally to the left colon in 33%, pancolitis in the remaining 33%
- Fevers to 39.5 °C in severe disease
- Anemia requiring transfusion
- Macro-ulcerations
- Pseudopolyps
- Oral aphthous ulcers
- Iritis, uveitis, episcleritis
- Seronegative arthritis, sacroiliitis
- Erythema nodosum, pyoderma gangrenosum
- Primary sclerosing cholangitis

The pathogenesis is not entirely clear but possibilities include [1, 2]:

- Likely components of autoimmune disease, and genetics
- Stress and environmental contributions

The pathology of mucosal biopsies can show [1, 3]:

- Gross: continuous colonic involvement with ulceration (see Fig. 49.1), loss of vascular markings, petechiae, exudates, friability, and hemorrhage
- Histological: distorted crypt architecture, crypt abscesses, cryptitis (see Fig. 49.2), inflammatory cells in the lamina propria

The diagnosis is made with a combination of [1–4]:

- Established with history and endoscopic findings
- Confirmed with histology on colonic biopsy
- Complete blood count, electrolytes, erythrocyte sedimentation rate, C-reactive protein, liver function tests
- Stool culture

The differential diagnosis of ulcerative colitis should include [1–4]:

- Crohn's disease
- Radiation colitis
- Ischemic colitis
- Infectious etiologies including *Escherichia coli, Shigella, Campylobacter, Salmonella*, and sexually transmitted diseases

Medical therapy does not cure the condition but offers symptomatic and ameliorative relief and includes [1–4]:

- 5-aminosalicylic acid rectally and/or orally
- Rectal steroids, oral steroids if no response
- Azathioprine, 6-mercaptopurine
- Infliximab, cyclosporine

Colectomy in steroid refractory disease offers definitive cure of the disease.

N. Selsky (✉)
Department of Medicine, University of Connecticut,
56 Kingswood Road, West Hartford, CT 06119, USA
e-mail: nselsky@resident.uchc.edu

G.Y. Wu et al. (eds.), *Atlas of Dermatological Manifestations of Gastrointestinal Disease*,
DOI 10.1007/978-1-4614-6191-3_49, © Springer Science+Business Media New York 2013

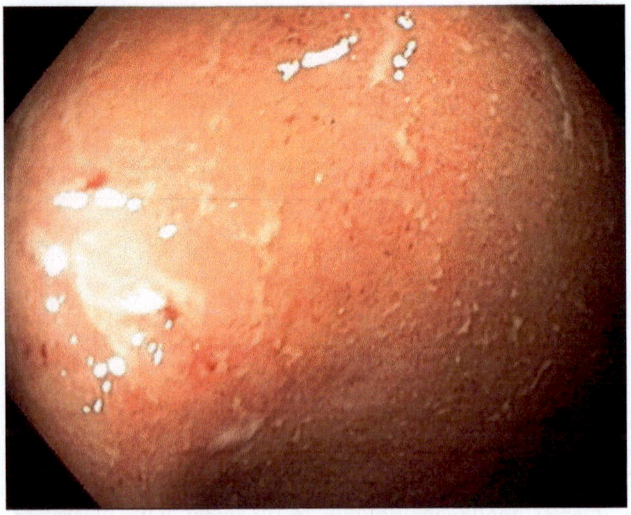

Fig. 49.1 An endoscopic view of showing multiple colonic mucosal ulcers in a patient with active ulcerative colitis

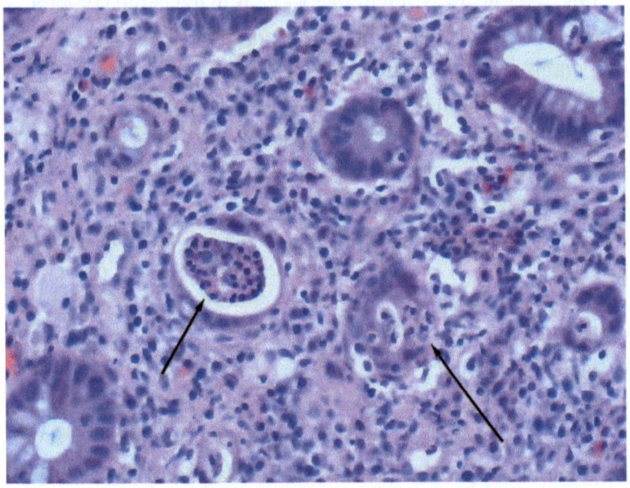

Fig. 49.2 A photomicrograph of a colonic mucosal biopsy from a patient with active ulcerative colitis. The increased edema and damage to the walls of the crypts (*arrow on the right*) as well as crypt abscesses seen as collections of inflammatory cells within crypts (*right arrow*). Hematoxylin and eosin; high power

References

1. Podolsky DK. Inflammatory bowel disease. N Engl J Med. 2002;347:417–29.
2. Baumgart DC, Sandborn WJ. Inflammatory bowel disease: clinical aspects and established and evolving therapies. Lancet. 2007;369:1641–57.
3. Leighton JA, Shen B, Baron TH, et al. ASGE guidelines: endoscopy in the diagnosis and treatment of inflammatory bowel disease. Gastrointest Endosc. 2006;63:558–65.
4. Kornbluth A, Sachar DB. Ulcerative colitis practice guidelines in adults. Am J Gastroenterol. 2004;99:1371–85.

Pyoderma Gangrenosum

50

Liam Zakko, Justin Finch, Marti J. Rothe, and Jane M. Grant-Kels

Clinical signs and features include:

- Four clinical varieties [1]:
  - Classical: painful deep ulcer with a violaceous, undermined border and necrotic, purulent center; can start as papule and progress to ulcer (see Fig. 50.1)
  - Pustular: painful, sterile pustule with no ulcerative progression
  - Bullous: presents as a tense bulla that rapidly progresses to an ulcer
  - Vegetative: superficial ulcer that progresses to a vegetative/exophytic lesion
- Seventy percent of lesions on lower extremity [1], but can be at any skin location (often peristomal) [2]
- Often exhibits pathergy [1, 2]
- Among patients with ulcerative colitis, 0.5–20% develop pyoderma gangrenosum (PG) usually during a flare [1, 2]
- Of those with PG, 33% have inflammatory bowel disease (IBD) [2]

Pathogenesis of this disease is unclear but hypotheses include:

- Appears to be related to autoantibodies that cross react between gut antigens and cytokeratins [1]

L. Zakko (✉)
Yale Department of Internal Medicine, 20 York Street,
Yale New Haven Hospital,
New Haven, CT 06510, USA
e-mail: liam.zakko@yale.edu

J. Finch • M.J. Rothe • J.M. Grant-Kels
Department of Dermatology,
University of Connecticut Health Center,
21 South Road, Farmington, CT 06030, USA
e-mail: finch@uchc.edu; rothe@uchc.edu; grant@uchc.edu

- Disease is most often seen with ulcerative colitis, but also seen with Crohn's, leukemia, myelodysplastic syndrome, monoclonal gammopathies, rheumatoid arthritis [1]

Histopathological features include:

- A neutrophilic dermatitis [1]
- Biopsy findings are dependent on the stage of the disease [2]
- Classically histological findings are characterized by a dense diffuse neutrophilic infiltrate of the dermis, central necrotizing ulceration; features of acute folliculitis, fibrinoid blood vessel changes (vasculitis), perivascular lymphocytic infiltrates, and fibrosis may be seen dependent on site of biopsy and stage of lesion [2] (see Fig. 50.2)

The diagnosis is made using a combination of [1]:

- Laboratory tests: complete blood county (CBC)/C-reactive protein (CRP)/erythrocyte-sedimentation rate (ESR)/basic electrolytes/urine and serum electrophoresis/bone marrow biopsy
- Tissue culture: bacterial, fungal, mycobacterial
- Endoscopy if bowel symptoms present
- Biopsy helps rule out other possible causes

The differential diagnosis should include:

- Sweet syndrome
- Cutaneous infection
- Cutaneous malignancy
- Vasculopathy
- Collagen vascular disease
- Halogenoderma
- Spider bite

Treatment options include:

- Treat underlying disease [1, 2]
- Pain control [1–3]
- Local care: topical steroids, intralesional steroids, topical tacrolimus, treatment of secondary infections, platelet-derived growth factors [1–3]

G.Y. Wu et al. (eds.), *Atlas of Dermatological Manifestations of Gastrointestinal Disease*,
DOI 10.1007/978-1-4614-6191-3_50, © Springer Science+Business Media New York 2013

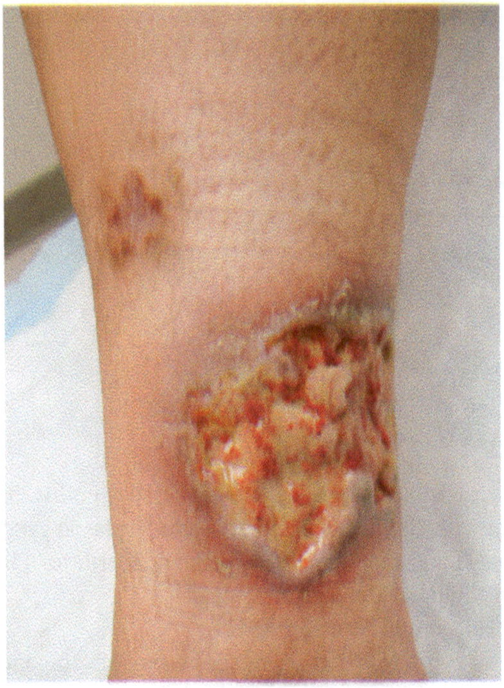

Fig. 50.1 Pyoderma gangrenosum. Purulent, undermined ulcer on the lower leg

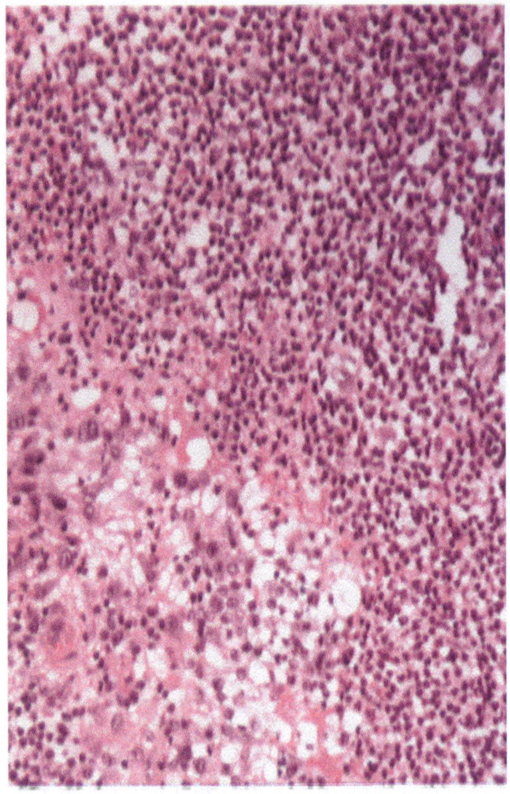

Fig. 50.2 Pyoderma gangrenosum. A photomicrograph of diffuse dermal infiltrate of predominantly neutrophils (400×)

- Systemic treatment with oral steroids, pulse IV steroids, colchicine, dapsone, sulfonamides, minocycline, cyclosporine, mycophenolate mofetil, methotrexate, azathioprine [1–3]
- Steroid refractory: tumor necrosis factor (TNF)-α inhibitors [2, 3]
- Surgical debridement is contraindicated [1]

Sweet Syndrome

Clinical signs and features include:

- Also named *acute febrile neutrophilic dermatosis*, classically in women 30–50 years old [1]
- Often follows an upper respiratory infection or gastrointestinal infection [1]
- Tender erythematous skin lesions (papules, nodules, plaques) appear on face, trunk, and extremities (see Fig. 50.3) [1]
- Lungs, bones, joints, liver, kidney, pancreas, eyes can also be affected [1, 3]
- Associated with abrupt onset of fever, leukocytosis, arthralgias, headache, fatigue, chronic cough, infiltrates on chest x-ray [1, 3]
- Recurs in 25–50% of cases [1]
- Rarely a cutaneous manifestation of IBD; only 35 IBD-associated cases reported and Sweet syndrome usually occurs during exacerbation of IBD [2]

Pathogenesis of this disease unclear [1], but involves

- Neutrophils are clearly central to the disease process [1]
- Causes include systemic inflammatory illness, myeloproliferative malignancy, drugs (granulocyte colony-stimulating factor, nonsteroid anti-inflammatory drugs [NSAIDs], propylthiouracil, trimethoprim-sulfamethoxazole, oral contraceptive pill, minocycline, furosemide, hydralazine, lithium, diazepam, vaccines), pregnancy, infection [3]

Histopathological features include:

- A neutrophilic dermatosis [1]
- Marked edema that can result in subepidermal vesiculation of the papillary dermis
- Dense reticular, dermal, perivascular, and interstitial inflammatory infiltrate composed of predominantly neutrophils with lymphocytes, histiocytes, and eosinophils (see Fig. 50.4) [1]. Late lesions can demonstrate many histiocytes. In addition, a histiocytoid variant has been described.
- Leukocytoclasis is common [1]
- Vasculitis is generally absent [1]

The diagnosis is made using a combination of [1]:

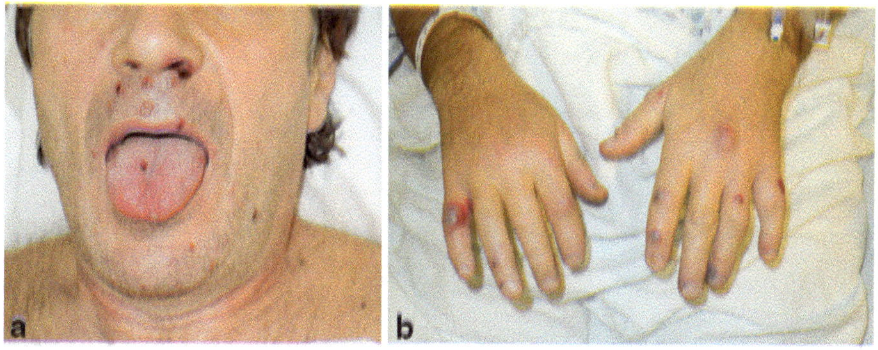

Fig. 50.3 Sweet's syndrome. Oral ulcers (**a**) and edematous, purulent papules (**b**)

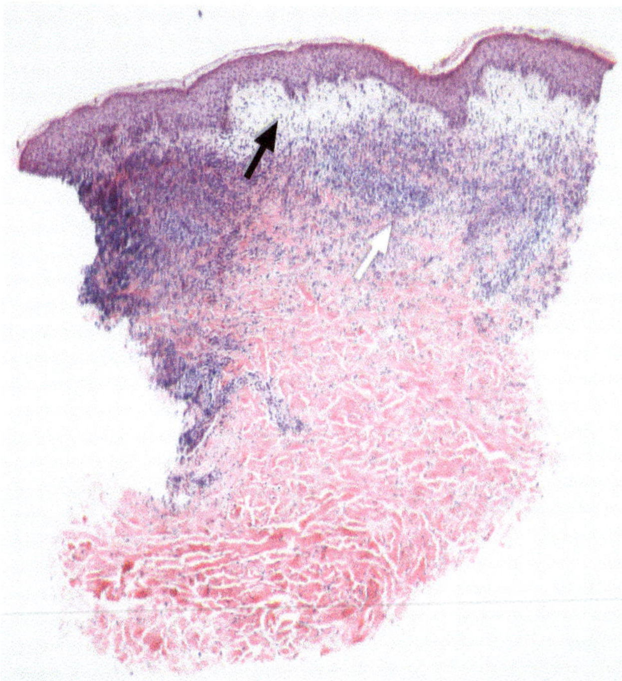

Fig. 50.4 Sweet's syndrome. A photomicrograph showing superficial dermal edema (*black arrow*) and a diffuse dermal neutrophilic infiltrate (*white arrow*)

- CBC/smear/bone marrow biopsy and aspirate/serum and urine protein electrophoresis/urinary analysis/liver enzymes/ESR/CRP
- Colonoscopy if symptoms of IBD
- Biopsy

The differential diagnosis should include:

- Pyoderma gangrenosum
- Erythema multiforme
- Urticarial vasculitis
- Bowel-associated dermatosis–arthritis syndrome
- Halogenoderma
- Neutrophilic eccrine hidradenitis
- Granulomatous disease
- Cutaneous infection
- Malignancy

Treatment options include:

- Treat underlying cause [3]
- Simple occurrence responds to topical steroids, NSAIDs [3]
- Severe disease may require oral corticosteroids, dapsone, potassium iodide, colchicine, cyclosporine A, anti-TNF-α antibodies [1–3]

References

1. Timani S, Mutasim DF. Skin manifestations of inflammatory bowel disease. Clin Dermatol. 2008;26:265–73.
2. Larsen S, Bendtzen K, Nielsen OH. Extraintestinal manifestations of inflammatory bowel disease: epidemiology, diagnosis, and management. Ann Med. 2010;42:97–114.
3. Dabade TS, Davis MD. Diagnosis and treatment of the neutrophilic dermatoses (pyoderma gangrenosum, Sweet's syndrome). Dermatol Ther. 2011;24:273–84.

Hereditary Nonpolyposis Colorectal Cancer or Lynch Syndrome: Gastrointestinal Features

51

Omar Shahbaz

Hereditary nonpolyposis colorectal cancer (HNPCC) is a genetic condition in which mutations result in defects in DNA mismatch repair (MMR). It portends a higher risk for colon cancer with approximately an 80% lifetime risk and is inherited in an autosomal dominant fashion. Approximately 2–7% of all colorectal cancer in the United States is caused by these mutations with an average age of diagnosis of 44 years old [1].

Gastrointestinal (GI) symptoms associated with this condition are [2]:

- Presentation of colon carcinoma: anorexia, malaise, rectal bleeding, unexplained weight loss, abdominal pain, diarrhea, constipation, abnormal rectal examination, abdominal tenderness, iron deficiency anemia without an identifiable cause, positive fecal occult blood
- Symptoms of advanced disease: abdominal distention, obstipation, peritonitis, weight loss, jaundice, cachexia
- Symptoms of metastasis: abdominal mass, hepatomegaly, groin, or supraclavicular lymphadenopathy, portal obstruction, obstruction, perforation, hemorrhage

Clinical signs and findings are [2]:

- Early age of onset and multiplicity of cancers
- In HNPCC, the mean age of initial colorectal cancer diagnosis is 45 compared to 65 years of age for sporadic colorectal cancer; some patients present with colorectal cancer in their twenties
- Greater than 10% of patients have had more than one cancer by time of diagnosis
- Increased incidence of the following cancers: colorectal (see Figs. 51.1 and 51.2) [3] endometrial, ovarian, upper urological tract, gastric, small bowel, biliary/pancreatic, skin (sebaceous adenomas, carcinomas, and keratoacanthomas), as well as brain tumors
- Synchronous or metachronous tumors

Pathogenesis involves specific genetic mutations [1, 4, 5]:

- Autosomal dominant, hereditary abnormality in the MMR genes
- Most common MMR genes involved are *MSH2* and *MLH1*; other MMR genes include *MSH6* and *PMS2*
- Tumors are thought to arise from preexisting adenomas, which are not more frequent but have increased potential for malignancy
- Subtypes:
  - Muir–Torre syndrome: HNPCC with associated sebaceous neoplasms, cutaneous keratoacanthomas, and visceral carcinomas
  - Turcot's syndrome: HNPCC with associated brain tumors, typically gliomas

Pathology can show [1, 2]:

- Adenomas, often villous, with components of high-grade dysplasia and demonstrating accelerated rate of malignant transformation
- More aggressive histology compared to sporadic colorectal cancer: increased frequency of poorly differentiated (see Fig. 51.3), mucinous and signet ring cells (see Fig. 51.4).

The diagnosis is made by considering [4–6]:

- Fulfillment of Amsterdam or Bethesda criteria; examination of tumor tissue is indicated. Tests include immunohistochemistry testing (IHC), microsatellite instability testing (MSI), and DNA analysis.
- Revised Bethesda Guidelines for Testing Colorectal Tumors for Microsatellite Instability [5]:
  - Colorectal cancer diagnosed before age 50
  - Presence of synchronous, metachronous colorectal, or other HNPCC-associated tumors regardless of age (colorectal, endometrial, stomach, ovarian, pancreas, ureter and renal pelvis, biliary tract [usually glioblastoma] tumors, sebaceous gland adenomas and keratoacanthomas in Muir–Torre syndrome and carcinoma of the small bowel

O. Shahbaz (✉)
Department of Internal Medicine,
University of Connecticut Health Center, Farmington, CT, USA
e-mail: omshahbaz@resident.uchc.edu

G.Y. Wu et al. (eds.), *Atlas of Dermatological Manifestations of Gastrointestinal Disease*,
DOI 10.1007/978-1-4614-6191-3_51, © Springer Science+Business Media New York 2013

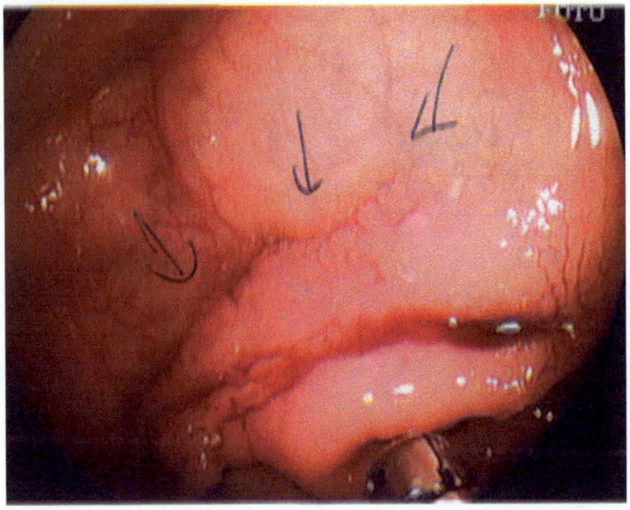

Fig. 51.1 An endoscopic view of an HNPCC found during screening colonoscopy. The polyp appeared as a small irregular area of mucosa in the cecum (*arrows*) (From Baiocchi et al. [3]; with permission)

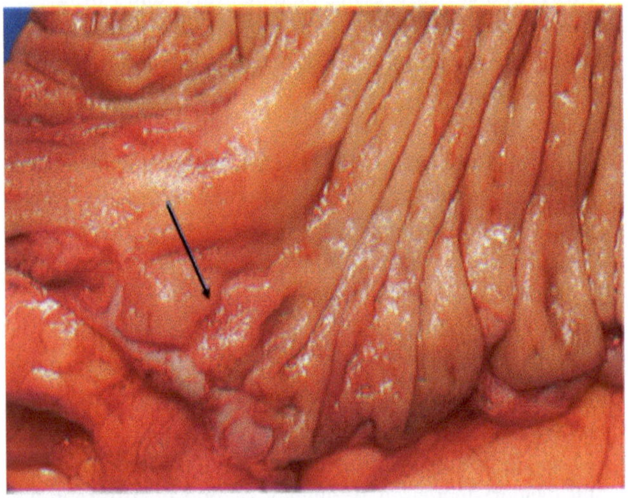

Fig. 51.2 The resected specimen showing the small irregular sessile nature of the lesion (*arrow*) (From Baiocchi et al. [3]; with permission)

- Colorectal cancer with MSI-high (MSI-H)-like histology diagnosed before age 60
- Colorectal cancer diagnosed in a patient with one or more first degree relatives with an HNPCC-related tumor, with one of the cancers diagnosed before age 50 years
- Colorectal cancer diagnosed in a patient with two or more first or second-degree relatives with HNPCC-related tumors, regardless of age

• Amsterdam II criteria for clinical identification of individuals with HNPCC:

- Three or more relatives with HNPCC-associated cancer (e.g., colorectal cancer, endometrial, small bowel,

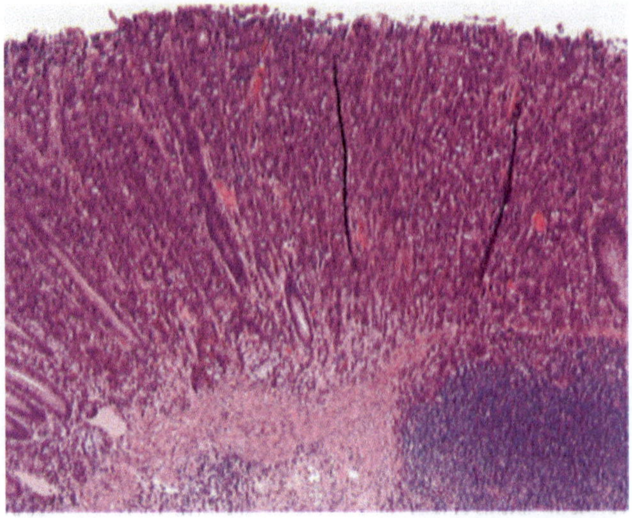

Fig. 51.3 A photomicrograph showing poorly differentiated adenocarcinoma with a signet ring cell component (hematoxylin and eosin [H and E] stain; low power) (From Baiocchi et al. [3]; with permission)

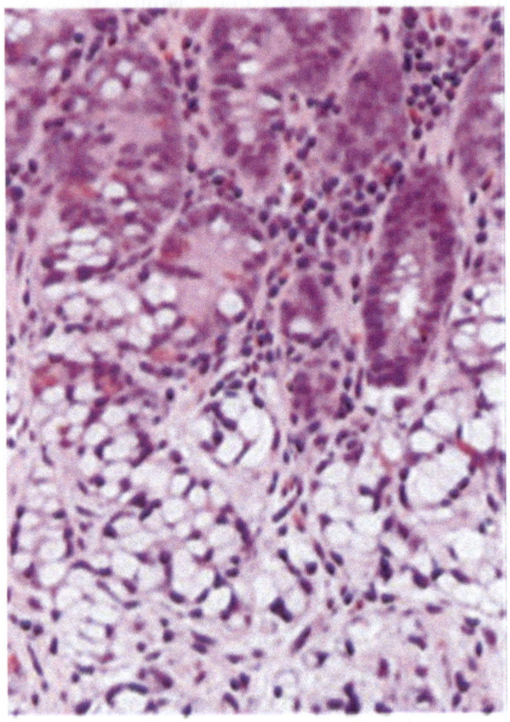

Fig. 51.4 A photomicrograph showing signet-ring cella (H and E stain; high power) (From Baiocchi et al. [3]; with permission)

ureter, renal–pelvis cancer); one should be first-degree relative of other two
- Two or more successive generations affected
- One or more relatives diagnosed before age 50
- Familial adenomatous polyposis should be ruled out in cases of colorectal carcinoma
- Tumors should be verified by pathological examination

The differential diagnosis of hereditary nonpolyposis colorectal cancer should include [4–6]:

- Familial polyposis coli
- Gardner's syndrome
- Other family cancer syndromes: Li-Fraumeni syndrome, Von Hippel Lindau disease, *BRCA1* gene, multiple endocrine neoplasia 2A and 2B

The treatment involves [7–10]:

- Diet
  - No specific dietary interventions (European Society for Medical Oncology [ESMO] grade C)
- Medications
  - No specific chemoprevention (ESMO grade A)
  - Aspirin associated with reduced risk of colorectal cancer in patients with Lynch syndrome (level 2 evidence)
- Surgery
  - Colectomy
    - Prophylactic colectomy not recommended for healthy mutation carriers (ESMO grade C)
    - Discuss option of extended colectomy versus need for intensive surveillance after standard surgery at time of diagnosis of colorectal cancer, especially in young patients with Lynch syndrome (ESMO grade C)
  - Hysterectomy and bilateral salpingo-oophorectomy
    - Prophylactic hysterectomy with bilateral salpingo-oophorectomy may prevent endometrial and ovarian cancer in women with Lynch syndrome (level 2 evidence)
- Follow-up
  - Smoking cessation
  - Cancer screening
    - ESMO recommendations for cancer surveillance
      - Start colonoscopy at age 20–25 years and repeat every 1–2 years; upper age limit not established (ESMO grade C, level III)
      - Endometrial and ovarian cancer screening
        - Annually starting at age 30–35 years including: gynecological examination, pelvic ultrasound, CA-125 analysis, aspiration biopsy
        - ESMO Grade C Level III
      - Tests for other associated cancers based on family history may include the following:
        - Upper endoscopy, abdominal ultrasound with urine cytology starting at age 30–35 years and repeated every 1–2 years (ESMO grade C, level III)
    - Recommendations based on systematic review
      - Colonoscopy recommended every 1–2 years starting at age 20–25 years (age 30 years if MSH6 mutations) or 10 years younger than youngest age of person diagnosed in family
      - Other recommendations despite no demonstrated efficacy:
        - Endometrial sampling and transvaginal ultrasound or uterus and ovaries annually starting at age 30–35 years
        - Urinalysis with cytology annually starting at age 25–35 years
        - History, examination, education, and genetic counseling annually starting at age 21 years
    - Screening guidelines from Johns Hopkins University
      - Colonoscopy every 1–3 years starting at age 25 years or 5–10 years earlier than youngest age of colorectal cancer in the family
      - Fecal occult blood testing every year starting with age of first colonoscopy

References

1. Ponti G, Ponz de Leon M. Muir-Torre syndrome. Lancet Oncol. 2005;6:980–7.
2. Hamilton W, Round A, Sharp D, Peters TJ. Clinical features of colorectal cancer before diagnosis: a population-based case-control study. Br J Cancer. 2005;93:399–405.
3. Baiocchi GL, Mazza G, Baronchelli C, et al. Right colon cancer missed by virtual colonoscopy in HNPCC patient. J Gastrointest Canc. 2011;43:518–20. Oct 11 (Epub ahead of print).
4. Vasen HF, Watson P, Mecklin JP, Lynch HT. New clinical criteria for hereditary nonpolyposis colorectal cancer (HNPCC, Lynch syndrome) proposed by the International Collaborative Group on HNPCC. Gastroenterology. 1999;116:1453–6.
5. Umar A, Boland CR, Terdiman JP, et al. Revised Bethesda guidelines for hereditary nonpolyposis colorectal cancer (Lynch syndrome) and microsatellite instability. J Natl Cancer Inst. 2004;96:261–8.
6. Balmaña J, Castells A, Cervantes A, ESMO Guidelines Working Group. Familial colorectal cancer risk: ESMO clinical practice guidelines. Ann Oncol. 2010;21:v78–81.
7. Burn J, Gerdes AM, Mecklin JP, et al. Long-term effect of aspirin on cancer risk in carriers of hereditary colorectal cancer: an analysis from the CAPP2 randomised controlled trial. Lancet. 2011;378:2081–7.
8. Schmeler KM, Lynch HT, Chen LM, et al. Prophylactic surgery to reduce the risk of gynecologic cancers in the Lynch syndrome. N Engl J Med. 2006;354:261–269.
9. Markowitz SD. Aspirin and colon cancer—targeting prevention? N Engl J Med. 2007;356:2195–8.
10. Lindor NM, Petersen GM, Hadley DW, et al. Recommendations for the care of individuals with an inherited predisposition to Lynch syndrome: a systemic review. JAMA. 2006;296:1507–17.
11. Screening guidelines from Johns Hopkins University. Cortlandt Forum. 2004;17:66.

Muir–Torre Syndrome: Dermatological Features

52

Liam Zakko, Justin Finch, Marti J. Rothe, and Jane M. Grant-Kels

Clinical signs and features include:

- Sebaceous neoplasms: particularly sebaceous adenomas, epitheliomas, and carcinomas
- Sebaceous adenomas are the most common sebaceous neoplasm associated with Muir–Torre syndrome (MTS) and appear as yellowish circumscribed papules or nodules, which most commonly present on the face but in MTS they are more often on the trunk [1]
- Sebaceous epitheliomas (sebaceoma): appear as yellow papules or nodules or plaques occasionally with rolled borders; usually are solitary; commonly ulcerate and bleed; some experts believe basal cell carcinoma with sebaceous differentiation is the same entity as sebaceous epithelioma [2]
- Sebaceous hyperplasia may be associated with MTS but is not specific for MTS and is very common in general population (see Fig. 52.1)
- Sebaceous carcinoma, except in patients with MTS, is usually periocular and may appear as a subcutaneous nodule, thickening of skin, or pedunculated tumor and often mimics chalazion; sebaceous carcinoma is more typically extraocular in MTS [3]
- May also see keratoacanthomas with sebaceous differentiation: firm, dome-shaped, erythematous nodule with a central keratin plug that grows rapidly and can be several centimeters in diameter (see Fig. 52.2)
- Visceral malignancy: nearly one half of patients have two or more visceral malignancies; the most common first malignancy is colon cancer accounting for nearly half of cancers; nearly one fourth of patients with MTS have colonic polyps; MTS can also be associated with other digestive tract cancers; genitourinary cancers account for nearly one fourth of visceral cancers; breast cancer, 12%; hematologic cancer, 9% [1, 2]
- Median age at diagnosis of cancer: 55 years; 22–32% of patients present with sebaceous neoplasm before the internal cancer; 9–12% are diagnosed simultaneously with sebaceous neoplasm and internal cancer; 56–59% are diagnosed with internal cancer before the sebaceous neoplasm [2]

Pathogenesis of this disease involves:

- Autosomal dominant with high penetrance but variable expression
- DNA mismatch repair gene is defective leading to microsatellite instability (MSI) [4]
- Appears to be a component of hereditary nonpolyposis coli cancer syndrome (Lynch syndrome), with loss of MSH-2 more common than MLH-1 and rarely MSH-6 mutations [4]

Histopathological features include:

- Sebaceous adenoma: well-circumscribed multilobulated neoplasm often in continuity with overlying squamous epithelium composed of predominantly (>50%) mature sebocytes centrally in addition to basaloid seboblastic cells noted in multiple layers at the periphery of each lobule. The distribution of the seboblastic cells and sebocytes as well as transitional cells can vary from within lobules (see Fig. 52.3)
- Sebaceous epithelioma or sebaceoma has a more irregularly shaped lobules or masses of cells with a

L. Zakko (✉)
Yale Department of Internal Medicine, 20 York Street, Yale New Haven Hospital, New Haven, CT 05610, USA
e-mail: liam.zakko@yale.edu

J. Finch • M.J. Rothe • J.M. Grant-Kels
Department of Dermatology, University of Connecticut Health Center, 21 South Road, Farmington, CT 06030, USA
e-mail: finch@uchc.edu; rothe@uchc.edu; grant@uchc.edu

G.Y. Wu et al. (eds.), *Atlas of Dermatological Manifestations of Gastrointestinal Disease*,
DOI 10.1007/978-1-4614-6191-3_52,

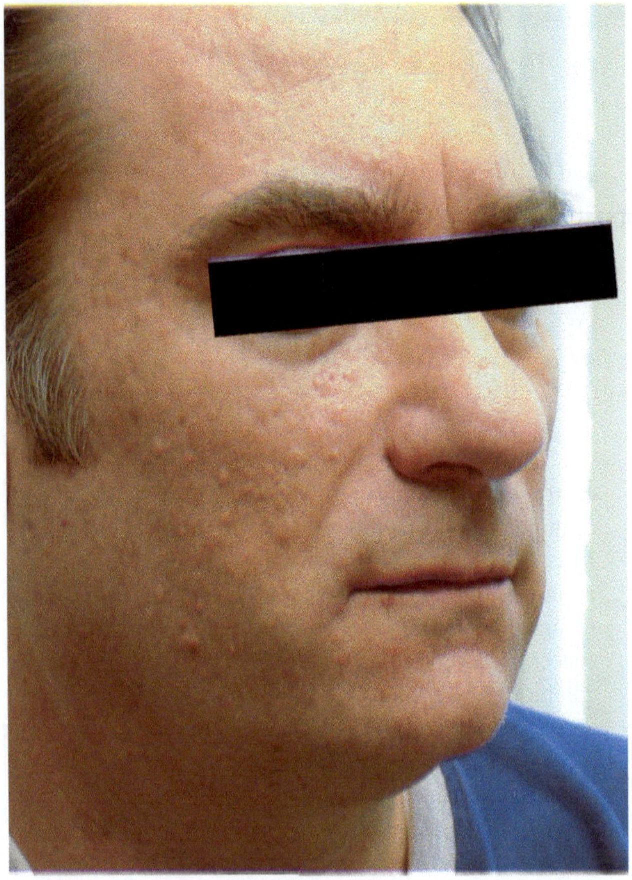

Fig. 52.1 Extensive sebaceous hyperplasia

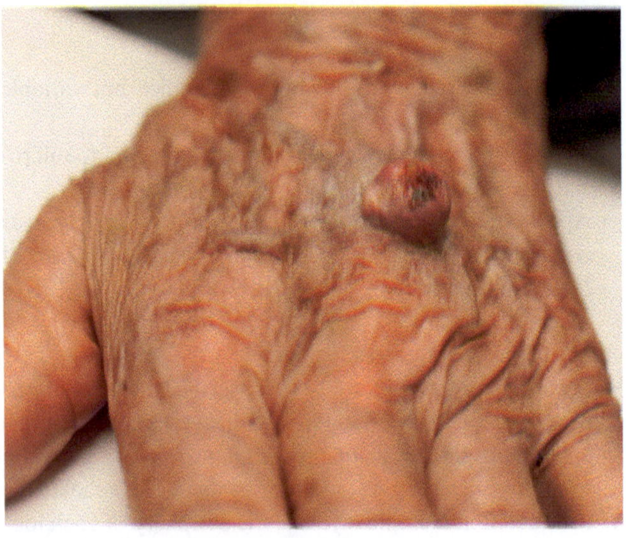

Fig. 52.2 Keratoacanthoma. Crateriform nodule on the dorsal hand, with hyperkeratotic core

preponderance (>50%) of undifferentiated germinative seboblastic cells plus scattered transitional cells and aggregates of central mature sebocytes

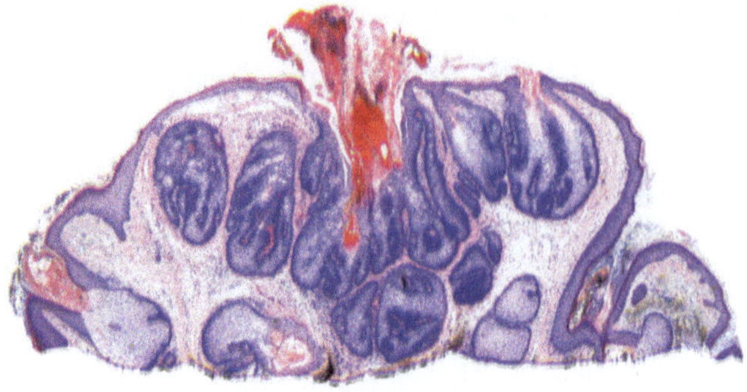

Fig. 52.3 Sebaceous adenoma. Circumscribed lobular tumor comprising sebaceous cells and basaloid cells (40×)

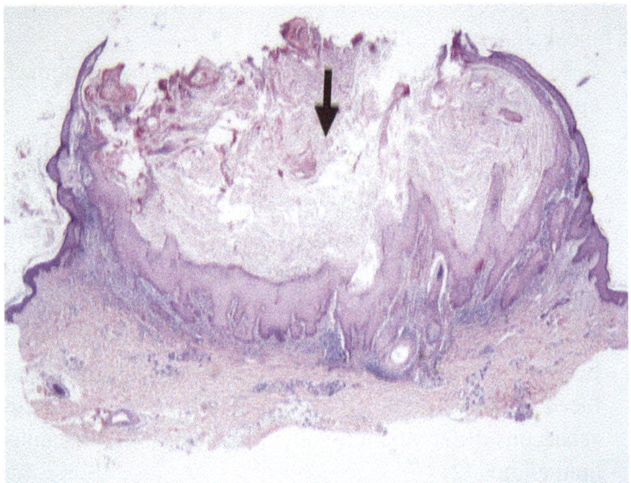

Fig. 52.4 Keratoacanthoma. Well-circumscribed keratin-filled crater (*arrow*) surrounded by pale, glassy keratinocytes (10×)

- Sebaceous carcinoma: asymmetrical, poorly circumscribed, infiltrating neoplasm composed of germinative cells plus some cells demonstrating sebaceous differentiation, evidence of mitotic figures as well as cellular/nuclear pleomorphism/hyperchromatism; more likely MTS if periocular
- Keratoacanthoma: atypical squamous neoplasm with an exo- and endophytic architecture and a central horn filled crater; if contains sebaceous differentiation more likely to be MTS (see Fig. 52.4)

The diagnosis is made using a combination of:

- One of A and B or all of C with no other etiology of the findings [5]:
  - Group A: sebaceous adenoma, sebaceous epithelioma, sebaceous carcinoma, keratoacanthoma with sebaceous differentiation
  - Group B: a visceral malignancy
  - Group C: multiple keratoacanthomas, multiple visceral malignancies, family history of MTS

- The identification of a sebaceous neoplasm on the trunk or extremities in a patient younger than 50 years old warrants additional work-up [4]
  - If immunohistochemistry testing of the neoplasm shows absence of expression of MSH-2, MSH-1, or MSH-6, then MSI analysis is recommended.
  - If MSI is detected, then the proband and family should have cancer surveillance
  - If MSI is not detected but there is a positive family history for MTS, then germline mutation analysis should be performed and, if positive, the proband and family should have cancer surveillance
  - If MSI is not detected and family history is negative for MTS, then no further testing is recommended

The differential diagnosis should include:

- Sebaceous hyperplasia
- Cowden's disease
- Multiple trichoepitheliomas
- Basal cell nevus syndrome
- Ferguson–Smith syndrome
- Tuberous sclerosis
- Extramammary Paget's disease
- Metastatic renal clear cell carcinoma
- Balloon cell melanoma
- Metastatic sebaceous carcinoma of the parotid gland

Treatment options include [1, 6]:

- Sebaceous adenoma and epithelioma: excision/cryosurgery
- Sebaceous carcinoma: wide excision or Mohs surgery
- Keratoacanthoma: excision or Mohs surgery
- Oral isotretinoin alone or in combination with interferon-α may prevent or partially treat cutaneous lesions

References

1. Ponti G, Ponz de Leon M. Muir–Torre syndrome. Lancet Oncol. 2005;6:980–7.
2. Eisen DB, Michael DJ. Sebaceous lesions and their associated syndromes: part II. J Am Acad Dermatol. 2009;61:563–78.
3. Shalin SC, Lyle S, Calonje E, Lazar AJF. Sebaceous neoplasia and the Muir–Torre syndrome: important connections with clinical implications. Histopathology. 2010;56:133–47.
4. Abbas O, Mahalingam M. Cutaneous sebaceous neoplasms as markers of Muir-Torre syndrome: a diagnostic algorithm. J Cutan Pathol. 2009;36:613–9.
5. Schwartz RA, Torre DP. The Muir–Torre syndrome: a 25 year retrospective. J Am Acad Dermatol. 1995;33:90–104.
6. Eisen DB, Michael DJ. Sebaceous lesions and their associated syndromes: part I. J Am Acad Dermatol. 2009;61:549–60.

Part IV

Abdominal Pain

Hereditary Angioedema: Gastrointestinal Features

53

Jameel Uddeen

Hereditary angioedema has a bimodal distribution with peak incidences in the second and fourth decades and is characterized by local swelling in subcutaneous tissues. Diagnosis must generally be made during an acute episode [1].

The most common gastrointestinal (GI) symptoms are [1–3]:

- Vomiting particularly early in attack
- Acute severe abdominal pain; <24 h up to 5 days
- Can also present with chronic recurring abdominal pain
- Diarrhea, usually watery
- Nausea
- Prodromal phase including increased irritability, aggressiveness, fatigue, hunger

Clinical signs and findings include [1–3]:

- Bowel edema (see Fig. 53.1a, c, e) [4]
- Usually hypoactive bowel sounds, can be hyperactive
- Tenderness and at times rebound tenderness
- Bowel edema can result in obstruction, limited biliary drainage resulting in gallbladder disease or pancreatitis
- Hypotension
- Ascites
- Skin edema, nonpitting, nonerythematous affecting face, extremities, and genitals
- Laryngeal edema

The pathogenesis appears to involve genetic mutations [5]:

- Mutation in one of two copies of the plasma protein C1 inhibitor, with the product of one gene unable to control generation of bradykinin. Low levels of C1 inhibitor and/or poorly functional C1 inhibitor, which is unable to bind the usual substrates and unable to inhibit activation of the contact/fibrinolytic and classical complement pathways. This results in vasodilation, increased capillary permeability, fluid extravasation, and edema.

The typical pathology will show [1, 5, 6]:

- Gross: edematous thickening of the intestinal wall (see Fig. 53.1b, d, f) [4]
- Histological: perivascular mononuclear cell infiltrate, moderate nonspecific inflammatory cell infiltration, and edema of lamina propria

The diagnosis is made by [1, 5, 6]:

- Laboratory: C1 inhibitor (C1-Inh) level, C2 level, C3 Level, C4 level, C1 esterase inhibitor function, complete blood count, electrolytes, liver enzymes,
- Imaging: abdominal ultrasound (see Fig. 53.1a, c, e) [4], CT abdomen (see Figs. 53.1 and 53.2) [7], abdominal radiograph

The differential diagnosis of hereditary angioedema includes [1, 3, 5]:

- Mesenteric vein thrombosis
- Irritable bowel syndrome
- Inflammatory bowel disease
- Vasculitis
- Intramural hemorrhage
- Acute ileitis (*Yersinia, Campylobacter* infections)
- Gastroesophageal reflux disease
- Peptic ulcer disease
- Peritoneal carcinomatosis
- Acquired angioedema
- Allergic angioedema
- Angiotensin-converting-enzyme inhibitor–induced angioedema
- Idiopathic angioedema

There is no cure but symptomatic treatment involves [3, 6]:

- Chronic long-term prophylaxis: 17 alpha-alkylated androgens (danazol, oxandrolone, stanozolol). Antifibrinolytic agents (epsilon-aminocaproic acid, tranexamic acid), C1-Inh
- Short-term prophylaxis: fresh frozen plasma (FFP) 1–12 h before provoking event, C1-Inh, 17 alpha-alkylated androgens 5–10 days before provoking event
- Acute attacks: epinephrine, C1-Inh, FFP

J. Uddeen (✉)
Department of Internal Medicine, University of Connecticut Health Center, Farmington, CT, USA

University of Connecticut, 2 Earls Court Unit E, Farmington, CT 06032, USA
e-mail: uddeen@resident.uchc.edu

G.Y. Wu et al. (eds.), *Atlas of Dermatological Manifestations of Gastrointestinal Disease*,
DOI 10.1007/978-1-4614-6191-3_53, © Springer Science+Business Media New York 2013

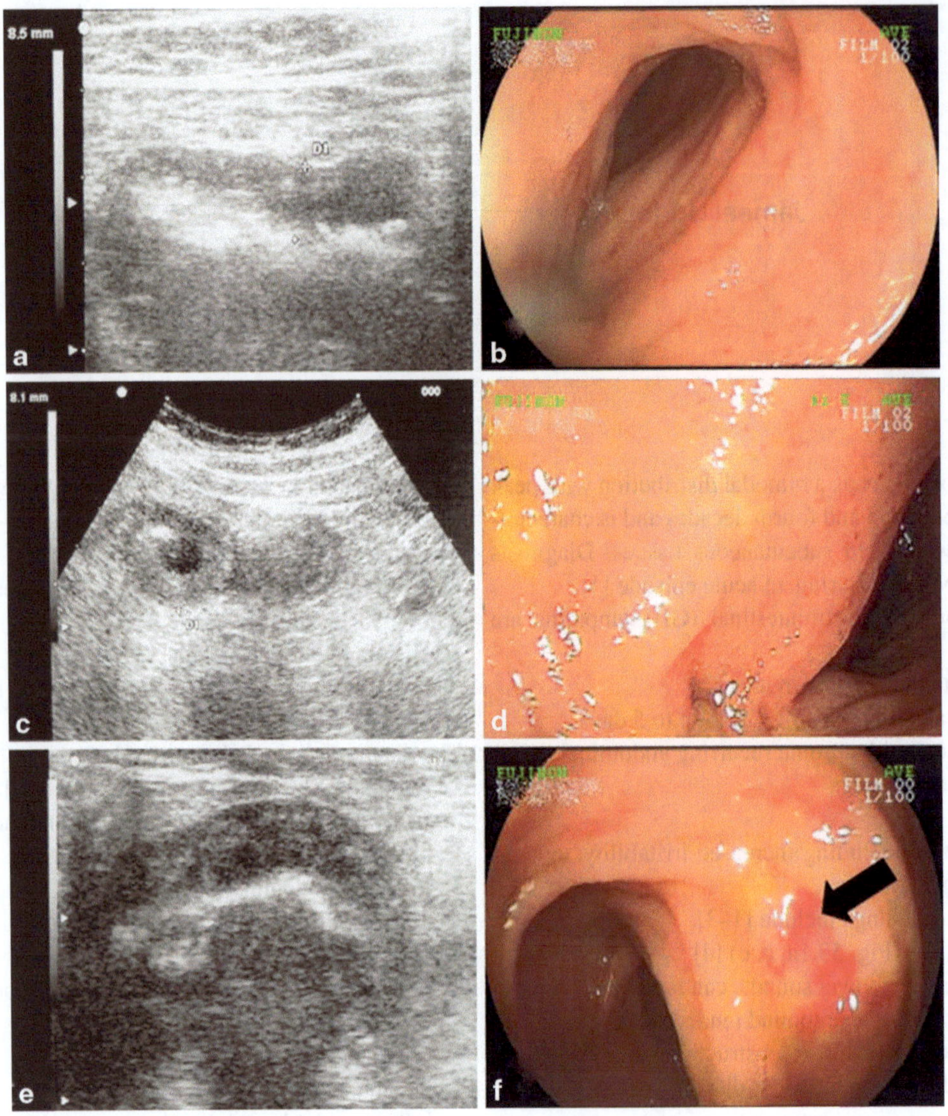

Fig. 53.1 Transabdominal ultrasound. Longitudinal (**a**) and transverse sections (**c** and **e**) of small bowel wall showing edema in a patient with hereditary angioedema during an episode of abdominal pain. (**b**) A double-balloon endoscopic view of edematous jejunum during an episode of abdominal pain without magnification. (**d**) With magnification. (**f**) Demonstrating petechial bleeding and generalized edema in the ileum with focal inflammatory lesions (*arrow*) (From Spahn et al. [4]; with permission)

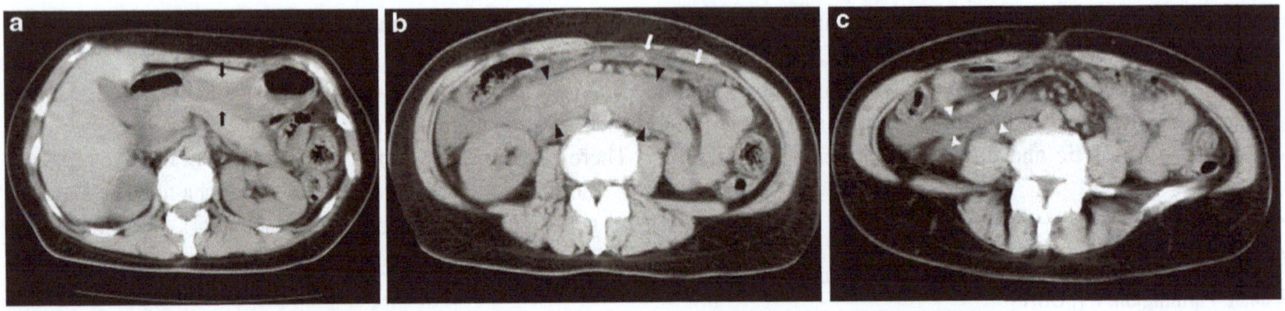

Fig. 53.2 Abdominal computed tomography images of circumferential wall thickening (**a**) of the gastric antrum (*arrows*). (**b**) Marked dilatation of the third part of the duodenum (*arrowheads*), with thickening of the omentum (*arrows*) also present. (**c**) Retroperitoneal edema (*arrowheads*) and thickening of the small bowel mesentery (From Wakisaka et al. [7]; with permission)

- Symptomatic treatment: narcotic analgesics, antiemetics, and aggressive fluids

References

1. Frank MM. Hereditary angioedema. J Allergy Clin Immunol. 2008;121:398–401.
2. Bork K, Staubach P, Eckardt AJ, Hardt J. Symptoms, course, and complications of abdominal attacks in hereditary angioedema due to C1 inhibitor deficiency. Am J Gastroenterol. 2006;101:619–27.
3. Nzeako UC, Frigas E, Tremaine WJ, et al. Hereditary angioedema as a cause of transient abdominal pain. J Clin Gastroenterol. 2002;34:57–61.
4. Spahn TW, Grosse-Thie W, Mueller MK. Endoscopic visualization of angiotensin-converting enzyme inhibitor-induced small bowel angioedema as a cause of relapsing abdominal pain using double-balloon enteroscopy. Dig Dis Sci. 2008;53:1257–60.
5. Agostoni A, Aygören-Pürsün E, Binkley KE, et al. Hereditary and acquired angioedema: problems and progress: proceedings of the third C1 esterase inhibitor deficiency workshop and beyond. J Allergy Clin Immunol. 2004;114:S51–S131.
6. Nzeako UC. Diagnosis and management of angioedema with abdominal involvement: a gastroenterology perspective. World J Gastroenterol. 2010;16:4913–21.
7. Wakisaka M, Shuto M, Abe H, et al. Computed tomography of the gastrointestinal manifestation of hereditary angioedema. Radiat Med. 2008;26:618–21.

54 Hereditary Angioedema: Dermatological Features

Liam Zakko, Justin Finch, Marti J. Rothe, and Jane M. Grant-Kels

Clinical signs and features include:

- Affects 1:10,000–1:50,000 persons; begins in childhood and worsens after puberty, although severity lessens after the sixth decade of life [1]
- Characterized by recurrent swelling attacks of the face, abdomen, extremities, genitalia, oropharynx, and/or larynx without urticaria and typically unilateral, nonpruritic, nonpitting, uncomfortable but painless (see Fig. 54.1)
- Fifty percent of patients have an episode of laryngeal edema at some point with a mortality rate as high as 30% [1]
- When affecting the gastrointestinal (GI) tract, attacks present with severe abdominal pain, nausea, vomiting, and diarrhea
- Without treatment, patients experience swelling episodes every 7–14 days [1]. Swelling episodes generally worsen for 12–36 h, peak, and then improve in 2–3 days [1]
- Aura/prodromal symptoms such as tingling, headache, mood changes, and anxiety are common and may be followed by erythema marginatum. This nonpruritic rash is characterized by serpiginous, slightly raised borders and affects the trunk and inner surfaces of the extremities. Attacks of angioedema may have triggers (trauma, especially dental procedures, surgery, menstruation, oral contraceptives, hormone replacement therapy, angiotensin-converting enzyme [ACE] inhibitors, infection, stress) but they often occur without an inciting event.
- Associated with autoimmune diseases, particularly glomerulonephritis, systemic lupus erythematosus, Sjögren syndrome, thyroiditis [2]

Pathogenesis of this disease involves:

- Autosomal dominant: 75% with a family history, 25% spontaneous mutations; mutation on chromosome 11; significant variability in penetrance [3]
- Functional deficiency of C1 esterase inhibitor (C1-Inh) results in increased bradykinin formation

Histopathological features include:

- Edema of deep dermis and underlying subcutaneous fat, fascia, muscles
- Separation of collagen bundles due to the edema (see Fig. 54.2)
- Vascular dilation with wide endothelial cell gaps and extravasation of vascular contents
- Scant mononuclear cells perivascularly but a paucity of immune cells compared with an allergic reaction
- Erythema marginatum: perivascular and interstitial neutrophils with lymphocytes but without vasculitis; dense deposits of bradykinin in stromal and endothelial tissue seen via immunofluorescence [4]

The diagnosis is made using a combination of:

- Clinical signs: attacks aggravated by estrogen and unresponsive to corticosteroids, antihistamines, and epinephrine
- Measurement of complement levels [5]:
  - Type 1 (85% of cases): C1-Inh deficiency; decreased C1-Inh antigen; C4 decreased between and during attacks
  - Type 2 (15% of case): C1-Inh functional abnormality; C1-Inh antigen normal to increased; C4 decreased between and during attacks
  - Type 3 occurs primarily in women and is often estrogen dependent; C1-Inh levels and function are normal; C4 and other complement levels are normal; factor XII mutation may be present

L. Zakko (✉)
Yale Department of Internal Medicine, 20 York Street, Yale New Haven Hospital, New Haven, CT 06510, USA
e-mail: liam.zakko@yale.edu

J. Finch • M.J. Rothe • J.M. Grant-Kels
Department of Dermatology, University of Connecticut Health Center, 21 South Road, Farmington, CT 06030, USA
e-mail: finch@uchc.edu; rothe@uchc.edu; grant@uchc.edu

G.Y. Wu et al. (eds.), *Atlas of Dermatological Manifestations of Gastrointestinal Disease*, DOI 10.1007/978-1-4614-6191-3_54, © Springer Science+Business Media New York 2013

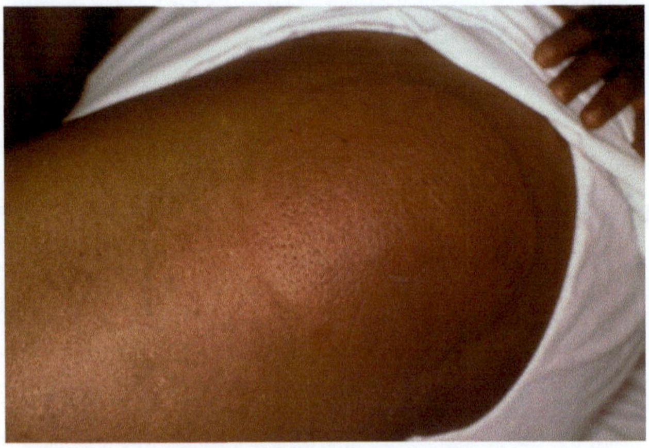

Fig. 54.1 Angioedema. Large, indurated erythematous plaque on the thigh with peau d'orange appearance of the surface (Image courtesy of Yale Residency Collection)

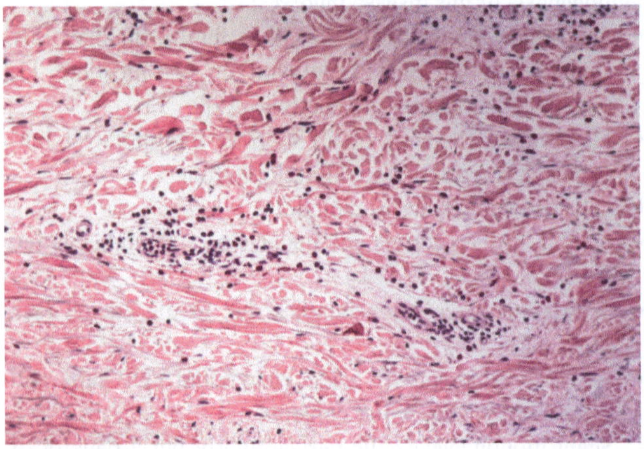

Fig. 54.2 Angioedema. Intense dermal edema causes separation of collagen bundles. Perivascular mast cells and eosinophils are sometimes seen (100×)

- Difficult to diagnose because symptoms overlap with common medical illnesses; diagnosis is often made after >10 years of symptoms

The differential diagnosis should include:

- ACE inhibitor-induced angioedema
- Acquired angioedema
- Acquired C1-Inh deficiency
- Type III angioedema
- Acute allergen angioedema
- Delayed pressure angioedema
- Nonsteroidal anti-inflammatory drug–associated angioedema
- Muckler–Wells syndrome
- Cytokine-induced angioedema
- Clarkson's syndrome
- Nonepisodic angioedema
- Episodic angioedema with eosinophilia
- Rheumatism

Treatment options include:

- Traditional: trigger avoidance; supportive measures especially airway management; androgens and antifibrinolytics agents for prophylaxis in patient with frequent attacks, although these have numerous side effects
- New treatments: C1-Inh replacement therapy (Cinryze, Berinert) to treat acute attacks and for prophylaxis; ecallantide: selective recombinant kallikrein inhibitor; given subcutaneously for treatment of acute attacks (carries black box warning because of allergy/anaphylaxis in 3.9%; Icatibant: bradykinin receptor blocker for treatment of acute attacks with much less allergy risk than ecallantide but can have injection site reactions [1, 3, 5]

References

1. Moellman JJ, Bernstein JA. Diagnosis and management of hereditary angioedema: an emergency medicine perspective. J Emerg Med. 2012;43(2):391–400. Epub ahead of print.
2. Kaplan AP, Greaves MW. Angioedema. J Am Acad Dermatol. 2005;53:373–88.
3. Kanani A, Schellenberg R, Warrington R. Urticaria and angioedema. Allergy Asthma Clin Immunol. 2011;7:S9.
4. Sheffer AL, Craig JM, Willms-Kretschmer K, et al. Histopathological and ultrastructural observations on tissues from patients with hereditary angioneurotic edema. J Allergy. 1971;47:292–7.
5. Firszt R, Frank MM. An overview of novel therapies for acute hereditary angioedema. Am J Clin Dermatol. 2010;11:383–8.

Part V

Metabolic Disturbances

Glucagonoma: Gastrointestinal Features

55

Marie Lourdes Ynson

Glucagonoma is a rare tumor of alpha cells in the pancreas. This disease results in glucagon overproduction of approximately 1,000 times normal. The incidence of this pathology is thought to be 1 in 20 million, although this is likely an underestimation given the lack of specific symptoms. The effect on long-term survival is not known because of the rarity of the condition. Although it originates in the pancreas, the effects of this disease are widespread and can affect multiple organ systems [1, 2].

Clinical signs and findings include [3]:

- This is associated with a *glucagonoma syndrome* with the following clinical findings:
  - Weight loss (80%)
  - Glucose intolerance (40–90%)
  - Normochromic, normocytic anemia (35–90%)
  - Hypoaminoacidemia (80%)
  - Diarrhea (25%)
  - Thromboembolism (15–25%)
  - Glossitis, cheilosis (15–40%)
  - Psychiatric symptoms (0–17%)

The pathogenesis is not entirely understood [1, 2]:

- Glucagonoma is a type of pancreatic neuroendocrine tumor that secretes excessive amounts of the hormone glucagon
- Most of these tumors occur sporadically, but 5–17% of cases are associated with multiple endocrine neoplasia (MEN-1) syndrome.
- Most tumors are localized to the tail of the pancreas (see Figs. 55.1 and 55.2)
- These tumors are malignant in up to 60% of cases and are usually large (mean, 6 cm) at presentation
- There is a mean delay in diagnosis of 7 years, with some reports of up to 18 years
- Eighty percent of sporadic tumors demonstrate hepatic metastases at time of diagnosis

Pathology from specimens typically show [1–3]:

- Firm, encapsulated tumors consisting of islet cells that demonstrate glucagon within the cells by immunoperoxidase staining

The diagnosis is made by considering [1–3]:

- It has been recommended that all of the following criteria should be satisfied to diagnose a glucagonoma [3]:
  - Demonstration of a tumor mass by direct visualization (see Fig. 55.1, 55.2, 55.3) [4] or radiographic techniques
  - Proof that the tumor shows a preponderance of glucagon-containing cells on appropriate staining and/or proof of increased tissue levels of immunoreactive glucagon; chromogranin staining can demonstrate the neuroendocrine origin of the cells (see Fig. 55.4) [4]
  - Elevation of basal-circulating immunoreactive glucagon and at least one of the following coincidental findings:
    - Skin rash
    - Glucose intolerance
    - Hypoaminoacidemia
- However, in most studies, the findings of a pancreatic tumor and increased serum glucagon at levels >500–1,000 pg/mL are enough for a diagnosis of glucagonoma
- To localize the tumor, different imaging modalities can be used such as ultrasound, computed tomography scan, magnetic resonance imaging, somatostatin receptor scintigraphy, endoscopic ultrasound

The differential diagnosis of glucagonoma should include [1–3, 5]:

- The hyperglucagonemia of a glucagonoma should be differentiated from other causes of hyperglucagonemia such as cirrhosis, pancreatitis, diabetes mellitus, prolonged fasting, sepsis, burns, renal failure, familial hyperglucagonemia, and acromegaly

The treatment involves removal of the tumor or suppression of its activity [1–3, 5]:

- Localized tumors may be treated with surgery alone

M.L. Ynson (✉)
Department of Internal Medicine, University of Connecticut Health Center, Farmington, CT, USA
e-mail: mynson@resident.uchc.edu

G.Y. Wu et al. (eds.), *Atlas of Dermatological Manifestations of Gastrointestinal Disease*,
DOI 10.1007/978-1-4614-6191-3_55, © Springer Science+Business Media New York 2013

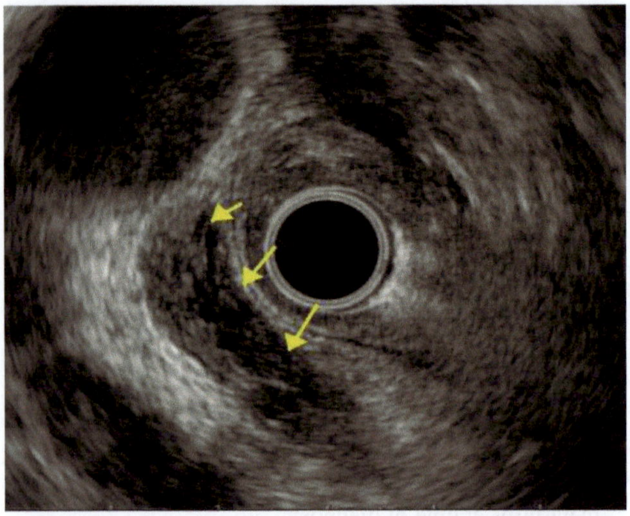

Fig. 55.1 A radial endoscopic ultrasound image showing mass (*arrows*) in pancreatic head

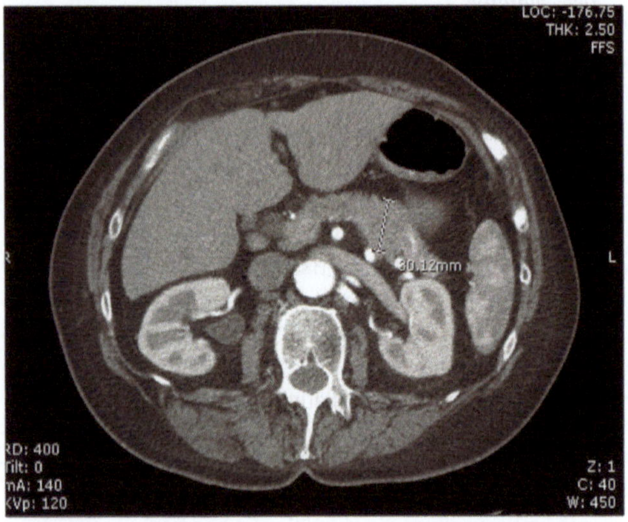

Fig. 55.2 A CT scan image showing mass in pancreatic tail, typical of glucagonoma

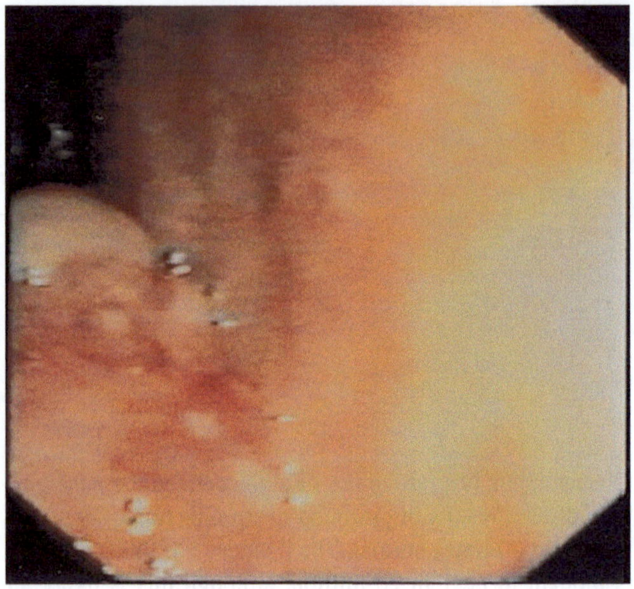

Fig. 55.3 Endoscopic image of the posterior portion of the duodenal bulb where a glucagonoma has eroded into mucosa (From Guirado et al. [4]; with permission)

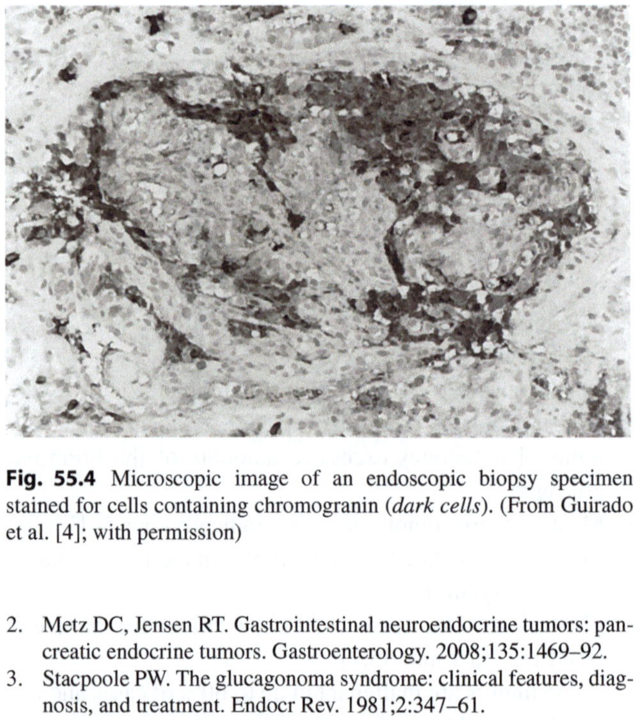

Fig. 55.4 Microscopic image of an endoscopic biopsy specimen stained for cells containing chromogranin (*dark cells*). (From Guirado et al. [4]; with permission)

- In metastatic disease, a combination of different treatment modalities can be used such as chemotherapy, α-interferon, somatostatin analogs, and liver chemoembolization
- Octreotide (somatostatin analog) given 100–500 μg subcutaneously three times a day decreases plasma glucagon levels in >80% of patients, which can reduce some glucagonoma syndrome symptoms

References

1. Simon P, Spilcke-Liss E, Wallaschofski H. Endocrine tumors of the pancreas. Endocrinol Metab Clin North Am. 2006;35:431–47.
2. Metz DC, Jensen RT. Gastrointestinal neuroendocrine tumors: pancreatic endocrine tumors. Gastroenterology. 2008;135:1469–92.
3. Stacpoole PW. The glucagonoma syndrome: clinical features, diagnosis, and treatment. Endocr Rev. 1981;2:347–61.
4. Guirado AG, Sanchez-Fayos P, Bosch O, et al. Endoscopic findings of a pancreatic glucagonoma. Dig Dis Sci. 2001;46:2779–82.
5. Kindmark H, Sundin A, Granberg D, et al. Endocrine pancreatic tumors with glucagon hypersecretion: a retrospective study of 23 cases during 20 years. Med Oncol. 2007;24:330–7.

Necrolytic Migratory Erythema

56

Liam Zakko, Justin Finch, Marti J. Rothe, and Jane M. Grant-Kels

Clinical signs and features include:

- Rare dermatitis that occurs mostly in patients with α-cell tumor of the pancreas (glucagonoma) that usually occurs in the fifth to sixth decade and presents with frequency of 1:20,000,000 persons/year [1]
- Rash comes in waves of irregular erythematous lesions with visible scale with subsequent necrosis and crusting of the epidermis in the center of the lesions leading to bullae [2]
- Central healing ultimately occurs giving the lesions an annular appearance; the process for development to healing is about 2 weeks
- Predilection for intertriginous sites and areas subject to pressure and frictions [2] (e.g., perineum, groin, buttocks, lower abdomen, and lower extremities) (see Fig. 56.1)
- Often superinfected with *Staphylococcus aureus* and *Candida Albicans*
- Lesions tend to be highly pruritic; occasionally associated with stomatitis, glossitis, angular cheilitis, and nail changes [2]
- Can be related to multiple endocrine neoplasia (MEN)-1 or MEN-2 (rare)
- By diagnosis, 50–100% have metastatic tumor but although it is incurable the slow-growing tumor is unlikely to cause death [3]
- May also occur in absence in the pseudoglucagonoma syndrome in which there is an absence of a pancreatic tumor. Causes include liver disease, malabsorption, inflammatory bowel disease, and other malignancies [1, 2]
- May occur secondary to glucagon cell adenomatosis [4]

Pathogenesis of this disease is unclear but hypotheses include:

- Possibly due to increased level of glucagon in blood: suggested by the apparent correlation of decreased symptom severity with decreased glucagon (via tumor resection or administration of somatostatin analogues); against this, however, is that patients with nonglucagonoma disease do not always have elevated glucagon [3]
- Nutritional deficiency: similar histology to other deficiencies; improvement in patients given amino acids, zinc, and fatty acids; glucagon may stimulate pathways leading to hypovitaminosis B (symptoms have many features of vitamin B deficiencies) and low levels of free fatty acids and amino acids [3]
- Liver disease may lead to decreased hepatic degradation of glucagon and hypoalbuminemia. Hypoalbuminemia can then cause a decrease in zinc and essential fatty acid levels [1, 2]

Histopathological features include:

- Classic: necrolysis of stratum spinosum ("sudden death") with intracellular edema and keratinocyte degeneration (dyskeratosis and necrosis) leading to subcorneal/midepidermal clefts and bullae; psoriasiform epidermal hyperplasia with confluent parakeratosis; hypergranulosis with pallor of the epidermis; often a lymphohistiocytic infiltrate around the dilated vessels in the edematous papillary dermis (see Fig. 56.2)

The diagnosis is made using a combination of:

- Evidence of glucagonoma: hyperglucagonemia, glucose intolerance, weight loss, normocytic anemia, malaise,

L. Zakko (✉)
Yale Department of Internal Medicine, 20, York Street, Yale New Haven Hospital, New Haven, CT 06510, USA
e-mail: liam.zakko@yale.edu

J. Finch • M.J. Rothe • J.M. Grant-Kels
Department of Dermatology, University of Connecticut Health Center, 21 South Road, Farmington, CT 06030, USA
e-mail: finch@uchc.edu; rothe@uchc.edu; grant@uchc.edu

G.Y. Wu et al. (eds.), *Atlas of Dermatological Manifestations of Gastrointestinal Disease*, DOI 10.1007/978-1-4614-6191-3_56, © Springer Science+Business Media New York 2013

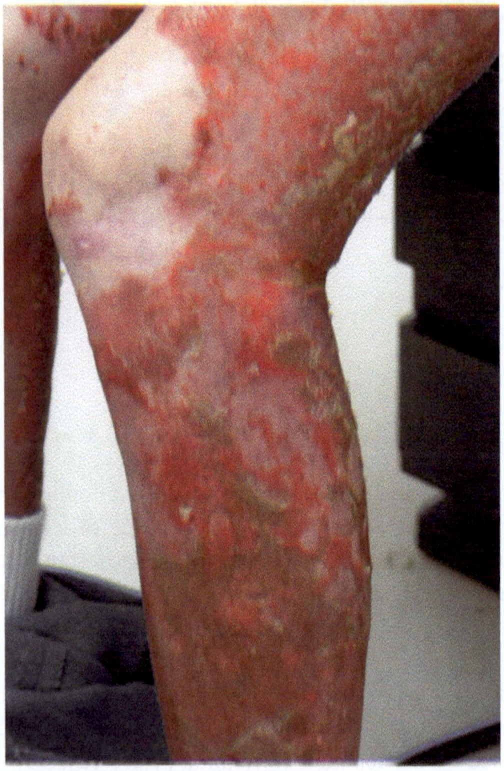

Fig. 56.1 Necrolytic migratory erythema. Erythematous, erosive, desquamating plaques

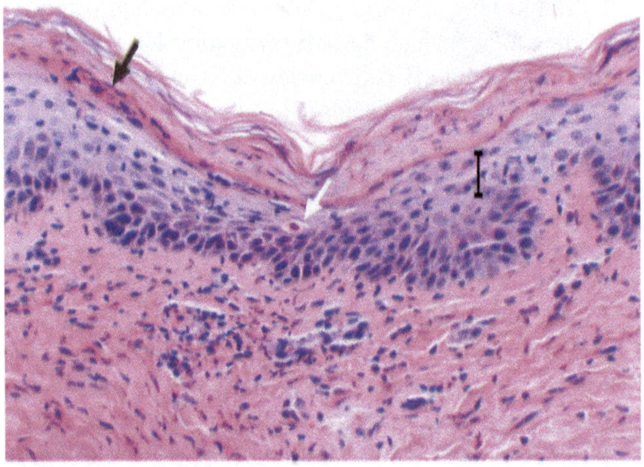

Fig. 56.2 Necrolytic migratory erythema. Pronounced pallor of the upper epidermis (*black bracket*), keratinocyte necrosis (*white arrow*), and confluent parakeratosis (*black arrow*) (200×)

venous thrombosis, diarrhea, neurological/psychological symptoms

- Studies: fasting glucagon level, hormone profile: insulin, gastrin, adrenocorticotropic hormone, vasoactive intestinal polypeptide, somatostatin, complete blood count, liver function tests, hepatitis C, erythrocyte-sedimentation rate, zinc level, essential amino acid levels, free fatty acid levels, computed tomography scan of abdomen/pelvis, ultrasound of abdomen

The differential diagnosis should include:

- Zinc deficiency
- Migratory acral erythema
- Pellagra
- Somatostatinoma
- Chronic candidiasis
- Psoriasis
- Pemphigus
- Eczema
- Pityriasis rosea
- Toxic epidermal necrolysis
- Erythema multiforme
- Cystic fibrosis
- Contact dermatitis

Treatment options include [1, 3]:

- Direct to skin: topical steroids, zinc, tar treatments
- Antiglucagon: somatostatin analogues, interferon-α
- Supplements: amino acids, zinc, essential fatty acids
- Tumor treatments: surgery to debulk/excise and perhaps chemotherapy

References

1. Chastain MA. The glucagonoma syndrome: a review of its features and a discussion of its perspectives. Am J Med Sci. 2001;321:306–20.
2. Fedeles F, Murphy M, Rothe MJ, Grant-Kels JM. Nutrition and bullous skin disease. Clin Dermatol. 2010;28:627–43.
3. van Beek AP, de Haas ER, van Vloten WA, et al. The glucagonoma syndrome and necrolytic migratory erythema: a clinical review. Eur J Endocrinol. 2004;157:531–7.
4. Otto AI, Marshalks M, Zalatnai A, et al. Glucagon cell adenomatosis: a new entity associated with necrolytic migratory erythema and glucagonoma syndrome. J Am Acad Dermatol. 2011;65:458–9.

Part VI

Infection

Typhoid Fever: Gastrointestinal Features

57

Marie Lourdes Ynson

Typhoid fever is a bacterial infection caused by *Salmonella*. The World Health Organization estimates the current incidence at 16–33 million cases annually. The incidence vastly decreased from its peak due to sanitation improvements. Gastrointestinal symptoms of the disease include [1–3]:

- Stepwise fever (initial low-grade fevers that rise progressively by the second week and remain at 39–40°C)
- Flu-like symptoms with chills
- Dull frontal headache (80%)
- Anorexia (55%)
- Myalgia and malaise (10%)
- Apathetic affect
- Poorly localized abdominal discomfort/pain (30–40%)
- Vomiting (18%)
- Marked constipation (13–16%)
- "Pea-soup" diarrhea (22–28%)
- Abdominal distention

The typical clinical signs and findings are [1–3]:

- High-grade fevers
- Coated tongue
- Relative bradycardia
- Abdominal tenderness
- Hepatosplenomegaly (3–6%)
- Gastrointestinal bleeding (10% of patients) due to erosion of a necrotic Peyer's patch through the wall of an enteric vessel (see Fig. 57.1)
- Intestinal (ileal) perforation (1–3% of hospitalized patients)

The pathogenesis of the disease is based on invasive infection [1, 2, 4]:

- Typhoid fever is a systemic infection caused by the bacterium *Salmonella enterica* serotype typhi
- It is contracted by ingestion of food or water contaminated by feces or urine
- It is common in developing countries where there is poor hygiene and sanitation facilities
- Asymptomatic incubation period: 7–14 days
- The bacteria enter the gastrointestinal tract through the mouth and must survive the low gastric pH of the stomach to reach the small intestine
- In the small intestine, the bacteria adhere to mucosal cells, invade the mucosa by transcytosis, then enter lymphoid tissue of the Peyer's patches through the M cells and replicate within the macrophages and spread to the intestinal lymphoid follicles, mesenteric lymph nodes, and even the liver and spleen

The gross pathology will show [1, 2, 4]:

- Small intestinal inflammation
- In complicated disease, bleeding sites and perforated areas may be seen in the small intestine

The diagnosis is made by laboratory tests [1, 2, 4]:

- Laboratory: hemoglobin, white blood cell count and platelet count are usually normal or reduced; liver enzymes are two to three times the upper limit of normal
- Isolation of bacteria in cultured specimens is the gold standard of diagnosis- blood cultures are positive in 60–80% of patients, bone marrow cultures are positive 80–95% of patients
- Widal test is controversial: detects agglutinating antibodies to the O and H antigen of *Salmonella enterica typhi*

Typhoid fever should be differentiated from other febrile illness with nonspecific gastrointestinal complaints and few localizing signs [3, 4] such as:

- Malaria
- Tuberculosis
- Dengue
- Leptospirosis
- Viral hepatitis
- Amebic liver abscess
- Deep abscesses
- Influenza
- Infectious mononucleosis
- Brucellosis
- Typhus

M.L. Ynson (✉)
Department of Internal Medicine, University of Connecticut Health Center, Farmington, CT, USA
e-mail: mynson@resident.uchc.edu

G.Y. Wu et al. (eds.), *Atlas of Dermatological Manifestations of Gastrointestinal Disease*,
DOI 10.1007/978-1-4614-6191-3_57, © Springer Science+Business Media New York 2013

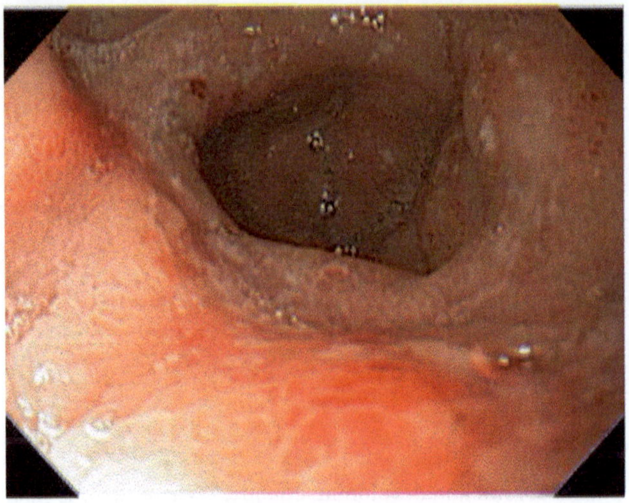

Fig. 57.1 Endoscopic image showing enteritis

The treatment involves eradication of the infecting organism [3, 4]:

- Empiric treatment: ceftriaxone 1–2 g/day intravenous (IV) for 7–14 days or azithromycin 1 g/day by mouth (PO) for 5 days
- Fully susceptible strains: ciprofloxacin (first line) 500 mg PO twice a day or 400 mg IV every 12 h for 5–7 days; second-line agents are: amoxicillin, chloramphenicol, trimethoprim-sulfamethoxazole for 14–21 days
- Multidrug resistant strains: ciprofloxacin (first-line) 500 mg PO twice a day or 400 mg IV every 12 h for 5–7 days, ceftriaxone 2–3 g/day IV for 7–14 days or azithromycin 1 g/day PO for 5 days

References

1. Parry CM, Tinh Hien T, Dougan G, et al. Medical progress typhoid fever. N Engl J Med. 2002;347:1770–80.
2. Lynch MF, Blanton EM, Bulens S, et al. Typhoid fever in the United States 1999–2006. JAMA. 2009;302:859–65.
3. Schwartz BS. Chapter 33. Bacterial and chlamydial infections. In: McPhee SJ, Papadakis MA, Rabow MW, editors. Current medical diagnosis and treatment 2012. New York: McGraw-Hill; 2011.
4. Pegues DA, Miller SI. Salmonellosis. In: Longo DL, Fauci AS, Kasper DL, Hauser SL, Jameson JL, Loscalzo J, editors. Harrison's principles of internal medicine. 18th ed. New York: McGraw-Hill; 2011.

Rose Spots

58

Liam Zakko, Justin Finch, Marti J. Rothe,
and Jane M. Grant-Kels

Clinical signs and features include:

- Most commonly associated with typhoid and paratyphoid fever, but may also be seen with *Shigella*, trichinosis, leptospirosis, brucellosis, psittacosis, rat bite fever, and miliary tuberculosis [1, 2]
- Seen in 10–50% of typhoid cases with usually 6–12 lesions at a time (more lesions are suggestive of paratyphoid disease) [2]; of note, lesions appear to be occurring less often with typhoid fever [3]
- Rose spots are 1–4 mm round, nonpruritic, erythematous papules that blanch, typically located on the upper chest and abdomen between the nipples and the umbilicus, occasionally on the back and proximal extremities, sparing the palms and soles (see Fig. 58.1) [2]
- Lesions usually develop 7–10 days into the illness and fade over the next 3–4 days, but new spots may occur over the next 1–2 weeks [2]

Pathogenesis of this disease is unclear but hypotheses include:

- Appear to be a local cutaneous inflammatory reaction to one or more bacterial products (suggested by studies showing reproduction of lesions by injecting salmonella endotoxin in the skin) [1]
- Lesions for the most part appear sterile; thus they are unlikely due to direct bacterial growth in the skin [1]
- Some postulate lesions due to bacterial emboli [2]

Histopathological features include:

- Dilated capillaries [4]
- Mild superficial perivascular mononuclear cell inflammatory infiltrate without leukocytoclastic vasculitis [4]

The diagnosis is made using a combination of:

- Need to diagnose underlying infection
- For typhoid fever, look for symptoms/signs of fever, headache, chills, cough, constipation, diarrhea, abdominal pain, nausea, myalgia, splenomegaly, lymphadenopathy [3]
- Laboratory findings include liver function abnormalities, anemia, leukocytosis/leukopenia, positive blood cultures, or high O-antigen titers for salmonella (although the latter is present in <50% of patients) [3]

The differential diagnosis should include:

- Other infections that cause rose spots, such as rickettsial typhus, paratyphoid fever, *Shigella* infection, trichinosis, leptospirosis, brucellosis, psittacosis
- Folliculitis/acne

Treatment options include:

- Treat underlying infection; for typhoid fever, first-line antibiotic treatment is a fluoroquinolone or a third-generation cephalosporin [3]

L. Zakko (✉)
Yale Department of Internal Medicine, 20 York Street, Yale New Haven Hospital, New Haven, CT 06510, USA
e-mail: liam.zakko@yale.edu

J. Finch • M.J. Rothe • J.M. Grant-Kels
Department of Dermatology,
University of Connecticut Health Center,
21 South Road, Farmington, CT 06030, USA
e-mail: finch@uchc.edu; rothe@uchc.edu; grant@uchc.edu

G.Y. Wu et al. (eds.), *Atlas of Dermatological Manifestations of Gastrointestinal Disease*,
DOI 10.1007/978-1-4614-6191-3_58, © Springer Science+Business Media New York 2013

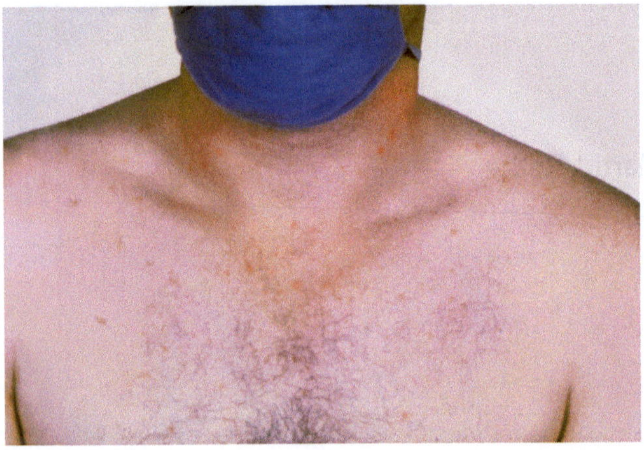

Fig. 58.1 Rose spots on the chest of a patient with typhoid fever (Image courtesy of Charles N. Farmer, MD)

References

1. Latwick KD, Hoke AW, Borchardt KA. Rose spots in typhoid fever. Arch Dermatol. 1972;105:252–5.
2. Belilos E, Tu RP, Sacks-Berg A, et al. Rose spots associated with enteric fever secondary to *Shigella sonnei*. Int J Dermatol. 1998;27:402–3.
3. Briedis DJ, Robson HG. Epidemiologic and clinical features of sporadic *Salmonella enteric* fever. Can Med Assoc J. 1978;119:1183–7.
4. Fine JD, Harrist TJ. Cutaneous leukocytoclastic vasculitis in the rose spot of paratyphoid fever. Int J Dermatol. 1982;21:216–7.

Part VII

Diarrhea

Cronkhite–Canada Syndrome: Gastrointestinal Features

59

Marie Lourdes Ynson

Cronkhite–Canada syndrome (CCS) is a sporadic, idiopathic syndrome characterized by multiple polyps in the gastrointestinal (GI) tract. First documented in 1955 by Drs. Cronkhite and Canada, only about 400 cases have been reported worldwide, 75% of which in Japan. Patients of European or Asian descent are most frequently affected, with an incidence of 1 per 1,000,000. Mean age of onset is the fifth to sixth decade with slight 3:2 predominance in men. An autoimmune process is suspected. Men are generally affected in a 2:1 ratio, with two thirds of all patients being of Japanese origin [1].

GI symptoms [2]:

- Symptoms appear in the sequence of GI symptoms, weight loss, weakness, edema then ectodermal changes
- Diarrhea
- Hypogeusia [3]
- Xerostomia
- Abdominal discomfort
- Weight loss and anorexia

The clinical signs and findings include [1, 2]:

- Skin hyperpigmentation
- Nail dystrophy
- Alopecia
- Findings in endoscopy of numerous nonadenomatous or juvenile type polyps or hamartomatous polyps throughout the GI tract except in the esophagus (see Fig. 59.1)

Although not understood completely, the pathogenesis includes [1, 2]:

- CCS is a rare disease characterized by the presence of nonadenomatous juvenile-type or hamartomatous polyps that occur throughout the GI tract (see Fig. 59.2) except in the esophagus with accompanying skin manifestations
- There is no strong evidence to suggest a familial disposition
- Autoimmunity is said to play a role
- Mental and emotional stress and physical fatigue are important risk factors because the stress acts on the GI mucosa, causing a local inflammatory reaction
- There also appears to be an increased risk for malignancy associated with this disease

The pathology is characterized by [1, 2]:

- The CCS polyp is characterized by its broad sessile base, expanded edematous lamina propria, and dilated cystic glands
- Some studies have also suggested that, histologically, CCS polyps are infiltrated with IgG4 plasma cells on immunohistochemistry staining

The diagnosis is made by considering the following [1, 2]:

- The presence of multiple nonadenomatous juvenile type or hamartomatous polyps in the GI tract except esophagus with the accompanying skin changes
- Laboratory results showing mild to moderate anemia, electrolyte disturbances, hypoproteinemia that reflects malabsorption, vitamin deficiencies (vitamin B_{12}, zinc, thiamine, folate)
- Findings consistent with protein-losing enteropathy are also present

The differential diagnosis of Cronkhite–Canada syndrome should include [1, 2]:

- Juvenile polyposis (JPS)
- Peutz-Jeghers syndrome (PJS)
- Familial adenomatous polyposis (FAP)
- Ménétrier's disease or hyperplastic hypersecretory gastropathy; enlarged gastric mucosal folds leads to protein loss and malabsorption
- Gardner's syndrome
- Turcot syndrome

Although not curative, the treatment entail [1, 2]:

- No guidelines or optimal therapy regimen available
- Goals of treatment: resolution of diarrhea, weight loss and ectodermal manifestations
- Treatment regimens include: corticosteroids, immunosuppressants (azathioprine), nutritional support (intravenous

M.L. Ynson (✉)
Department of Internal Medicine, University of Connecticut Health Center, Farmington, CT, USA
e-mail: mynson@resident.uchc.edu

G.Y. Wu et al. (eds.), *Atlas of Dermatological Manifestations of Gastrointestinal Disease*,
DOI 10.1007/978-1-4614-6191-3_59, © Springer Science+Business Media New York 2013

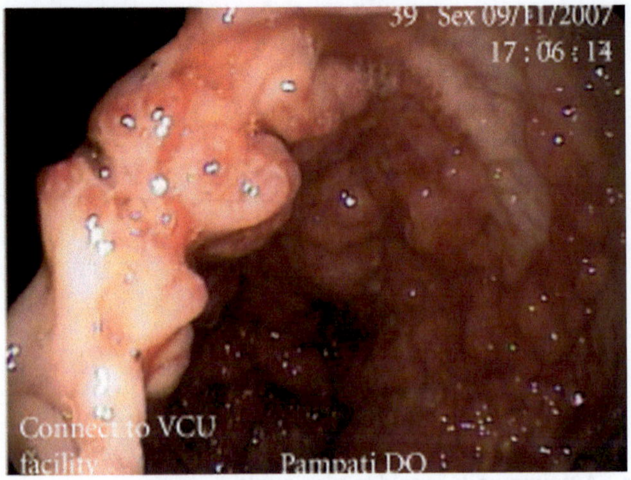

Fig. 59.1 An endoscopic view of diffuse sessile polypoid lesions within the stomach with mucosal edema (From Kao et al. [1])

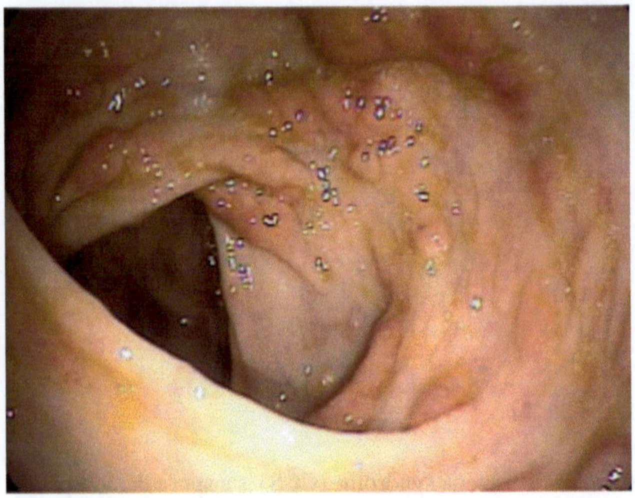

Fig. 59.2 An colonoscopic view showing sessile, strawberry-like polypoid lesions with normal appearing surrounding colonic mucosa (From Kao et al. [1])

fluids, vitamin supplements, electrolytes, amino acids, total parenteral nutrition).

- Some studies have also shown remission of disease after eradication of *Helicobacter pylori* infection [4]

References

1. Kao KT, Patel JK, Pampati V. Cronkhite–Canada syndrome: a case report and review of literature. Gastroenterol Res Pract. 2009;2009:619378.
2. Sweetser S, Ahlquist DA, Osborn NK, et al. Clinicopathologic features and treatment outcome in Cronkhite–Canada syndrome: support for autoimmunity. Dig Dis Sci. 2012;57:496–502.
3. Blonski WC, Furth EE, Kinosian BP, et al. A case of Cronkhite–Canada syndrome with taste disturbance as a leading complaint. Digestion. 2005;71:201–5.
4. Chandrashekar UK, Gnanadev NC, Acharya V, et al. Cronkhite–Canada syndrome with Helicobacter pylori infection. Calicut Med J. 2010;8:e7.

Cronkhite–Canada Syndrome: Dermatological Features

60

Liam Zakko, Justin Finch, Marti J. Rothe, and Jane M. Grant-Kels

Clinical signs and features include:

- Dermatological triad:
  - Hyperpigmentation: macules and papules (lentigo-like), light to dark brown, a few mm to 10 cm in diameter, diffusely located but most commonly on the hands, feet, face, lips, buccal mucosa
  - Nail changes: dystrophy, onycholysis, unique inverted triangle of inverted normal nail bordered by dystrophic nail (see Fig. 60.1)
  - Alopecia: rapidly progressive, patchy but leading to complete hair loss: also facial, axillary, extremity, and pubic hair loss (see Fig. 60.2)
- Median age diagnosis, 59 years old [1]
- Males > females
- Since 1955, there have been 400 cases, 75% in Japan, 15% develop malignancy most commonly of the sigmoid colon and rectum [2]
- Incidence of one patient per million population

Pathogenesis unknown:

- Possible autoimmune etiology with increased antinuclear antibodies and IgG4 in polyps and association with hypothyroidism, systemic lupus erythematous, rheumatoid arthritis, scleroderma [2, 3]
- Stress and fatigue may also contribute

Histopathological features include [4]:

- Light microscopy of skin lesions shows elongated epidermal rete ridges with an increased number of melanocytes in the basal cell layer, epidermal hyperpigmentation, and melanophages, with a mild superficial perivascular lymphohistiocytic infiltrate
- Electron microscopy demonstrates increased melanocytes, increased dendritic processes with melanin granules, and an increased number of melanin granules within keratinocytes
- Mucosal lesions demonstrate acanthosis with hyperpigmentation with or without melanocytic hyperplasia

The diagnosis is made using a combination of:

- Clinical diagnosis based on dermatologic triad (hyperpigmentation, alopecia, nail changes) and gastrointestinal (GI) manifestations

The differential diagnosis should include:

- Other multiple syndromes with lentigines, including Peutz–Jeghers syndrome and Lynch syndrome
- Autoimmune pancreatitis

Treatment options include [3]:

- Supportive: fluid, electrolytes, nutrition, total parenteral nutrition/bowel rest in severe cases
- Often there is a favorable response to steroids
- Proton pump inhibitor/H2 blocker; cromolyn sodium can improve GI symptoms
- If mast cells/eosinophils seen on biopsy, then may see a response to antihistamine agents
- Azathioprine
- Surgery only for catastrophic conditions

L. Zakko (✉)
Yale Department of Internal Medicine, 20, York Street, Yale New Haven Hospital, New Haven, CT 06510, USA
e-mail: liam.zakko@yale.edu

J. Finch • M.J. Rothe • J.M. Grant-Kels
Department of Dermatology, University of Connecticut Health Center, 21 South Road, Farmington, CT 06030, USA
e-mail: finch@uchc.edu; rothe@uchc.edu; grant@uchc.edu

G.Y. Wu et al. (eds.), *Atlas of Dermatological Manifestations of Gastrointestinal Disease*, DOI 10.1007/978-1-4614-6191-3_60, © Springer Science+Business Media New York 2013

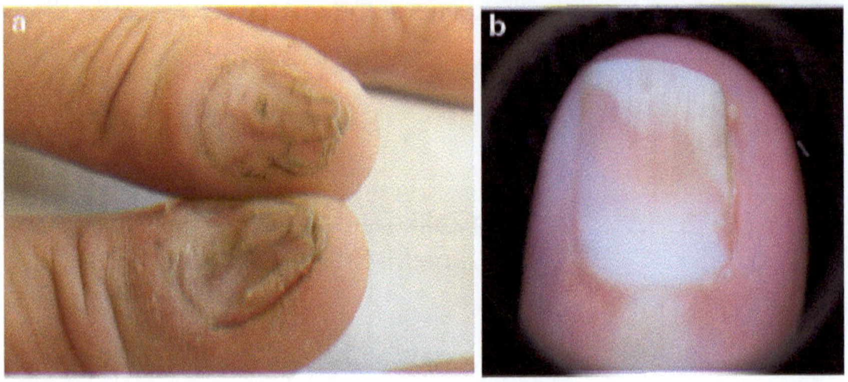

Fig. 60.1 (**a**), Nail dystrophy. (**b**), Onycholysis

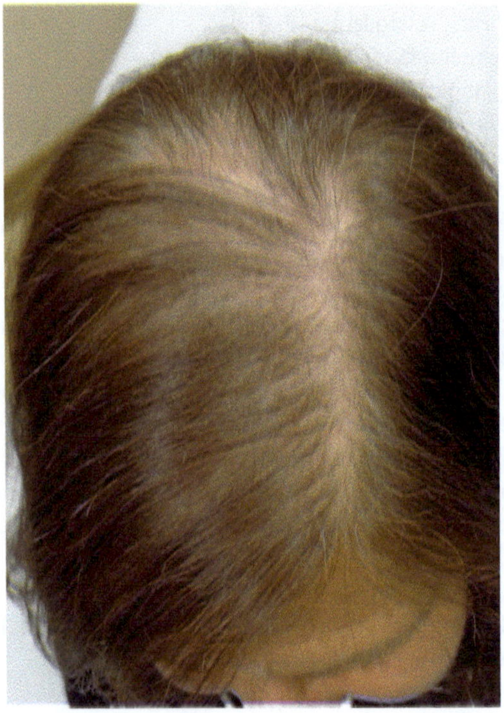

Fig. 60.2 Diffuse nonscarring alopecia

References

1. Ward EM, Wolfsen HC. Pharmacologic management of Cronkhite–Canada syndrome. Expert Opin Pharmacother. 2003;4:385–9.
2. Kao KT, Patel JK, Pampati V. Cronkhite-Canada syndrome: a case report and review of the literature. Gastroenterol Res Pract. 2009:619378. Epub 2009 Aug 25.
3. Sweetser S, Ahlquist DA, Osborn NK, et al. Clinicopathologic features and treatment outcomes in Cronkhite–Canada syndrome: support for autoimmunity. Dig Dis Sci. 2012;57:496–502.
4. Herzberg AJ, Kaplan DL. Cronkhite-Canada syndrome: light and electron microscopy of the cutaneous pigmentary abnormalities. Int J Dermatol. 1990;29:121–5.

Part VIII

Pancreatic Conditions

61 Von Hippel–Lindau Syndrome: Gastrointestinal Features

Marcy Qureshi

Von Hippel–Lindau (VHL) syndrome is an autosomal dominant genetic disorder. It is characterized by hemangioblastomas in the cerebellum, spinal cord, kidneys, and retinas, and results from a mutation in a tumor suppressor gene [1, 2].

The gastrointestinal symptoms include [1, 2]:

- Development of pancreatic cysts and cystadenomas (see Figs. 61.1 and 61.2) may cause pain as they expand inside the pancreas
- Development of pancreatic neuroendocrine tumor may cause symptoms depending on the various neuroendocrine substances secreted

Some clinical signs and findings are [1, 2]:

- Development of various benign and malignant tumors and cysts:
  - Hemangioblastoma in the central nervous system (CNS)
  - Retinal hemangioblastoma
  - Pheochromocytoma
  - Renal cell carcinoma
  - Renal cyst
  - Pancreatic cystadenoma
  - Pancreatic neuroendocrine tumors

The pathogenesis: a genetic defect in a tumor suppressor gene [1, 2]:

- Autosomal dominant disorder
- VHL tumor suppressor gene on chromosome 3p25–26 is affected in this disease
  - Loss of the VHL tumor suppressor gene leads to loss of the VHL protein and elongin B, C (VBC) complex leading to dysfunction of the ubiquitination of hypoxia-inducible factors and other proteins for VBC complex
  - The failure in degradation of hypoxia inducible factors leads to development of highly vascular tumors

The diagnosis is made by considering the following criteria [1, 2]:

- The following criteria are used for the diagnosis of VHL disease:
  - Patients with a family history of developing hemangioblastoma in the CNS or retina, renal cell carcinoma (RCC), pheochromocytoma or pancreatic tumors or cysts, epididymal cystadenoma
  - Patients without a family history of VHL disease but who develop hemangioblastoma in the CNS or retina in combination with other tumors such as RCC, pheochromocytoma, pancreatic tumors or cysts, or epididymal cystadenoma
- Genetic testing
  - Once diagnosed, complete genetic sequencing to identify the mutation in the VHL gene can benefit family members

The differential diagnosis of VHL syndrome should include [1, 2]:

- VHL 1: those patients who do not have pheochromocytoma
- VHL 2: those patients who do have pheochromocytoma
  - Type 2A: pheochromocytoma with other hemangioblastoma in the CNS but not with RCC
  - Type 2B: pheochromocytoma, RCC, and other CNS tumors
  - Type 2C: pheochromocytoma alone

There is no cure for this disease; treatment involves alleviating and preventing complications [1, 2]:

- Complex multisystem disorder that requires input from multiple medical subspecialties
- At-risk relatives should be entered into a comprehensive screening program in childhood
  - Retinal angioma: ophthalmic examination every 12 months beginning in infancy/childhood
  - CNS hemangioblastoma: magnetic resonance imaging (MRI) scans of the head and spine every 12–36 months in adolescence
  - Renal cell carcinoma: MRI scans of abdomen every 12 months from age 16 years

M. Qureshi (✉)
Department of Internal Medicine, University of Connecticut Health Center, Farmington, CT, USA
e-mail: mQureshi@echn.org

G.Y. Wu et al. (eds.), *Atlas of Dermatological Manifestations of Gastrointestinal Disease*,
DOI 10.1007/978-1-4614-6191-3_61,

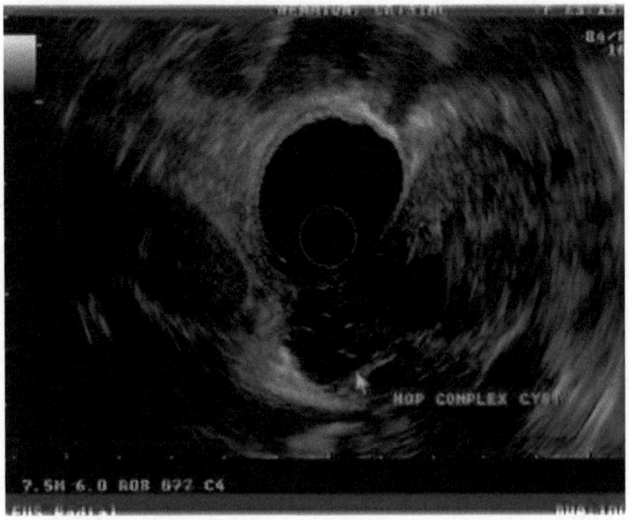

Fig. 61.1 A radial endoscopic ultrasound view of a complex cyst in the head of the pancreas in a patient with Von Hippel–Lindau syndrome

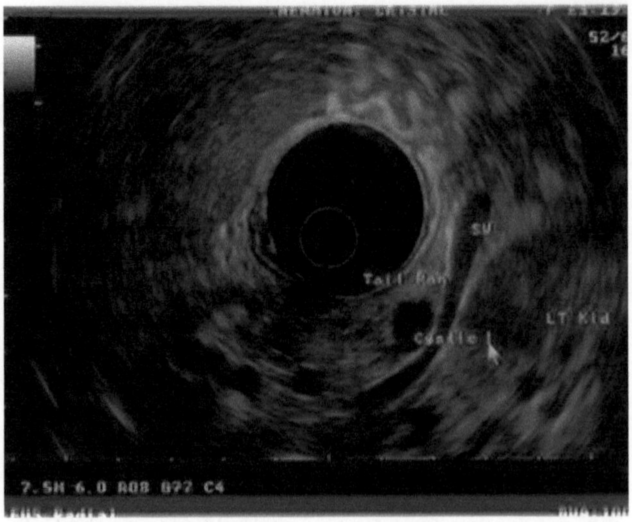

Fig. 61.2 A radial endoscopic ultrasound view of a simple cyst in the tail of the pancreas in a patient with Von Hippel–Lindau syndrome

- Pheochromocytoma: yearly screening beginning in childhood with 24-h urine for catecholamine metabolites or measurement of plasma nor-metanephrine levels
- Annual blood pressure screening

References

1. Maher ER, Neumann HPH, Richard S. Von Hippel–Lindau disease: a clinical and scientific review. J Hum Genet. 2011;19:617–23.
2. Shuin T, Yamasaki I, Tamura K, et al. Von Hippel–Lindau disease: molecular pathological basis, clinical criteria, genetic testing, clinical features of tumors and treatments. Jpn J Clin Oncol. 2006;36:337–43.

Von Hippel–Lindau Syndrome: Dermatological Features

62

Liam Zakko, Justin Finch, Marti J. Rothe, and Jane M. Grant-Kels

Von Hippel–Lindau (VHL) syndrome occurs in 1/36,000 live births and typically presents before age 40 years. The disease progresses with multiple tumors and death in the fourth decade of life [1].

Clinical features include:

- Central nervous system (CNS) hemangiomas and other visceral tumors [2]:
  - Retinal hemangioblastomas (25–60% of patients)
  - Endolymphatic sac tumors (10%)
  - Craniospinal hemangioblastomas : cerebellar (44–72%), brainstem (10–25%), spinal cord (13–50%)
  - Renal cell carcinoma or cysts (25–60%)
  - Pheochromocytomas (10–20%)
  - Pancreatic tumor or cyst (35–70%)
  - Epididymal cystadenoma (25–60%)
  - Broad ligament cystadenoma (rare)
- Fewer than 5% have cutaneous manifestations
- Capillary malformations are the most common finding and often affect the head and neck [1]
- Café-au-lait spots (well-circumscribed, evenly pigmented macules/patches 1 mm to 20 cm in diameter) (*see* Fig. 62.1)

L. Zakko (✉)
Yale Department of Internal Medicine, 20 York Street, Yale New Haven Hospital, New Haven, CT 06510, USA
e-mail: liam.zakko@yale.edu

J. Finch • M.J. Rothe • J.M. Grant-Kels
Department of Dermatology,
University of Connecticut Health Center,
21 South Road, Farmington, CT 06030, USA
e-mail: finch@uchc.edu; rothe@uchc.edu; grant@uchc.edu

Classification by presence or absence of different tumors [3]:

- Type 1: retinal/CNS hemangioblastomas and renal cell carcinoma; no pheochromocytoma
- Type 1 B: retinal/CNS hemangioblastomas with low risk for renal cell carcinoma; no pheochromocytoma
- Type 2A: pheochromocytomas and hemangioblastomas; low risk for renal cell carcinoma
- Type 2B: pheochromocytomas, hemangioblastomas, and renal cell carcinoma
- Type 2C: only pheochromocytomas

Pathogenesis is related to [1, 4]:

- Autosomal dominant genetic mutation to the VHL suppressor gene on chromosome 3p25–26 with 80% of cases being hereditary and 20% sporadic
- The VHL suppressor gene codes for a ubiquitin ligase that degrades hypoxia-inducible factors (HIF)
- Mutations in the gene lead to a lack of functioning ligase and a buildup of HIF, leading to an increase in signaling molecules, such as vascular endothelial growth factor (VEGF), platelet derived growth factor (PDGF), transforming growth factor (TGF)-alpha, and carbonic anhydrase IX, which cause neoangiogenesis and tumor formation

Pathology findings include:

- Capillary malformations: extensive and occasionally dilated capillary vessels in the dermis
- Café-au-lait spots: increased melanin content of both melanocytes and basal keratinocytes; may see macromelanosomes or large pigment granules; adnexal epithelium uninvolved

Differential diagnosis includes:

- Sporadic tumor formation

Treatment measures include:

- Screening to detect tumors early and excise when necessary including [3]:
- Annual eye examinations beginning in infancy or early childhood to screen for retinal angioma

G.Y. Wu et al. (eds.), *Atlas of Dermatological Manifestations of Gastrointestinal Disease*,
DOI 10.1007/978-1-4614-6191-3_62, © Springer Science+Business Media New York 2013

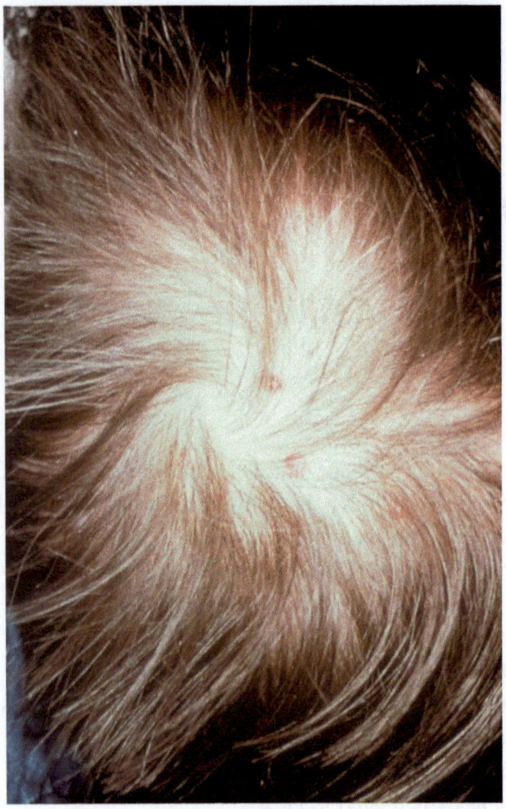

Fig. 62.1 Von Hippel–Lindau syndrome. Port wine stain of the scalp

- Magnetic resonance imaging (MRI) scans of head every 12–36 months beginning in adolescence to screen for CNS hemangioblastoma
- Annual MRI or ultrasound examinations of abdomen beginning at age 16 years to screen for renal cell carcinoma and pancreatic tumors
- Annual blood pressure monitoring and 24-h urine studies for catecholamine metabolites; for patients at high risk for pheochromocytoma, annual measurement of plasma normetanephrine levels and adrenal imaging, beginning at age 8 years
- Cosmetic treatment for cutaneous features

References

1. Ferzli PG, Millett CR, Newman MD, et al. The dermatologist's guide to hereditary syndromes with renal tumors. Cutis. 2008;81:41–8.
2. Lonser RR, Glenn GM, Walther M, et al. Von Hippel-Lindau disease. Lancet. 2003;361:2059–67.
3. Maher ER, Neumann HP, Richard S. Von Hippel-Lindau disease: a clinical and scientific review. Eur J Hum Genet. 2011;19:617–23.
4. Linehan WM, Vaselli J, Srinivasan R, et al. Genetic basis of cancer of the kidney: disease-specific approaches to therapy. Clin Cancer Res. 2004;10:6282S–9.

Part IX

Liver Conditions

Hepatitis C Virus: Gastrointestinal Features

63

Liam Zakko

Hepatitis C is caused by the hepatitis C virus (HCV) and affects the liver primarily. Although the infection itself is usually asymptomatic, long-term infection can ultimately lead to cirrhosis and subsequent liver failure, cancer, and varices. It is spread by blood contact and thought to affect 130–170 million people worldwide. Liver failure due to hepatitis C is the most common indication for liver transplantation in the United States, and no vaccine is currently available [1].

Gastrointestinal symptoms [1, 2] include:

- Often asymptomatic
- Acute symptoms (15% of infections): decreased appetite, fatigue, nausea, muscle/joint aches, weight loss, and right-sided abdominal pain

Clinical signs and findings [1, 2] include:

- Ascites, jaundice, bleeding varices, encephalopathy, sometimes liver cancer can be present
- Risk factors: drug use (45% prevalence in 20–59 year olds with any illegal drug use); blood transfusion before 1992; increased number of sex partners; iatrogenic (possibly from dialysis); HIV infection, children born to infected mothers, individuals born between the years 1945–65
- Fifteen percent–30% of patients report no risk factors

Pathogenesis [1, 3] involves:

- An enveloped flavivirus (with positive stranded viral RNA) that binds to cells and enters via receptor-mediated endocytosis
- Cells recognize pathogen-associated molecular patterns, which leads to increased interferon (IFN)-γ and proinflammatory cytokines, leading to IFN-β, interferon regulatory factor-3, and λ interferons that activate adaptive immunity
- Chronic infection due to mutation of epitopes of cytotoxic CD8+ T-cells and the increase of inhibitory receptors on chronically active T-cells leading to functional impairment. This and a rapid mutation rate allows the virus to escape immune clearance
- Much of the liver disease from chronic infection is due to chronic inflammation

Pathology may show typical features [1, 3]:

- Lymphocyte infiltration of the parenchyma (see Fig. 63.1)
- Lymphoid follicles in portal area (see Fig. 63.2)
- Bile duct reactive changes
- Worsening fibrosis as disease progresses

Diagnostic factors [1, 2]:

- Screening tests for those with risk factors or increased liver enzymes include serum assay for antibodies to hepatitis C and then polymerase chain reaction assay (PCR) for RNA of HCV to confirm active infection
- Once infection is confirmed, determine the viral load and genotype; there are six genotypes: genotype 1 is more prevalent in North America, South America, and Europe
- Screen for cirrhosis and hepatocellular carcinoma
- Clinically significant liver fibrosis has a gold-standard diagnosis with liver biopsy but serum assays may be used to identify fibrosis without the risks of a biopsy

Differential diagnosis [1, 2]:

- Nonalcoholic steatohepatitis
- Autoimmune hepatitis
- Alcohol hepatitis
- Other viral hepatitis infections

Various treatment options [2]:

- Treatment should be pursued in those with symptomatic HCV infection and those with moderate-to-severe fibrosis
- Standard treatment is pegylated interferon and ribavirin plus a protease inhibitor (telaprevir or boceprevir): this clears 65–70% of genotype I infections; dual therapy, pegylated interferon, and ribavirin clears virus in 70–80% of genotype II infections; better outcomes are associated with lower initial HCV count IL-2b CC host genotype,

L. Zakko (✉)
Yale Department of Internal Medicine, Yale New Haven Hospital, New Haven, CT, USA

Yale Primary Care Clinic, 789 Howard Avenue, New Haven, CT 06519-1304, USA
e-mail: liam.zakko@yale.edu

G.Y. Wu et al. (eds.), *Atlas of Dermatological Manifestations of Gastrointestinal Disease*,
DOI 10.1007/978-1-4614-6191-3_63,

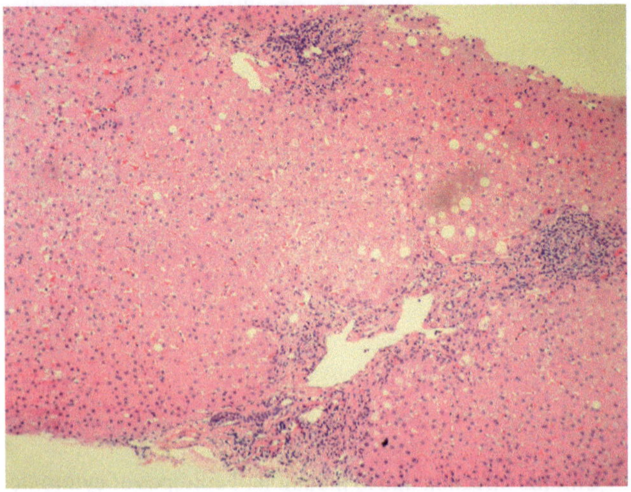

Fig. 63.1 A photomicrograph of a liver biopsy specimen showing a primarily pericentral lymphocytic inflammatory infiltrate and a moderate amount of steatosis that is typical of HCV infection. Hematoxylin and eosin (H and E) stain, low power

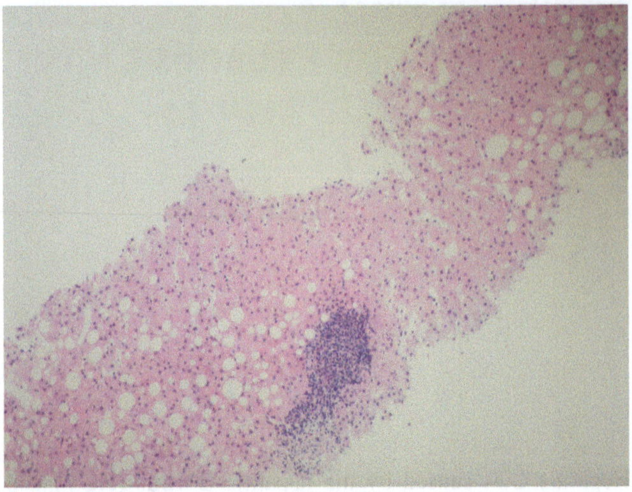

Fig. 63.2 A photomicrograph of a liver biopsy specimen showing a typical lymphoid aggregate or nodule composed of mononuclear cells. Steatosis is more extensive than in Fig. 63.1, which would be consistent with a genotype 3 infection. H and E stain, low power

and better adherence to treatment; side effects include fever, influenza-like illness, headache, cytopenia, fatigue, anorexia, depression, anxiety

- Rapid viremic response: clearance of virus by 4 weeks can lead to shorter therapy
- Early viremic response: decrease in viral count 100-fold or clearance by 12 weeks; if this does not occur, there is a 97% failure of treatment
- Side effects include rash, pruritus, anemia, gastrointestinal upset
- In the future, hope for treatment without pegylated interferon

References

1. Rosen HR. Chronic hepatitis C infection. N Engl J Med. 2011;364:2429–38.
2. Ghany MG, Strader DB, Thomas DL, Seeff LB, American Association for the Study of Liver Diseases. Diagnosis, management, and treatment of hepatitis C: an update. Hepatology. 2009;49:1335–74.
3. Houghton M. The long and winding road leading to identification of the hepatitis C virus. J Hepatol. 2009;51:939–48.

Hepatitis C Virus: Dermatological Features

64

Liam Zakko, Justin Finch, Marti J. Rothe, and Jane M. Grant-Kels

Lichen Planus

Clinical signs and features:

- 0.1–4% of the population, more often in women and those 30–60 years old
- Planar, purple, polygonal, pruritic, papules/plaques
- Acute onset on the flexor surfaces of the wrist, forearm, and leg
- May also occur on the oral mucosa (see Fig. 64.1), genital mucosa, scalp, nails, and rarely the esophagus
- Wickham striae: lesions covered by lacy, reticular, white lines (see Fig. 64.1)
- Clearing lesions often leave postinflammatory hyperpigmentation
- Linear lichen planus: lesions may be linear and arise via Koebner phenomenon (see Fig. 64.1)
- Annular lichen planus: arcuate groups of individual papules that develop rings or papules that extend peripherally with central clearing, often occurring on male genitalia and buccal mucosa
- Atrophic lichen planus: well-demarcated white, pink, bluish papules
- Hypertrophic lichen planus: usually occurs on the extremities, ankles, shins, and interphalangeal joints, and is very pruritic
- Vesiculobullous lichen planus: vesicles/bullae form on preexisting lesions

Differential diagnosis:

- Nummular eczema
- Papular atopic dermatitis
- Lichen simplex chronicus
- Pityriasis rosea
- Prurigo nodularis
- Psoriasis

Pathogenesis of this disease, although unclear, is immune-mediated:

- Statistically significant association with hepatitis C infection, although the reason for the association is unclear

Histopathological features:

- Irregular "saw-tooth" pattern of epidermal hyperplasia (see Fig. 64.2a)
- Compact hyperkeratosis with wedge-shaped thickening of the granular cell layer
- Vacuolar alteration of the basal layer of the epidermis (*see* Fig. 64.2b)
- Dense, bandlike, T-cell infiltrate obscuring the dermal-epidermal junction

Diagnostic factors:

- Clinical diagnosis if classic case
- Biopsy can be used to confirm especially atypical cases

Treatment options:

- Screen all patients for hepatitis C
- High-potency topical corticosteroids
- Topical calcineurin inhibitors
- Oral corticosteroids
- Oral antihistamines for itch
- Intralesional triamcinolone used to treat hypertrophic lichen planus
- Phototherapy

L. Zakko (✉)
Yale Department of Internal Medicine, Yale New Haven Hospital, New Haven, CT, USA

Yale Primary Care Clinic, 789 Howard Avenue, New Haven, CT 06519-1304, USA
e-mail: liam.zakko@yale.edu

J. Finch • M.J. Rothe • J.M. Grant-Kels
Department of Dermatology, University of Connecticut Health Center, 21 South Road, Farmington, CT 06030, USA
e-mail: finch@uchc.edu; rothe@uchc.edu; grant@uchc.edu

G.Y. Wu et al. (eds.), *Atlas of Dermatological Manifestations of Gastrointestinal Disease*, DOI 10.1007/978-1-4614-6191-3_64, © Springer Science+Business Media New York 2013

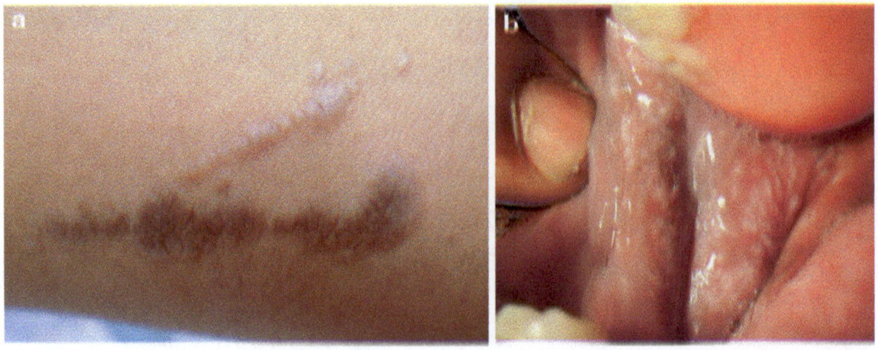

Fig. 64.1 (**a**) Cutaneous lichen planus. Flat, violaceous, polygonal papules on the forearm, in a linear array due to Koebnerization in an area of prior trauma. (**b**) Mucosal lichen planus. Violaceous plaque on the buccal mucosa, with lacy white reticulated pattern

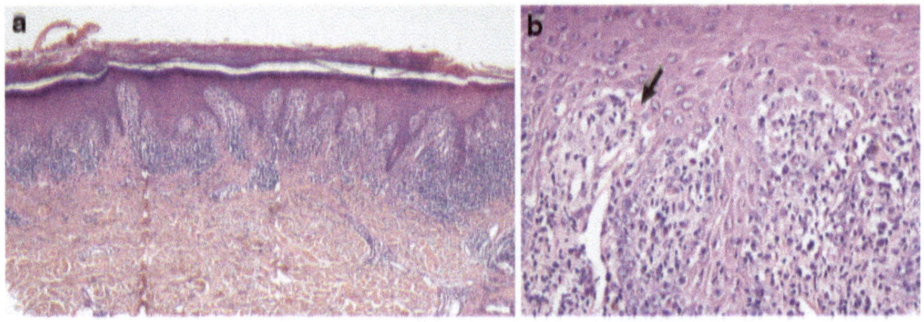

Fig. 64.2 Lichen planus. (**a**) Pathology demonstrates hypergranulosis, sawtooth-shaped rete ridges, with a lichenoid lymphocytic infiltrate (20×). (**b**) High-magnification image shows liquefactive degeneration of the basal layer (*white arrow*) with colloid bodies (*black arrow*)

- Systemic retinoids
- Methotrexate

Porphyria Cutanea Tarda

Clinical signs and features [1]:

- Cutaneous bullae and milia on dorsal surface of the hands (see Fig. 64.3): from exposure to sun and as an area of constant trauma; also see hyperpigmentation and hypertrichosis on the face—nonvirilizing type—particularly on the checks and temples and more common in females
- Classically increased photosensitivity, skin fragility, blistering, erosions, crusts, and milia in sun-exposed areas
- Rarely: sclerodermoid changes with waxy, yellow to white, indurated plaques resembling scleroderma; purplish red heliotropic suffusion of the central part of the face
- Most common porphyria worldwide, one in 10,000 people
- Average onset in middle age
- Hepatoerythropoietic porphyria: presents much earlier in infancy, with dark urine in diapers

Differential diagnosis:

- Variegate porphyria
- Hereditary co-porphyria
- Congenital erythropoietic purpura
- Epidermolysis bullosa acquisita
- Polymorphous light eruption
- Phototoxic drug eruption
- Hydroa vacciniforme

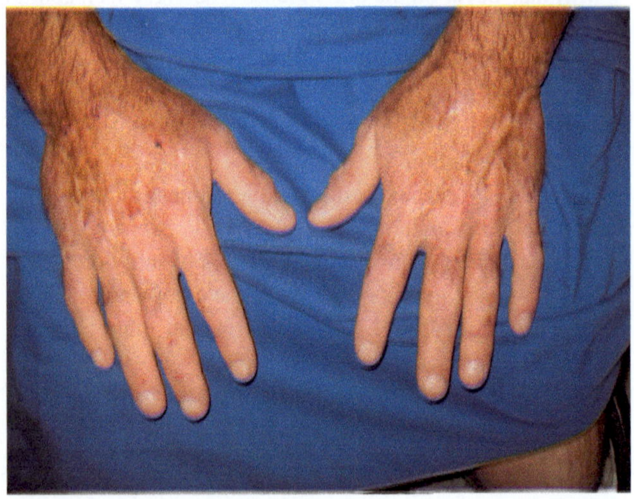

Fig. 64.3 Porphyria cutanea tarda. Erosions and vesicles on dorsal, sun-exposed hands

- Pseudoporphyria cutanea tarda

Pathogenesis [2]:

- Urophyrinogen decarboxylase (UROD) is mapped to chromosome region 1p34
- Type I—sporadic or acquired—UROD is only deficient in the liver
- Type II—autosomal dominant with incomplete penetrance; enzyme is deficient in all tissue
- Enzyme activity of ~25% of normal leads to a buildup of uroporphyrin and other carboxylated porphyrins in vari-

ous organs including the skin and liver. The buildup in the skin leads to the photochemical reaction in the skin

- Type I and II are associated with liver disease. Symptoms are often induced by alcohol, estrogens (oral contraceptive pills), hemochromatosis/iron overload, polychlorinated hydrocarbons, and liver disease, particularly HCV. Occurs due to iron increasing the oxidation of uropyrinogen to uroporphomethene, which decreases UROD by competitive inhibition
- Type III: autosomal recessive variant; primary relatives with disease but normal UROD levels in erythrocytes
- Hepatoerythropoietic porphyria (HEP): severe clinical features, early in life but otherwise similar to types I and II
- Pseudoporphyria cutanea tarda (PCT): similar clinical findings to PCT in patients with chronic kidney disease and/or hemodialysis, as well as drug-induced (nonsteroidal anti-inflammatory drugs, tetracyclines, nalidixic acid, furosemide, systemic retinoids)

Histopathological features:

- In the presence of uroporphyrin, photoactivation of the complement system leads to activation of mast cells and then proteases, resulting in a dermal-epidermal split. Histologically, one notes a subepidermal blister with retention of the dermal papillae and no significant inflammation. Periodic acid-Schiff (PAS) stain highlights the increased hyalin-like material around superficial dermal vessels. Later increased fibroblast activity leads to fibrosis and sclerodermoid skin changes (see Fig. 64.4).

Diagnostic factors [2]:

- Urine changes to red/brown within hours of exposure to natural light or pink to red fluorescence with an ultraviolet light source; no longer recommended because of low sensitivity and specificity
- Biochemical analysis: increased uroporphyrin (type I isomer > type III isomer), hepta-carboxylated porphyrins (type III isomer > type I isomer), and coproporphyrin in urine; increased coproporphyrin and isocoproporphyrin in feces

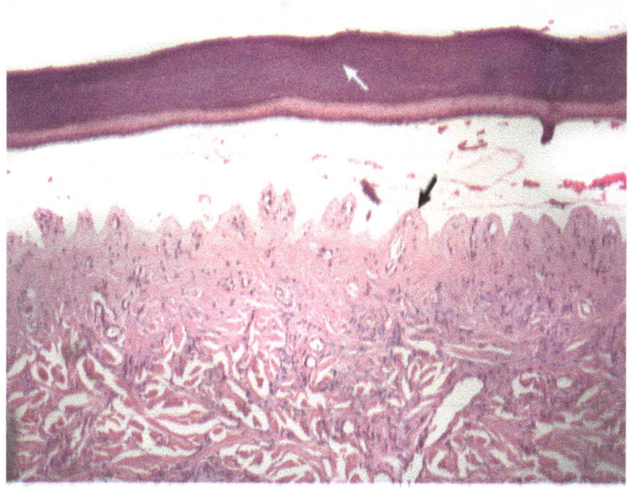

Fig. 64.4 Porphyria cutanea tarda. Pauci-inflammatory subepidermal blister with festooning of the dermal papillae (*black arrow*). Note the thick stratum corneum (*white arrow*), indicating acral location

Treatment options [2]:

- Avoid sunlight, skin protection (must block 400–410 nm light—use titanium dioxide or zinc oxide–based sunscreens)
- Minimize skin trauma
- Avoid triggers such as alcohol and estrogen
- Phlebotomy to reduce iron load
- Chloroquine: increased porphyrin excretion and decrease synthesis
- Phlebotomy and antimalarials are ineffective for HEP

References

1. Usatine RP, Tinitigan M. Diagnosis and treatment of lichen planus. Am Fam Physician. 2011;84:53–60.
2. Frank J, Poblete-Gutiérrez P. Porphyria cutanea tarda: when skin meets liver. Best Pract Res Clin Gastroenterol. 2010;24:735–45.

65 Primary Biliary Cirrhosis: Gastrointestinal Features

Liam Zakko

Primary biliary cirrhosis (PBC) is an autoimmune disease characterized by destruction of the small bile ducts in the liver. This ultimately leads to cholestasis followed by fibrosis and cirrhosis. There is a 9:1 female to male ratio, with prevalence as high as one in 4,000 [1].

The gastrointestinal (GI) symptoms include [1–3]:

- There are four stages of disease clinically: (1) preclinical (only increased antimitochondrial antibody); (2) asymptomatic (increased alkaline phosphatase and gamma glutamyl-transpeptidase); (3) symptomatic; (4) liver insufficiency
- Fifty percent–60% of patients present without symptoms, with most developing symptoms over 2–4 years, although some may remain asymptomatic for up to 20 years; it is unclear why there is a difference in progression and how to predict those who will progress rapidly
- Common symptoms include fatigue (65–80%), pruritus (20–70%), anicteric cholestasis, hyperlipidemia (usually with high-density lipoprotein [HDL] > low-density lipoprotein [LDL] and not requiring therapy), abdominal pain (particularly right upper quadrant pain; etiology often unknown, occasionally secondary to gallstone disease, rarely due to hepatocellular carcinoma, jaundice, hepatomegaly)
- Jaundice usually occurs prior to hepatic decompensation with ascites, encephalopathy, coagulopathy

The clinical signs and findings are [1–3]:

- Twenty percent of patients have more severe disease in the presence of an autoimmune hepatitis picture
- Five percent–10% of patients have a premature ductopenic variant with rapid onset of ductopenia leading to severe icteric cholestasis and cirrhosis within 5 years
- Portal hypertension is often due to presinusoidal presence of nodular regenerative hyperplasia, not cirrhosis; variceal hemorrhage can occur but is often not an indication for immediate transplant
- Disease associations include lichen planus, scleroderma, CREST (calcinosis; Raynaud syndrome; esophageal dysmotility; sclerodactyly; telangiectasia), systemic lupus erythematosus, Sjögren syndrome, Raynaud syndrome, autoimmune thyroid disease, celiac disease, ulcerative colitis, pulmonary fibrosis, glomerulonephritis, sarcoidosis, recurrent tubular acidosis, recurrent urinary tract infection, rheumatoid arthritis, periostitis
- Decreased survival is associated with jaundice, irreversible bile duct loss, cirrhosis, other autoimmune diseases

The pathogenesis appears to involve autoimmune abnormalities [1–4]:

- A genetic component is suggested as the disease in more common in Northern Europeans, more common in those with relatives with disease (one sixth have an affected relative), 63% concordance in monozygotic twins, and more common in women (10:1 female:male ratio)
- Most commonly accepted hypothesis is that the disease represents molecular mimicry immune response due to bacteria (*Escherichia coli, Novosplingobium aromaticivorans*), tobacco use, viruses, and chemicals
- Immune targets appear to be a family of 2-oxo-acid dehydrogenase complexes with infiltrating autoreactive T-cells reactive against these proteins
- Intense immune response against biliary epithelial cells appears caused by the way bile duct cells handle these proteins versus the way other cells modify them

The pathology seen in liver biopsies can show [3, 4]:

- Four stages of the disease (may all be present in same sample, disease staged by most advanced stage present in the sample)
  - Stage I: localization of inflammation in the portal triads
  - Stage II: decreased number of bile ducts, inflammation extends into surrounding parenchyma
  - Stage III: fibrous septa link adjacent portal triads
  - Stage IV: end-stage liver disease, frank cirrhosis with regenerative nodules

The diagnosis is made based on [1–4]:

L. Zakko (✉)
Yale Department of Internal Medicine, Yale New Haven Hospital, New Haven, CT, USA

Yale Primary Care Clinic, 789 Howard Avenue, New Haven, CT 06519-1304, USA
e-mail: liam.zakko@yale.edu

G.Y. Wu et al. (eds.), *Atlas of Dermatological Manifestations of Gastrointestinal Disease*, DOI 10.1007/978-1-4614-6191-3_65, © Springer Science+Business Media New York 2013

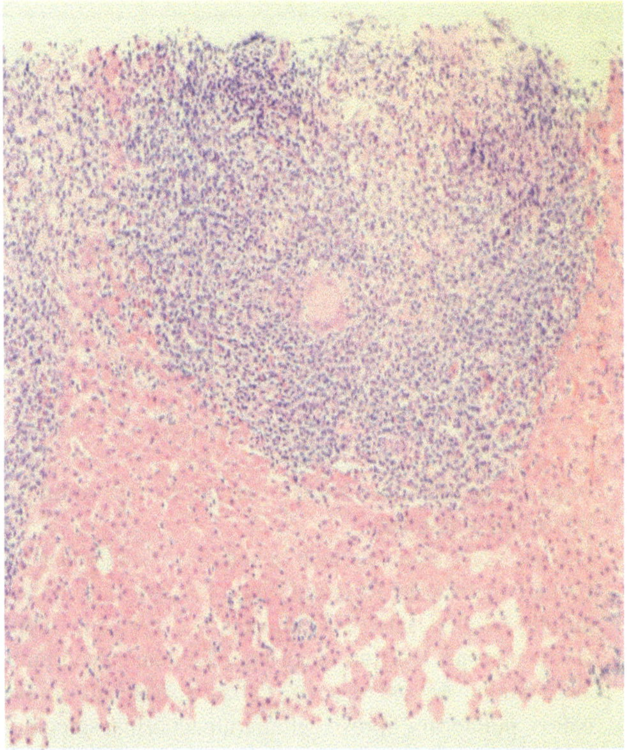

Fig. 65.1 A photomicrograph of a liver specimen from a patient with primary biliary cirrhosis showing a dense mononuclear infiltrate surrounding and damaged bile ducts. Hematoxylin and eosin stain, low power

- Three criteria for PBC diagnosis: if all three criteria are positive, the diagnosis is definite; if two criteria are positive, the diagnosis is probable
  - Detectable antimitochondrial antibodies
  - Elevated liver enzymes (alkaline phosphate most common) for 6 months
  - Histologic findings in the liver compatible with the disease (see Fig. 65.1)

The differential diagnosis of primary biliary cirrhosis should include [1–4]:

- Nonalcoholic liver disease
- Primary sclerosing cholangitis
- Lymphoma
- Cystic fibrosis
- Drug-induced liver injury
- Thyrotoxicosis

There is no cure but symptomatic treatment involves [1–4]:

- Ursodeoxycholic acid (UDCA) is first-line therapy with 25–30% complete response, 20% with no progression histologically if treatment started in stage I and II disease
- Budesonide can be used with UDCA to improve histology and biochemical tests, but has no effect on survival
- Colchicine: use if there is an incomplete response to UCDA
- Methotrexate: use if there is an incomplete response to UCDA and colchicine
- Liver transplant: definitive treatment, 92% survival at 1 year, 85% survival at 5 years; however, does not change antibody status and recurrent at 3 years is 15% and at 10 years is 30%

References

1. Bhandari BM, Bayat H, Rothstein KD. Primary biliary cirrhosis. Gastroenterol Clin North Am. 2011;40:373–86.
2. Crosignani A, Battezzati PM, Invernizzi P, et al. Clinical features and management of primary biliary cirrhosis. World J Gastroenterol. 2008;14:3313–27.
3. Heathcote J. The clinical expression of primary biliary cirrhosis. Semin Liver Dis. 1997;17:23–33.
4. Kaplan MM, Gershwin ME. Primary biliary cirrhosis. N Engl J Med. 2005;353:1261–73.

Primary Biliary Cirrhosis: Dermatological Features

66

Liam Zakko, Justin Finch, Marti J. Rothe, and Jane M. Grant-Kels

Clinical signs and features include:

- Dermatologic disease is the presenting symptom in 38% of patients [1]
- Xanthoma (5–10%): most commonly presents around eyes, xanthelasma (*see* Fig. 66.1a) may affect hands, elbows, knees, ankles (may be more likely in sites of minor trauma) (*see* Fig. 66.1b); rarely develops xanthoma striatum palmare or xanthomatous neuropathy [1–3]
- Pruritus: second most common complaint of patients (fatigue is most common complaint); pruritus disrupts sleep and contributes to fatigue; left untreated skin becomes scarred and hyperpigmented; worse in winter with decreased ultraviolet light to breakdown bilirubin [3–5]
- Earlier diagnosis of primary biliary cirrhosis (PBC) has resulted in decrease in severity of symptoms [2, 6]. Disease associations include lichen planus, scleroderma, CREST (calcinosis; Raynaud syndrome; esophageal dysmotility; sclerodactyly; telangiectasia), systemic lupus erythematous, Sjögren syndrome, Raynaud, thyroiditis, celiac disease, ulcerative colitis, pulmonary fibrosis [5]

The differential diagnosis should include:

- Nonalcoholic liver disease
- Primary sclerosing cholangitis
- Lymphoma
- Cystic fibrosis
- Drug-induced liver injury
- Thyrotoxicosis

Pathogenesis of this disease involves:

- Xanthoma: histiocytes that take-up lipid component of lipoproteins deposited in dermis and subcutaneous tissue [3, 4]
- Pruritus: etiology unclear, likely secondary to bile salts (suggested by response to cholestyramine) but unclear how they lead to disease; may be due to balance of intrahepatic bile acids, level of serum opioids (responds to opioid antagonists), maybe centrally mediated due to serum contents [2, 3]
- Primary biliary cirrhosis (PBC) is an autoimmune disease of the biliary ducts with a female:male ratio of 9:1; patients are presumed to have a genetic predisposition, which is triggered by environmental factors such as smoking and infection [5, 6]

Histopathological features include:

- Xanthoma in PBC: lipid laden or foamy histocytes in a diffuse and/or nodular pattern in the upper dermis (*see* Figs. 66.2 and 66.3)
- Lichen planus in PBC: irregular epidermal hyperplasia with compact hyperkeratosis, wedge shaped hypergranulosis, vacuolar alteration and a bandlike inflammatory infiltrate obscuring the dermal-epidermal interface and composed of predominantly lymphocytes.
- Hyperpigmented skin in PBC: due to increased melanin in the epidermis and dermis.

The diagnosis is made using a combination of:

- Three criteria for diagnosis of PBC: if all three criteria positive, then diagnosis is definite; if two criteria positive, then diagnosis is probable [2]

L. Zakko (✉)
Yale Department of Internal Medicine, Yale New Haven Hospital, New Haven, CT, USA

Yale Primary Care Clinic,
789 Howard Avenue, New Haven, CT 06519-1304, USA
e-mail: liam.zakko@yale.edu

J. Finch • M.J. Rothe • J.M. Grant-Kels
Department of Dermatology,
University of Connecticut Health Center,
21 South Road, Farmington, CT 06030, USA
e-mail: finch@uchc.edu; rothe@uchc.edu; grant@uchc.edu

G.Y. Wu et al. (eds.), *Atlas of Dermatological Manifestations of Gastrointestinal Disease*,
DOI 10.1007/978-1-4614-6191-3_66, © Springer Science+Business Media New York 2013

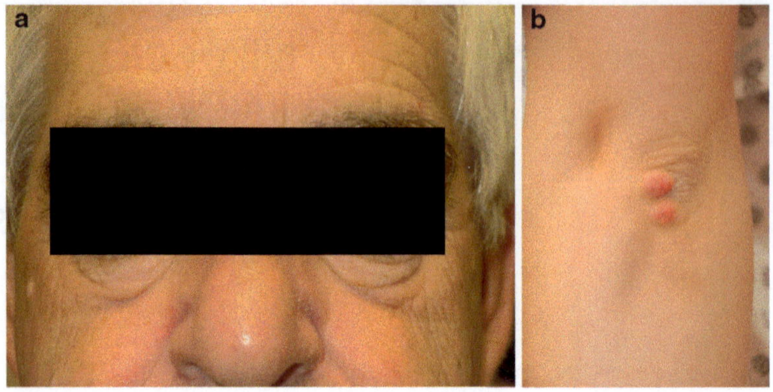

Fig. 66.1 Primary biliary cirrhosis. (**a**) Xanthelasma. (**b**) Tuberous xanthoma

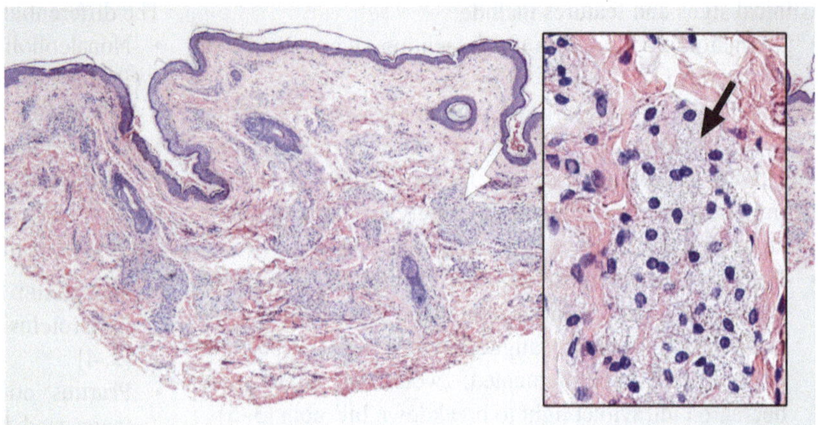

Fig. 66.2 Xanthelasma. A photomicrograph of a section of thin epidermis (eyelid skin) showing foam cells in the dermis. (Hematoxylin and eosin [H and E] stain, 40×; *inset* 1000×)

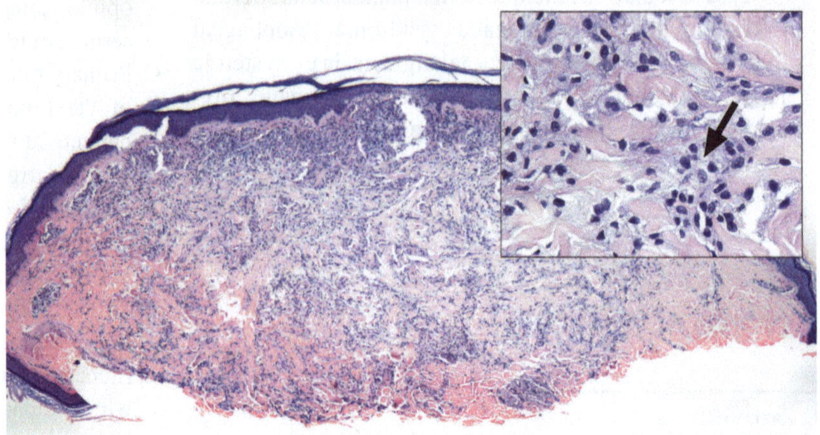

Fig. 66.3 Tuberous xanthoma. A photomicrograph of a section of a nodular lesion showing foam cells in the dermis. (H and E stain, 20×; *inset* 1000×)

- Detectable antimitochondrial antibodies
- Elevated liver enzymes (alkaline phosphate most common) for 6 months
- Histologic findings in the liver compatible with the disease

Treatment options include:

- Disfiguring xanthoma can be surgically resected [3]
- Pruritus responds to cholestyramine, rifampin, antihistamines, sertraline, naltrexone, ultraviolet light, ursodeoxycholic acid, plasmapheresis, liver transplant [2, 3, 7]
- Ultimately primary biliary cirrhosis requires direct treatment [2, 3, 5–7]

References

1. Koulentaki M, Ioannidou D, Stefanidou M, et al. Dermatological manifestations in primary biliary cirrhosis patients: a case control study. Am J Gastroenterol. 2006;101:541–6.
2. Kaplan MM, Gershwin ME. Primary biliary cirrhosis. N Engl J Med. 2005;353:1261–73.
3. Heathcote J. The clinical expression of primary biliary cirrhosis. Semin Liver Dis. 1997;17:23–33.
4. Hsu JC, Su TC, Chen MF, et al. Xanthoma striatum palmare in a patient with primary biliary cirrhosis and hypercholesterolemia. J Gastroenterol Hepatol. 2005;20:1799–1800.
5. Bhandari BM, Bayat H, Rothstein KD. Primary biliary cirrhosis. Gastroenterol Clin North Am. 2011;40:373–86.
6. Kumagi T, Heathcote EJ. Primary biliary cirrhosis. Orphanet J Rare Dis. 2008;3:I.
7. Crosignani A, Battezzati PM, Invernizzi P, et al. Clinical features and management of primary biliary cirrhosis. World J Gastroenterol. 2008;14:3313–27.

Cirrhosis: Gastrointestinal Features

67

Marcy Qureshi and Faripour Forouhar

Cirrhosis is the end stage of chronic liver disease characterized by the presence of fibrosis and scar tissue. This stage of liver disease is associated with multiple complications and causes poor quality of life, increased risk of infection, and has a poor prognosis. Although the disease is centered in the liver, it has myriad effects in other organ systems. Cirrhosis has a 10-year mortality of 34–66%. The wide range is due to differences in the various etiologies of disease.

Gastrointestinal (GI) symptoms include [1]:

- Increasing abdominal girth from ascites
- Upper GI bleeding or rectal bleeding

Clinical signs and findings include [1]:

- Development of portal hypertension
  - Hepatic encephalopathy
  - Esophageal (see Fig. 67.1), gastric, or rectal varices (see Fig. 67.2)
  - Portal hypertensive gastropathy (see Fig. 67.3)
  - Ascites/fluid retention
- Development of hepatocellular carcinoma

The pathogenesis stems from increased deposition of extracellular matrix components in sensitive areas of the liver [1]:

- Diffuse process characterized by tissue fibrosis and conversion of normal liver architecture into abnormal nodules
- Numerous causes
  - Chronic hepatitis B or C
  - Alcohol consumption
  - Obesity associated with nonalcoholic steatohepatitis
  - Autoimmune liver disease
  - Iron or copper storage diseases
  - Genetic deficiencies

On pathology examination, typical findings are [1]:

- Diffuse fibrosis (stage 4 on Metavir scoring system) (see Fig. 67.4)
- Regenerative nodules (see Figs. 67.5 and 67.6)
- Altered lobular architecture and establishment of intrahepatic vascular shunts between afferent and efferent vessels of the liver
- Capillarization of sinusoids and perisinusoidal fibrosis
- Vascular thrombosis and obliterative lesions in portal tracts and hepatic veins
- Underperfusion of lobular parenchyma and tissue hypoxia

The diagnosis is made by considering [1]:

- Imaging with ultrasound/computed tomography scan consistent with altered hepatic architecture
- Physical examination findings of portal hypertension
- Ascites fluid analysis consistent with portal hypertension
- Liver biopsy

The differential diagnosis of cirrhosis should include [1]:

- Chronic viral hepatitis
- Autoimmune
- Alcohol abuse
- Genetic disease: Wilsons disease, Hemochromatosis, alpha-1 antitrypsin deficiency
- Thyroid disease
- Celiac disease

The treatment involves:

- Treatment of underlying cause of cirrhosis
- Liver transplant
- Treatment of symptoms of portal hypertension
  - Diuretic therapy
  - Paracentesis
  - Variceal band ligation/nonselective beta blockade
  - Lactulose therapy to prevent hepatic encephalopathy

M. Qureshi
Department of Internal Medicine, University of Connecticut Health Center, Farmington, CT, USA

Eastern Connecticut Medical Professionals, 945 Main Street Suite 202/203, Manchester, CT 06040, USA
e-mail: mqureshi@echn.org

F. Forouhar (✉)
Department of Pathology, University of Connecticut Health Center, 21 South Road, Farmington, CT 06030, USA
e-mail: forouhar@nso1.uchc.edu

G.Y. Wu et al. (eds.), *Atlas of Dermatological Manifestations of Gastrointestinal Disease*,
DOI 10.1007/978-1-4614-6191-3_67, © Springer Science+Business Media New York 2013

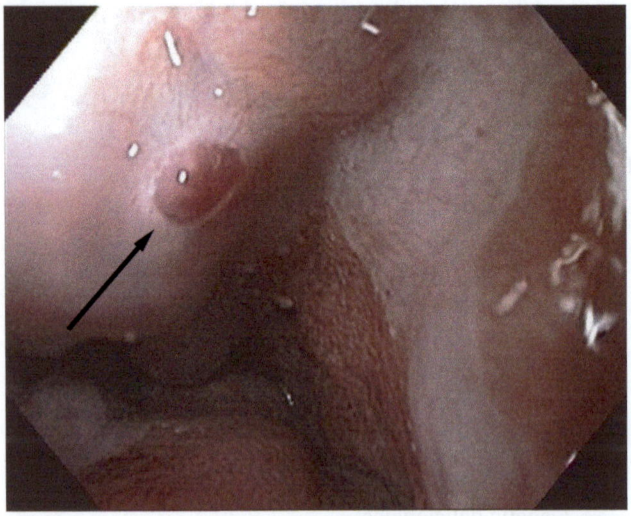

Fig. 67.1 An endoscopic view of large esophageal varices in the distal esophagus in a patient with cirrhosis due to hepatitis C. A "nipple sign" (*arrow*) on a varix is considered to be evidence of recent bleeding

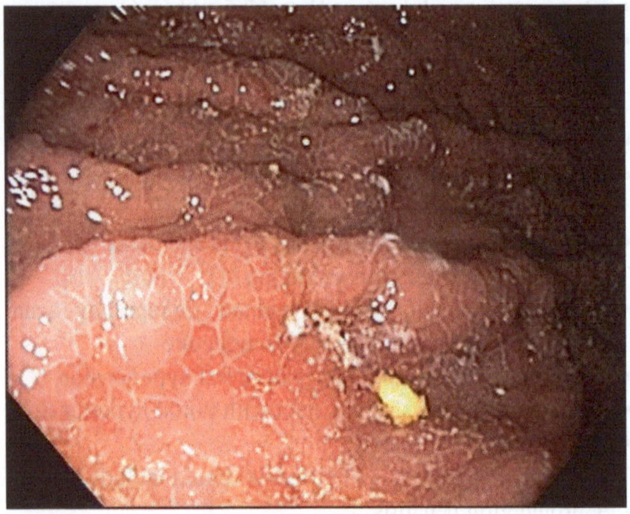

Fig. 67.2 An endoscopic, retroflexed view of the rectum showing dilated internal hemorrhoidal veins that have become rectal varices (*arrow*)

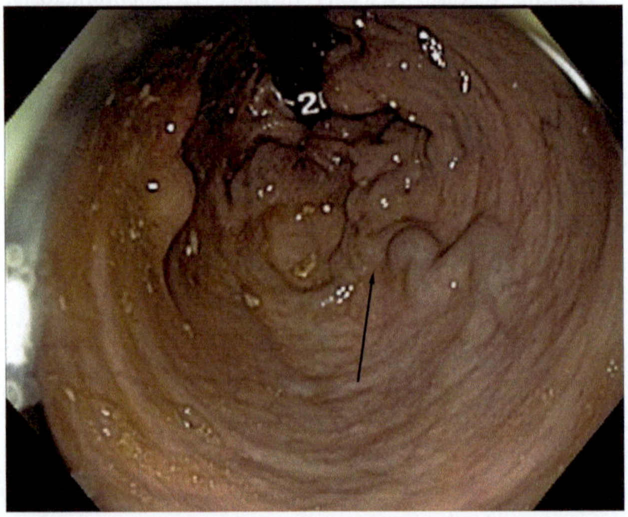

Fig. 67.3 An endoscopic view of portal gastropathy. Hyperemic edematous mucosa with a "fish scale" appearance is characteristic of this feature of portal hypertension

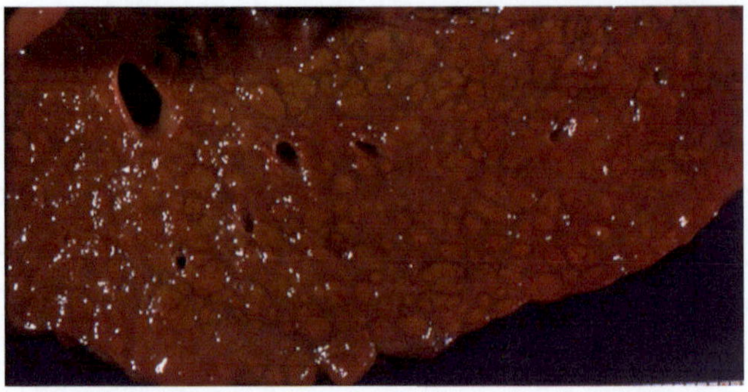

Fig. 67.4 The cut surface of a cirrhotic liver demonstrating a grossly nodular appearance

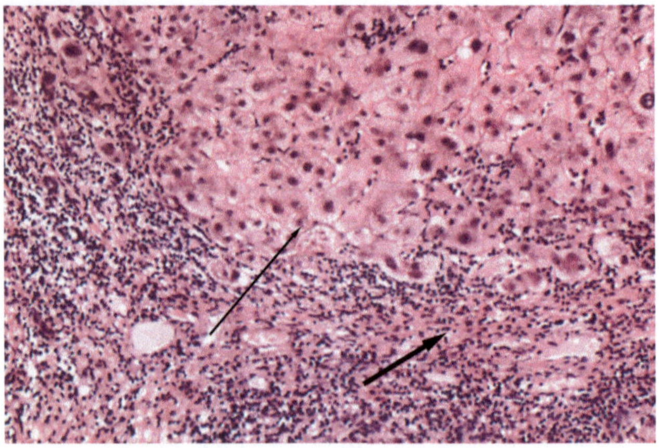

Fig. 67.5 A photomicrograph of a liver biopsy section from a cirrhotic patient. A regenerative nodule is shown (*thin arrow*) surrounded by fibrous septae (*thick arrow*) and a severe inflammatory response. Hematoxylin and eosin stain, high power

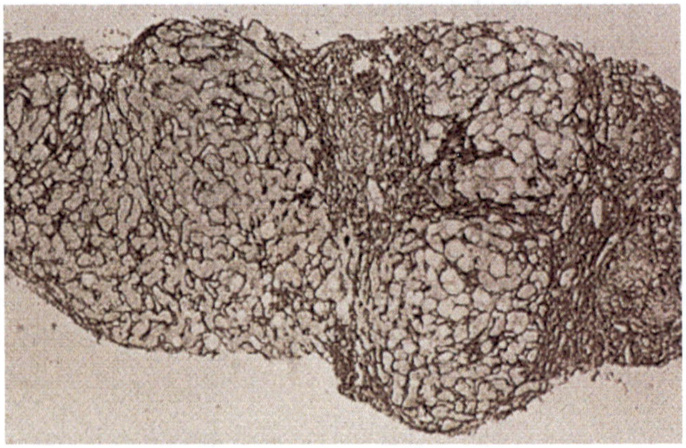

Fig. 67.6 A photomicrograph of a liver biopsy section from a cirrhotic patient. Regenerative nodules are shown clearly outlined by fibrotic septae. Reticulin stain, high power

Reference

1. Pinzani M, Rosselli M. Liver cirrhosis. Best Pract Res Clin Gastroenterol. 2011;25:281–90.

Cirrhosis: Dermatological Features 68

Liam Zakko, Justin Finch, Marti J. Rothe,
and Jane M. Grant-Kels

Clinical characteristics include:

- Liver disease often presents with cutaneous findings: chronic alcoholism, 43% have cutaneous findings; alcohol cirrhosis, 72% have spider angioma, palmar erythema, or Dupuytren's contractures [1]
- Jaundice: occurs when serum bilirubin >2.5–3.0 mg/dL; if mild, skin is yellow; if severe, skin is brown [1]
- Pruritus of cholestasis: tends to be generalized, worse in hands and feet [1]
- Prurigo nodularis: associated especially with cirrhosis due to hepatitis C; firm, pruritic hyperkeratotic nodules 1 mm–2 cm in diameter; usually on the extremities although no part of the body is exempt, often with xerotic/lichenified skin between nodules and excoriations/crusting on the lesions [1, 2]
- Spider angiomas (spider nevi) (*see* Fig. 68.1): occur in vascular area drained by superior vena cava [3–5] in 33% of cirrhotics; the more present, the worse the cirrhosis; on examination, they will disappear with pressure [1] and if large enough, they will pulsate [3]; they are closely associated with esophageal varices [3]
- Bier spots: hypopigmented, small irregular-shaped patches on the arms and legs; on examination, the lesions will disappear with pressure and with limb elevation [1]
- Paper money skin: upper trunk with scattered, needle-thin superficial capillaries; common in alcoholic cirrhosis [1]
- Palmar erythema: florid, crimson color of palms and fingertips [1] (most common on the thenar or hypothenar eminences), characteristically bilateral and symmetrical in 23% of cirrhotics [4] (*see* Fig. 68.2)
- Xanthelasma: can be a feature of cholestatic liver disease; localized cholesterol deposits beneath the skin (especially the eyelids); painless, yellow, soft plaques with well-defined borders that often grow over weeks [1]
- Hair and/or nail Loss; clubbing of nails; flat nails; Terry's nails (*see* Fig. 68.3), a nail finding in which the proximal two thirds of the nail appear white, with preservation of a normal 1–3 mm band of color at the distal nail bed [1, 5]
- Dupuytren's contracture: progressive fibrosis and thickening of the tendons in the palmar fascia that over time leads to stiffness in the joints to the point that a patient's fingers cannot fully extend or flex (*see* Fig. 68.4) [1]
- Disseminated superficial porokeratosis: multiple pink, tan flat annular papules and plaques with a slightly elevated keratotic margin (the process is more commonly seen in cirrhotics); of concern because these lesions can progress rarely to squamous cell carcinoma [1]
- Dilated superficial abdominal veins due to diversion of blood away from the portal venous system is exemplified by the caput medusa (*see* Fig. 68.5)

Pathogenesis is based on abnormalities caused by liver dysfunction:

- Pruritus: failure to metabolize toxins and filter bile salts; somewhat centrally mediated due to increased central nervous system opioids [1]

L. Zakko (✉)
Yale Department of Internal Medicine, Yale New Haven Hospital, New Haven, CT, USA

Yale Primary Care Clinic,
789 Howard Avenue, New Haven, CT 06519-1304, USA
e-mail: liam.zakko@yale.edu

J. Finch • M.J. Rothe • J.M. Grant-Kels
Department of Dermatology,
University of Connecticut Health Center,
21 South Road, Farmington, CT 06030, USA
e-mail: finch@uchc.edu; rothe@uchc.edu; grant@uchc.edu

G.Y. Wu et al. (eds.), *Atlas of Dermatological Manifestations of Gastrointestinal Disease*,
DOI 10.1007/978-1-4614-6191-3_68, © Springer Science+Business Media New York 2013

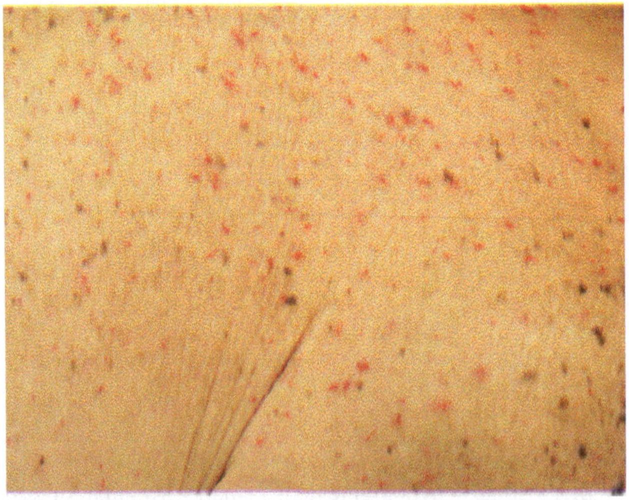

Fig. 68.1 Spider angiomata. A florid case on the chest. Telangiectatic "arms" extending radially from a central vessel is characteristic

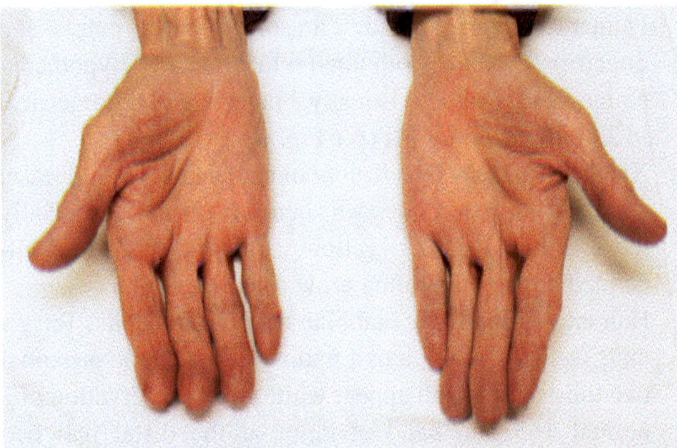

Fig. 68.2 Palmar erythema. Crimson color of palms, fingertips, thenar, and hypothenar eminences

- Prurigo nodularis: postulated that it may be due to increased neuropeptides, electrolyte abnormalities, changes in growth factors, or deposition of immune complexes [2]
- Spider nevi: associated with increased estrogen and estrogen/androgen ratio, although unclear if due to estrogen or elevations in growth factors, vascular endothelial growth factor (VEGF)/basic fibroblast growth factor (bFGF) [5]
- Palmar erythema: also associated with increased estrogen and estrogen/androgen ratio; due to vasodilation from increased prostacyclins and nitric oxide that accumulate in patients with liver disease [1]; may be increased in those with alcoholic cirrhosis due to phytoestrogen content of alcohol, acetaldehyde (an ethanol metabolite), and calcitonin gene-related peptide [5]

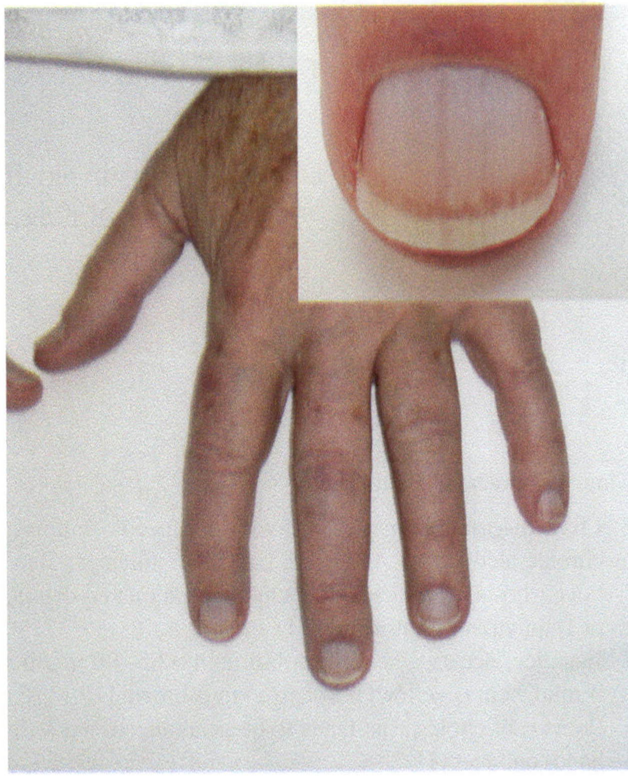

Fig. 68.3 Terry's nails. Apparent leukonychia (whitish nails) of all fingernails, obscuring the lunulae and sparing the distal 2–3 mm

- Xanthelasma: secondary to dyslipidemia; increased triglycerides and decreased high-density lipoprotein (HDL) are most common [1]
- Dupuytren's contracture: etiology unknown but associated with alcoholic cirrhosis [1]
- Porokeratosis: likely due to decreased humoral and cell-mediated responses [1]

The pathology of the skin is varied:

- Spider angioma: small dilated arterioles (0.5 cm in diameter) from which small telengiectatic vessels radiate [5]
- Terry's nails: distal band with telangiectasia; proximal area with hyperplasia of connective tissue between nail and bone [5]
- Porokeratosis: presence of cornoid lamella [5]
- Prurigo nodularis: compact hyperkeratosis with focal parakeratosis and marked acanthosis often of pseudoepithiliomatous proportions; thickening of papillary dermal collagen often in vertical orientation; hypertrophy and increased proliferation of dermal nerves; lymphocytes, histiocytes, mast cells and occasional eosinophils within the dermis [2]

Diagnosis is made on the basis of clinical features, imaging, blood tests, and pathology:

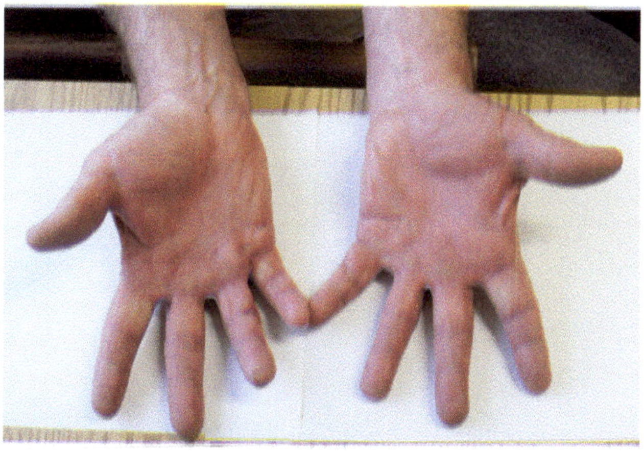

Fig. 68.4 Dupuytren's contractures. Progressive fibrosis and thickening of the tendons in the palmar fascia that prevents complete extension or flexion of the fingers

Fig. 68.5 Distended superficial abdominal veins due to diversion of blood from the portal venous system and is exemplified by the caput medusa

- Above findings in adults merit a workup for liver disease including liver function tests, tests for hepatic injury, and hepatic imaging

  The differential diagnosis includes:
- Variable depending on the skin findings but includes the differential for cirrhosis as well as a number of rheumatologic diseases, particularly rheumatoid arthritis and lupus, and high estrogen states such as pregnancy

  Treatment is largely symptomatic:
- Pruritus: resin cholestyramine, rifampin, naltrexone, and in severe/refractory cases consider plasmapheresis; responds to liver transplantation [1]
- Prurigo nodularis: first line, topical antipruritics (corticosteroids, pramoxine, menthol), intralesional steroids; second: ultraviolet light treatment, cryotherapy, vitamin D, capsaicin; third: naltrexone, cyclosporine, low-dose thalidomide [1, 2]
- Dupuytren contractures: surgical fasciectomy [1]
- Porokeratosis: clears with improved liver function [1]

References

1. Hazin R, Abu-Rajab Tamimi TI, Abuzetun JY, Zein NN. Recognizing and treating cutaneous signs of liver disease. Cleveland Clin J Med. 2009;76:599–606.
2. Lee MR, Shumack S. Prurigo nodularis: a review. Australas J Dermatol. 2005;46:211–20.
3. Ruocco V, Psilogenis M, Schiavo AL, Wolf R. Dermatologic manifestations of alcoholic cirrhosis. Clin Dermatol. 1999;17:463–8.
4. Serrao R, Zirwas M, English JC. Palmar erythema. Am J Clin Dermatol. 2007;8:347–56.
5. Ghosn SH, Kibbi AG. Cutaneous manifestations of liver diseases. Clin Dermatol. 2008;26:274–82.

Wilson's Disease: Gastrointestinal Features

69

Marcy Qureshi and Faripour Forouhar

Wilson's disease is an autosomal recessive disorder that causes copper to accumulate in various tissues throughout the body. Carriers occur at a rate of approximately one in 100, but the disease occurs in 1–4 per 100,000. Disease found early can be treated, but advanced disease may require a liver transplant [1].

Gastrointestinal symptoms associated with the disease are [1, 2]:

- Combination of liver disease with neuropsychiatric disturbances
- Symptoms related to end-stage liver disease or acute liver failure

Clinical signs and findings include [1, 2]:

- Elevated aminotransferases
- Acute or chronic hepatitis
- Fulminant hepatic failure
- Cirrhosis/end-stage liver disease with portal hypertension
  - Ascites/fluid retention
  - Esophageal/rectal varices
  - Portal hypertensive gastropathy
  - Hemorrhagic diathesis
  - Hepatic encephalopathy
- Kayser–Fleischer rings
- Sunflower cataracts
- Skin manifestations of chronic liver disease
  - Spider telangiectasias
  - Gynecomastia
  - Jaundice/icterus
  - Muehrcke's lines, Terry's nails
  - Palmar erythema
- Osteoarthritis
- Cardiac findings
- Nephrocalcinosis
- Chondrocalcinosis
- Hypercalciuria
- Depression
- Mood lability
- Psychosis
- Cognitive decline
- Tremor
- Dysarthria/aphasia
- Ataxia/bradykinesia
- Infertility/increased risk of miscarriage
- Hypoparathyroidism

The pathogenesis is based on a genetic defect in the excretion of copper [3]:

- Autosomal recessive
- Mutations in the *ATP7B* gene on chromosome 13
  - Reduction in the *ATP7B* function results in decreased biliary copper excretion
  - Increased copper accumulation in hepatic and extrahepatic tissues
  - Excess copper released into circulation and taken up by central nervous system

Typical liver pathology shows [3]:

- Liver biopsy dry weight 75 μg/g copper
- Liver biopsy histology varies with stage (see Fig. 69.1)
  - Early: hepatic steatosis, mitochondria with crystalline deposits and dilated cristae with advancing fibrosis
  - Later: lysosomal deposits of copper and copper metallothionein
  - Late stage: hepatocellular disruption with advanced cirrhosis and fibrosis
  - Acute liver failure: apoptosis and necrosis on the background of advanced fibrosis
- Copper staining of liver biopsy

M. Qureshi
Department of Internal Medicine, University of Connecticut Health Center, Farmington, CT, USA

Eastern Connecticut Medical Professionals, 945 Main Street Suite 202/203, Manchester, CT 06040, USA
e-mail: mqureshi@echn.org

F. Forouhar (✉)
Department of Pathology, University of Connecticut Health Center, 21 South Road, Farmington, CT 06030, USA
e-mail: forouhar@nso1.uchc.edu

G.Y. Wu et al. (eds.), *Atlas of Dermatological Manifestations of Gastrointestinal Disease*, DOI 10.1007/978-1-4614-6191-3_69, © Springer Science+Business Media New York 2013

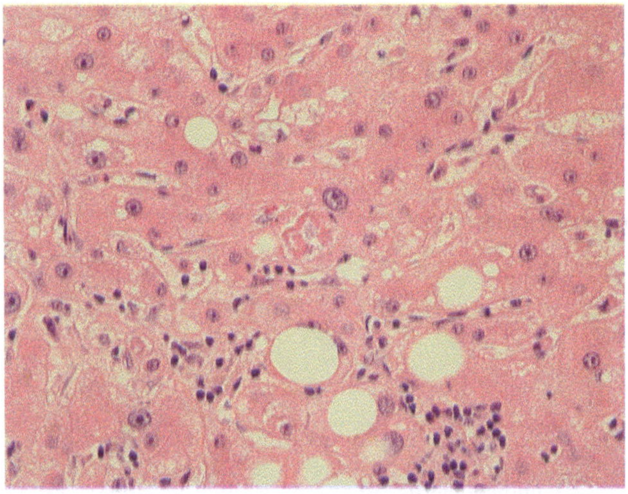

Fig. 69.1 Photomicrograph of liver biopsy specimen from a patient with Wilson's disease showing periportal region with spotty necrosis (focal inflammatory cell infiltration and hepatocellular pleomorphism indicating focal hepatocellular necrosis). There is also fatty change and a large Mallory body in the center. Hematoxylin and eosin, ×400

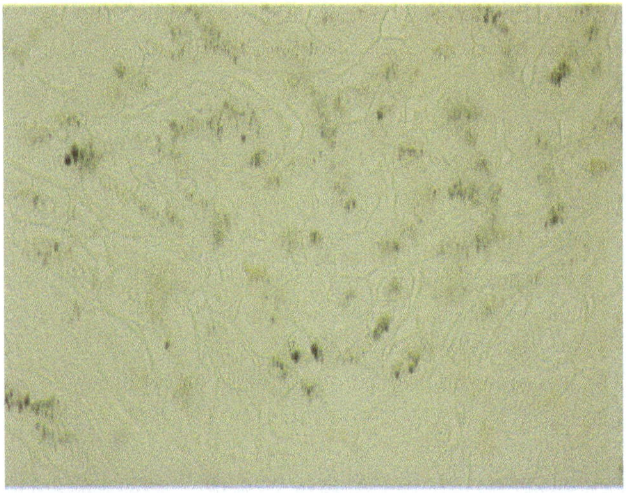

Fig. 69.2 Photomicrograph of liver biopsy specimen a periportal region showing copper deposition (*black granules*) in the hepatocytes. Copper stain ×400

- Copper staining positive nodules with nearby areas absent for copper staining (regenerative areas)(see Fig. 69.2)

The diagnosis is made by considering [3]:

- Family history
- Genetic testing with two mutations of *ATP7B*
- Physical examination
  - Kayser–Fleischer rings
  - Neuropsychiatric disturbances
- Imaging
  - MRI/CT brain detects changes in the basal ganglia or pons or thalamus
- Laboratory testing
  - Depressed levels of serum alkaline phosphatase for the degree of jaundice
  - Alkaline phosphatase:bilirubin level ratio <4
  - Aspartate aminotransferase/alanine aminotransferase (AST:ALT) >2.2
  - Serum copper >200 μg/dL
  - Serum free copper >20 μg/dL
  - Low ceruloplasmin <20 mg/dL
  - 24 h urinary copper
    - o One hundred micro grams per 24 h (in the presence of Kayser–Fleischer rings)
    - o Forty micro grams per 24 h (in the presence of liver biopsy consistent with Wilson's disease)
- Liver biopsy with hepatic copper >75 μg/g dry weight

The differential diagnosis of Wilson's disease should include [2, 3]:

- Nonalcoholic fatty liver disease
- Acute or chronic hepatitis
  - Viral hepatitis
  - Autoimmune hepatitis/overlap syndromes
- Fatty acid oxidation metabolism disorder
- Mitochondrial disorder

The treatment involves [2, 3]:

- Penicillamine 20 mg/kg/day by mouth to a maximum of 2 g/day
- Trientine 750–1,500 mg by mouth three to four times a day (adults)
- Zinc salts 150 mg by mouth three times a day (adults)
- Liver transplant

References

1. Ferenci P. Pathophysiology and clinical features of Wilson disease. Metab Brain Dis. 2004;19:229–39.
2. Schilsky M. Wilson disease: current status and the future. Biochimie. 2009;91:1278–81.
3. Rosencrantz R, Schilsky M. Wilson disease: pathogenesis and clinical considerations in diagnosis and treatment. Sem Liver Dis. 2011;31:245–59.

Wilson's Disease (Hepatolenticular Degeneration): Dermatological Features

70

Liam Zakko, Justin Finch, Marti J. Rothe, and Jane M. Grant-Kels

Clinical features include:

- Prevalence thought to be 1 in 30,000 [1, 2], although now with improved diagnostic techniques it may be determined that Wilson's is more common than previously thought [2]
- Most patients present with cirrhosis; usual onset is childhood to young adult but can present in patients as old as age 70 years [2]
- In children, 70% have at least one skin or mucosal finding including xerosis (46%) and white bands on the nails (19%) [3]
- In adults, classically associated with blue lunulae of the nails (10%), gray-brown macular hyperpigmentation especially of the lower extremities where it may have a rippled appearance, and vague greenish discoloration of the skin of the face, neck, and genitalia [1, 3, 4]
- Kayser-Fleischer rings: copper deposits in the cornea are the cardinal sign of the disease (reported in various series of patients with Wilson's as being present in 85–100% of patients with neurological/psychiatric symptoms, 33–86% with hepatic disease, and 0–59% with asymptomatic disease) (see Fig. 70.1) [2]
- Hepatic disease (nodular cirrhosis, fulminant liver failure, or aminotransferase elevations) can have associated dermatologic symptoms of pruritus, spider angiomas, palmar erythema, and jaundice. Skin findings are more likely in patients with longer duration of disease: spider angiomas are present in 5.3% of patients with disease less than 2 years in duration and in 33% of patients with disease less than 6 years in duration [3]
- Neurologic disease includes psychiatric symptoms (e.g., depression), tremor, chorea, and parkinsonism (from basal ganglia and surrounding area disease) [2, 5]
- Note: penicillamine treatment can also cause skin disease (degenerative dermatoses, lichenoid eruption, and mouth ulcers) [1]

The differential diagnosis should include:

- Other causes of liver disease
- Menkes' disease
- Protein calorie malnutrition
- Nephrotic syndrome
- Protein losing enteropathy
- Acquired copper deficiency

Pathogenesis of this disease has been delineated:

- Autosomal recessive disease in which copper pathologically accumulates in the liver and then the central nervous system and other tissues [3]
- Copper accumulation is caused by mutations in the *ATP7B* gene leading to defective copper incorporation into ceruloplasmin and a reduction in biliary excretion of copper [2]

Pathologic features include:

- Hyperpigmentation: due to increased melanin in basal cell layer; otherwise normal skin structure and no copper deposits [4]
- Kayser-Fleischer rings: fine granular deposits in Descemet's membrane at the periphery extending inward from Schwalbe's line [5]

L. Zakko (✉)
Yale Department of Internal Medicine, Yale New Haven Hospital, 20 York Street, New Haven, CT 06510, USA
e-mail: liam.zakko@yale.edu

J. Finch • M.J. Rothe • J.M. Grant-Kels
Department of Dermatology, University of Connecticut Health Center, 21 South Road, Farmington, CT 06030, USA
e-mail: finch@uchc.edu; rothe@uchc.edu; grant@uchc.edu

G.Y. Wu et al. (eds.), *Atlas of Dermatological Manifestations of Gastrointestinal Disease*, DOI 10.1007/978-1-4614-6191-3_70, © Springer Science+Business Media New York 2013

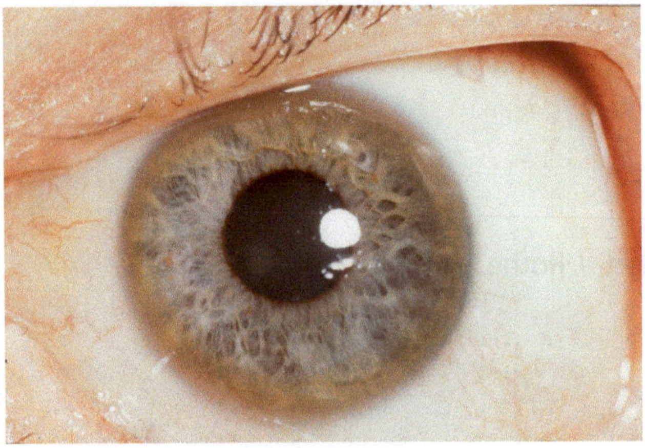

Fig. 70.1 A slit-lamp view of a typical example of pigment deposition encircling the iris of the eye. Kayser-Fleischer rings are characteristic but not pathognomonic for Wilson's disease

Diagnosis is made by a combination of the following [2]:

- Laboratory evidence of liver disease with low ceruloplasmin and high 24-h urinary copper excretion (increased urinary output after penicillamine challenge may be a better way to diagnose)
- Typical neurological findings or hepatic dysfunction with low plasma ceruloplasmin and/or the presence of Kayser-Fleischer rings
- If the patient has typical neurologic and hepatic dysfunction findings without typical lab or physical examination evidence of disease, then in certain populations genetic testing can be pursued

Treatment approach includes [2]

- If found before significant liver disease, copper chelation is the preferred treatment although it is lifelong
- Zinc/trientine is the treatment of choice as there are fewer side effects than with penicillamine; major concern is to watch for excessive chelation
- In advanced disease, liver transplant is often necessary

References

1. Al Mohizea S. Rippled hyperpigmentation in Wilson's disease. Int J Dermatol. 2010;49:67–9.
2. Mak CM, Lam CW. Diagnosis of Wilson's disease: a comprehensive review. Crit Rev Clin Lab Sci. 2008;45:263–90.
3. Seyhan M, Erdem T, Selimogu MA, et al. Dermatological signs in Wilson's disease. Pediatr Int. 2009;51:395–8.
4. Leu ML, Stickland GT, Wang CC, et al. Skin pigmentation in Wilson's disease. JAMA. 1970;211:1542–3.
5. Harry J, Tripati R. Kayser-Fleischer ring: a pathological study. Br J Ophthalmol. 1970;54:794–800.

71 Hereditary Hemochromatosis: Gastrointestinal Features

Marcy Qureshi and Faripour Forouhar

Hemochromatosis is a disease defined by iron overload. Hereditary hemochromatosis is an autosomal recessive disease with a prevalence of 2 per 1,000 in those of European ancestry. It most commonly presents with liver disease but can also affect many other organ systems [1].

Gastrointestinal symptoms often include [1]:

- Abdominal pain
- Symptoms related to complications of cirrhosis and portal hypertension
- Hepatomegaly
- Cirrhosis/end-stage liver disease with portal hypertension
  - Ascites/fluid retention
  - Esophageal/rectal varices
  - Portal hypertensive gastropathy
  - Hemorrhagic diathesis
  - Hepatic encephalopathy
- Diabetes mellitus/"bronze diabetes"
- Cardiomyopathy
- Impotence from hypogonadotropic hypogonadism due to pituitary involvement
- Development of hepatocellular carcinoma
- Elevated aminotransferase levels

The pathogenesis is based on genetic mutations that affect transport of iron. The most common involve HFE, a regulator of hepcidin, the major serum signaling protein [2–4]

- Autosomal recessive
- Mutation of *HFE* gene
  - Homozygous at *C282Y* (80% of cases have mutations at this locus)
  - Compound heterozygote mutation of *C282Y* and *H63D* plus another risk factor for iron overload
  - Homozygous H63D not clinically significant for development of iron overload
  - Leads to inappropriately high levels of iron absorption and deposition in the liver and other organs

The pathology of iron overload of the liver can show [1]:

- Liver biopsy (see Fig. 71.1)
  - Two to 4+ or more hepatocellular iron stores on staining with higher density in the periportal area
  - Severe iron storage shows 4+ staining with fibrosis
  - Hepatic iron index of 1.9 μmol/g/year
  - Hepatic iron concentration of >71 μmol/g/dry weight

The diagnosis is made with [1]:

- Transferrin saturation >45%
- Elevated ferritin
- C282Y and H63D mutation genetic testing
- Abnormal liver enzymes
- Hepatomegaly
- Liver biopsy
- Hepatic magnetic resonance imaging

The differential diagnosis of hemochromatosis should include [1]:

- Secondary iron overload
  - Sideroblastic anemia
  - Thalassemia major
  - Sickle cell anemia
  - Excess alcohol consumption
  - Parenteral iron overload from transfusions
- Nonalcoholic steatohepatitis

The treatment involves removal of iron and reduction of iron body stores [1]:

- Phlebotomy to remove excess iron stores performed weekly until
  - Ferritin is <50 ng/mL
  - Transferrin iron saturation <50%

M. Qureshi
Department of Internal Medicine, University of Connecticut Health Center, Farmington, CT, USA

Eastern Connecticut Medical Professionals, 945 Main Street Suite 202/203, Manchester, CT 06040, USA
e-mail: mqureshi@echn.org

F. Forouhar (✉)
Department of Pathology, University of Connecticut Health Center, 21 South Road, Farmington, CT 06030, USA
e-mail: Forouhar@nso1.uchc.edu

G.Y. Wu et al. (eds.), *Atlas of Dermatological Manifestations of Gastrointestinal Disease*, DOI 10.1007/978-1-4614-6191-3_71, © Springer Science+Business Media New York 2013

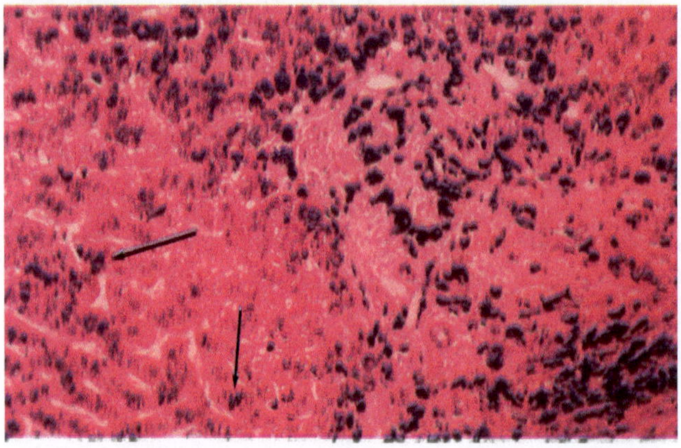

Fig. 71.1 A photomicrograph of a liver biopsy specimen stained with Prussian Blue showing iron overload liver parenchymal (hepatocytes) (*arrows*) typical of hemochromatosis. In addition, because of heavy overload, there is also iron present in epithelium of bile educts, Kupffer cells, and stroma of portal areas (High-power magnification)

- Chelation with deferoxamine, deferasirox, or deferiprone, if anemia and iron overload are present concomitantly
- Avoidance of vitamin C, which enhances iron toxicity
- Liver transplant; screen for hepatocellular carcinoma if cirrhosis is present

References

1. Gan EK, Powell LW, Olynyk JK. Natural history and management of HFE-hemochromatosis. Semin Liver Dis. 2011;31:293–301.
2. Alexander J, Kowdley K. HFE-associated hereditary hemochromatosis. Genet Med. 2009;11:307–11.
3. Deugnier Y, Brissot P, Loreal O. Iron and the liver: update 2008. J Hepatol. 2008;48:S113–23.
4. Babitt JL, Lin HY. The molecular pathogenesis of hereditary hemochromatosis. Semin Liver Dis. 2011;31:280–92.

Hemochromatosis: Dermatological Features

72

Liam Zakko, Justin Finch, Marti J. Rothe, and Jane M. Grant-Kels

Clinical characteristics include:

- Also called "bronze diabetes" [1]
- Multisystem disease due to iron deposition that usually presents in 30–40 year olds as iron stores increase to 15–40 g (normal is usually 4 g) [1, 2]; besides skin changes, patient can have cirrhosis, diabetes, and hypogonadism
- Increased discoloration of skin exposed to the sun (persons often report tanning with minimal sun exposure) [1] (see Fig. 72.1); occurs in mucous membranes/conjunctival membranes in 15–20% of patients [3]
- Hyperpigmentation is an early sign found in 90% of patients; often grayish due to iron deposits (heme2) and brownish (due to increased melanin production) bronze hue [1]
- Loss of body hair (particularly pubic and axillary due to hypogonadism) [1, 3]
- Koilonychia [1]
- Ichthyosiform alterations: fish-scale skin due to extremely dry skin [1]
- Forty percent of patients with hemochromatosis are alcoholics, although that is likely just hemochromatosis potentiated by ethanol; ethanol may increase iron uptake and absorption, decrease iron utilization secondary to decreased erythropoiesis, repeated bursts of hemolysis, and increased iron deposition due to liver damage [4]

L. Zakko (✉)
Yale Department of Internal Medicine, Yale New Haven Hospital, 20 York Street, New Haven, CT 06510, USA
e-mail: liam.zakko@yale.edu

J. Finch • M.J. Rothe • J.M. Grant-Kels
Department of Dermatology, University of Connecticut Health Center, 21 South Road, Farmington, CT 06030, USA
e-mail: finch@uchc.edu; rothe@uchc.edu; grant@uchc.edu

Pathogenesis is based on genetic defects that affect regulation of iron absorption:

- One of the most common autosomal recessive genetic diseases (1:400 prevalence) in which there is a defect in intestinal iron absorption due to a mutation on chromosome 6 (60–93% homozygous for mutation C282Y) [1–3]
- Cutaneous iron deposits injure vital skin structures culminating in increased melanin production (increased in sun exposed areas due to the synergistic effects of ultraviolet light on melanin production) [3]

Pathology of the skin can be varied:

- Broken elastic fibers with decreased numbers of fibers presenting as dermal atrophy in one quarter of patients and epidermal atrophy in 62% of patients with decreased thickness of the stratum malpighii [5]
- Ichthyosis: orthokeratotic hyperkeratosis and reduction/disappearance of the stratum granulosum [5]
- Hyperpigmented areas with increased melanin noted within the basal cell layer of the epidermis; iron deposits and siderophages especially around blood vessels and eccrine sweat glands as well as within the basement membrane zone of eccrine glands [5] highlighted by an iron stain, such as Perl's Prussian blue stain (see Fig. 72.2).

Diagnosis is made by a combination of clinical features and laboratory tests:

- Significantly under diagnosed; it is estimated that a primary care physician sees a patient with the disorder every 2 weeks [2]
- Increased serum transferrin saturation with increased ferritin [2]
- Early diagnosis by analysis of the *HFE* gene [3]
- Gold standard is liver biopsy [2]

The differential diagnosis includes:

- Diabetes mellitus
- Secondary iron overload

G.Y. Wu et al. (eds.), *Atlas of Dermatological Manifestations of Gastrointestinal Disease*,
DOI 10.1007/978-1-4614-6191-3_72,

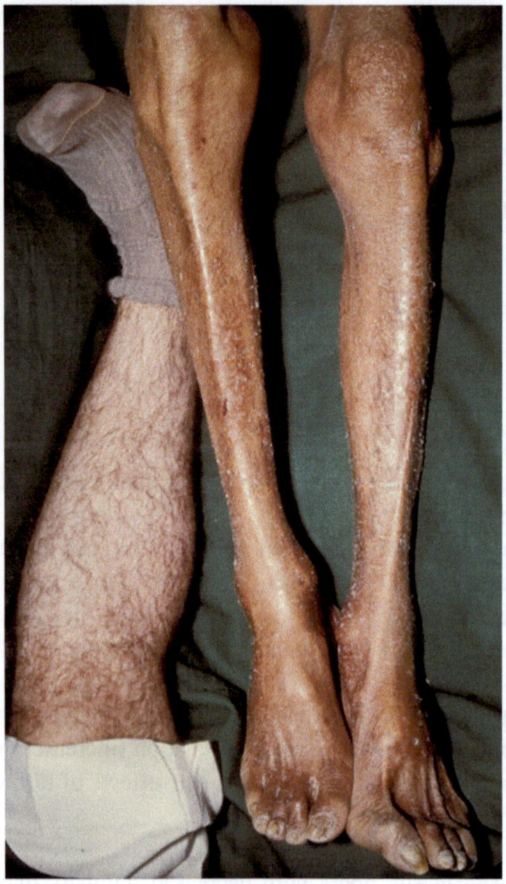

Fig. 72.1 Bronzing of the skin

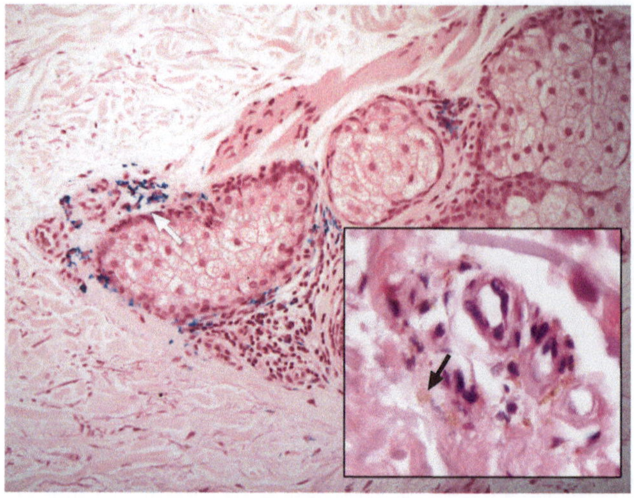

Fig. 72.2 Hemochromatosis. A photomicrograph showing iron deposition around the sebaceous glands is highlighted in blue with Perl's stain (100×). High-power hematoxylin and eosin stain (*inset*) shows perivascular iron deposition (*arrow*) (1000×)

Treatment consists of removal of iron:

- Decrease serum iron through phlebotomy (500 mL/week until hemoglobin <12 g/dL) [2]
- Ichthyosiform alterations: hydrating creams and ointments and avoid sunlight [1]
- Do not allow patients to handle raw seafood because patients at increased risk of *Vibrio vulnificus* and *Yersinia enterocolitica* infection [2]
- Avoid iron supplements, eat red meat in moderation, avoid or minimize alcohol [2]

References

1. Hazin R, Abu-Rajab Tamimi TI, Abuzetun JY, Zein NN. Recognizing and treating cutaneous signs of liver disease. Cleveland Clin J Med. 2009;76:599–606.
2. Brandhagen DJ, Fairbanks VF, Baldus W. Recognition and management of hemochromatosis. Am Fam Physician. 2002;65:853–61.
3. Köstler E, Porst H, Wollina U. Cutaneous manifestations of metabolic diseases: uncommon presentations. Dermatol. 2005;23:457–64.
4. Ruocco V, Psilogenis M, Schiavo AL, Wolf R. Dermatologic manifestations of alcoholic cirrhosis. Clin Dermatol. 1999;17:463–8.
5. Chevrant-Brenton J, Simon M, Bourel M, Ferrand B. Cutaneous manifestations of idiopathic hemochromatosis. Arch Dermatol. 1997;113:161–5.

Index

G.Y. Wu et al. (eds.), *Atlas of Dermatological Manifestations of Gastrointestinal Disease*,
DOI 10.1007/978-1-4614-6191-3, © Springer Science+Business Media New York 2013